New Frontiers in Bladder Cancer Research

New Frontiers in Bladder Cancer Research

Editor: Trinity Schell

STATES
ACADEMIC PRESS
www.statesacademicpress.com

www.statesacademicpress.com

STATES ACADEMIC PRESS

Cataloging-in-Publication Data

New frontiers in bladder cancer research / edited by Trinity Schell.
p. cm.
Includes bibliographical references and index.
ISBN 978-1-63989-795-7
1. Bladder--Cancer. 2. Bladder--Cancer--Research. 3. Bladder--Cancer--Diagnosis.
4. Bladder--Cancer--Treatment. 5. Bladder--Diseases. I. Schell, Trinity.
RC280.B5 N49 2023
616.994 62--dc23

States Academic Press,
109 South 5th Street,
Brooklyn, NY 11249, USA

ISBN 978-1-63989-795-7 (Hardback)

Contents

Preface

Bladder cancer refers to numerous types of cancer that can develop in the tissues of the urinary bladder. The signs and symptoms of bladder cancer include low back pain, blood in the urine and pain during urination. The epithelial cells lining the bladder become malignant and cause bladder cancer. There are various risk factors associated with this type of cancer, such as recurrent bladder infections, smoking, prior radiation therapy, exposure to specific chemicals and family history. The most prevalent type of bladder cancer is transitional cell carcinoma that starts in the cells of the deepest tissue layer in the bladder. Other types of bladder cancer include adenocarcinoma, squamous cell carcinoma and small cell carcinoma. Treatment for bladder cancer is determined by the type of cancer and the stage of the disease, and may include immunotherapy, surgery, chemotherapy and radiation therapy. This book contains some path-breaking studies in bladder cancer research. It will serve as a reference to a broad spectrum of readers.

Significant researches are present in this book. Intensive efforts have been employed by authors to make this book an outstanding discourse. This book contains the enlightening chapters which have been written on the basis of significant researches done by the experts.

Finally, I would also like to thank all the members involved in this book for being a team and meeting all the deadlines for the submission of their respective works. I would also like to thank my friends and family for being supportive in my efforts.

Editor

1

Mutant Kras as a Biomarker Plays a Favorable Role in FL118-Induced Apoptosis, Reactive Oxygen Species (ROS) Production and Modulation of Survivin, Mcl-1 and XIAP in Human Bladder Cancer

Sreevidya Santha [1,2], Xiang Ling [1,2,*], Ieman A. M. Aljahdali [1,3], Sailee S. Rasam [4], Xue Wang [5,6], Jianqun Liao [1,2], Jue Wang [7], Christos Fountzilas [8], Qingyong Li [9], Jun Qu [5] and Fengzhi Li [1,10,*]

1 Department of Pharmacology and Therapeutics, Roswell Park Comprehensive Cancer Center, Elm and Carlton Streets, Buffalo, New York, NY 14263, USA; sreevidya.gp@gmail.com (S.S.); Ieman.Aljahdali@RoswellPark.org (I.A.M.A.); Jian.Liao@RoswellPark.org (J.L.)
2 Canget BioTekpharma, LLC, Buffalo, New York, NY 14203, USA
3 Department of Cellular & Molecular Biology, Roswell Park Comprehensive Cancer Center, Buffalo, New York, NY 14263, USA
4 Department of Biochemistry, Jacobs School of Medicine, University at Buffalo, State University of New York, Buffalo, New York, NY 14203, USA; saileesu@buffalo.edu
5 Department of Pharmaceutical Sciences, School of Pharmacy, University at Buffalo, State University of New York, Buffalo, New York, NY 14214, USA; xwang79@buffalo.edu (X.W.); junqu@buffalo.edu (J.Q.)
6 Department of Cell Stress Biology, Roswell Park Comprehensive Cancer Center, Buffalo, New York, NY 14263, USA
7 Department of Interdisciplinary Oncology, University of Arizona Cancer Center, Phoenix Arizona, AZ 85004, USA; juewang@email.arizona.edu
8 Department of Medicine, Roswell Park Comprehensive Cancer Center, Buffalo, New York, NY 14263, USA; Christos.Fountzilas@RoswellPark.org
9 College of Pharmaceutical Science, Zhejiang University of Technology, Hangzhou 310014, China; liqy@zjut.edu.cn
10 Developmental Therapeutics (DT) Program, Roswell Park Comprehensive Cancer Center, Buffalo, New York, NY 14263, USA
* Correspondence: Xiang.Ling@RoswellPark.org (X.L.); fengzhi.li@roswellpark.org (F.L.);

Simple Summary: FL118 is a novel orally available small molecule anticancer drug. We found that bladder cancer cells with a mutant Kras is highly sensitive to FL118-induced cell growth inhibition and cell death induction through inhibiting the anti-cancer cell death and drug resistance factors (survivin, Mcl-1, XIAP). In the Kras-mutation bladder cancer cells, FL118 can stimulate the reactive oxygen species (ROS) over-production for killing bladder cancer cells and inhibiting bladder cancer cell-established tumor growth. Elimination of mutant Kras by Kras-specific shRNA technology in mutant Kras-containing bladder cancer cell-established tumor decreased FL118 effectiveness to inhibit bladder cancer tumor growth. In this regard, mutant Kras is a potential favorable biomarker for FL118. This finding is significant because mutant Kras is known to be a formidable challenge treatment resistant factor in various types of cancer. Thus, FL118 could use mutant Kras as favorable biomarker for patient selection to carry out precision medicine.

Abstract: Tumor heterogeneity in key gene mutations in bladder cancer (BC) is a major hurdle for the development of effective treatments. Using molecular, cellular, proteomics and animal models, we demonstrated that FL118, an innovative small molecule, is highly effective at killing T24 and UMUC3 high-grade BC cells, which have Hras and Kras mutations, respectively. In contrast,

HT1376 BC cells with wild-type Ras are insensitive to FL118. This concept was further demonstrated in additional BC and colorectal cancer cells with mutant Kras versus those with wild-type Kras. FL118 strongly induced PARP cleavage (apoptosis hallmark) and inhibited survivin, XIAP and/or Mcl-1 in both T24 and UMUC3 cells, but not in the HT1376 cells. Silencing mutant Kras reduced both FL118-induced PARP cleavage and downregulation of survivin, XIAP and Mcl-1 in UMUC3 cells, suggesting mutant Kras is required for FL118 to exhibit higher anticancer efficacy. FL118 increased reactive oxygen species (ROS) production in T24 and UMUC3 cells, but not in HT1376 cells. Silencing mutant Kras in UMUC3 cells reduced FL118-mediated ROS generation. Proteomics analysis revealed that a profound and opposing Kras-relevant signaling protein is changed in UMUC3 cells and not in HT1376 cells. Consistently, in vivo studies indicated that UMUC3 tumors are highly sensitive to FL118 treatment, while HT1376 tumors are highly resistant to this agent. Silencing mutant Kras in UMUC3 cell-derived tumors decreases UMUC3 tumor sensitivity to FL118 treatment. Together, our studies revealed that mutant Kras is a favorable biomarker for FL118 targeted treatment.

Keywords: FL118; bladder cancer; apoptosis; survivin; Mcl-1; XIAP; mutant Kras; reactive oxygen species (ROS); proteomics analysis; human bladder tumor mouse models

1. Introduction

Bladder cancers are a heterogeneous group of neoplasms in terms of clinical behavior and response to chemotherapy [1]. Most are urothelial carcinomas, which are subdivided into non-muscle-invasive bladder cancer (NMIBC) and muscle-invasive bladder cancer (MIBC) with distinct molecular features and clinical outcome [1]. NMIBCs frequently recur and, in some cases, progress to invasive and metastatic disease, while the MIBCs frequently metastasize [2]. Therefore, this is an expensive disease to treat. For NMIBC, transurethral resection is the initial treatment followed by intravesical administration of immunomodulating or chemotherapeutic agents [3], while radical cystectomy, preceded by neoadjuvant chemotherapy in most cases, is the current standard approach to manage and treat patients with MIBCs [1,4].

Current combination chemotherapies for MIBC are based on methotrexate, vinblastine, adriamycin and cisplatin (MVAC) or gemcitabine plus cisplatin, which are highly toxic with severe side effects [5]. Although various types of targeted drugs for bladder cancer are in clinical development [4–7], it remains to be seen if the clinical trials with targeted therapies hold promise for the treatment of this disease. In addition, the prognosis of patients with MIBC has not been improved in the past two decades, and bladder cancer still is one of the most expensive cancers to treat [8,9]. The median survival of patients with metastases is 15.2 months and a 5-year survival rate of 15.3% [10]. Up to date, Erdafitinib (Balversa, an FGFR inhibitor) is the first targeted drug approved by FDA for metastatic urothelial cancer. However, there are major concerns about its shorter duration of response and toxicity profile (e.g., ocular toxicity) [11]. Therefore, the development of new and effective anti-bladder cancer therapeutic agents is still a high unmet need for patients with bladder cancer, especially for those with advanced, high-grade bladder cancer.

As mentioned early, the highly heterogeneous nature of bladder cancer is a major hurdle for the development of successful therapies. Current studies indicate that activation of fibroblast growth factor receptor 3 (FGFR3) and Ras gene mutations are frequent in NMIBCs, while MIBC develops predominantly through the inactivation of the p53, retinoblastoma (RB), phosphatase and tensin homolog (PTEN) tumor suppressor pathways [12–14]. Oncogenic activation of both FGFR3 and Ras genes results in the stimulation of the mitogen-activated protein kinase (MAPK) and AKT pathways [15]. However, based on our studies reported here, this is unlikely the entire mechanism of this disease.

We have initially reported on a novel anticancer small molecule named FL118 [16]. However, its detailed mechanism of action continues to be investigated to determine FL118's breadth of efficacy against a wide variety of cancers. This report continues to build on our previously published findings (refer to the Discussion section for more information) as we further advance our understanding of whether FL118 can be an effective treatment for advanced high-grade bladder cancer. Our studies reveal that mutant Kras is a favorable biomarker that can be potentially used in the stratification of cancer patients for FL118 treatment. This finding is significant because Kras mutation was a difficult target in many types of cancer, including pancreatic and colorectal cancers.

2. Materials and Methods

2.1. Reagents and Antibodies

Antibodies for poly (ADP-ribose) polymerase (PARP) (9542S), Ras^{G12V} (14412S), Ras^{G12D} (14429S), phospho-AKT (4060S), phospho-ERK1/2 (4370S), cIAP2 (3130S), XIAP (2042S), Mcl-1 (4572S) and survivin (2803S) were purchased from Cell Signaling. The antibody for Kras (101667-T32) was purchased from Sino Biological (Southeastern, PA, USA). The antibodies for survivin were also purchases from Santa Cruz Biotechnology ((sc-10811) and from Epitomics (2565-1). Antibodies for GAPDH (sc-25778/sc-47724), AKT (sc-8312) and ERK1/2 (sc-292838) were purchased from Santa Cruz. The second antibodies of goat anti-mouse IgG (G21040) and goat anti-rabbit IgG (G21234) were purchased from Invitrogen/ThermoFisher. Antibodies for topoisomerase 1 were purchased from BD Biosciences (556597) and TopoGEN (TG2012-4). All primary antibodies were diluted in the range of 500× to 1000×. In this study, secondary antibodies were diluted 5000× to 10,000×. Dulbecco's modified eagle's medium (DMEM), penicillin–streptomycin solution, trypsin EDTA and phosphate-buffered saline (PBS) were from Mediatech, Inc. (Manassas, VA, USA); Opti-MEM was from Gibco. Lipofectamine 2000 was from Invitrogen/ThermoFisher. Fetal bovine serum (FBS) was from Atlanta Biologicals. The 3-(4,5-dimethylthiazol-2-yl)-2,5-diphenyltetrazolium bromide (MTT) was from Affymetrix. The protease inhibitor cocktail was from Sigma-Aldrich; the reactive oxygen species (ROS) assay kit was from Abcam; the BCA™ protein assay kit was from Pierce and Western lightning plus ECL was from PerkinElmer (Shelton, CT, USA).

2.2. Cell Culture

Human bladder cancer cell lines HT1376, T24, UMUC3, RT112 and TCCSUP were originally from ATCC and were kindly provided by Drs. Yuesheng Zhang and Candace Johnson, Roswell Park Comprehensive Cancer Center. Dr. Johnson's lab also provided human bladder cancer cell line 253 J B-V for this study. Human colorectal cancer (CRC) cell lines SNU-C2B and HCT117 were purchased from ATCC. Cells were grown under standard culture conditions at 37 °C in a humidified atmosphere containing 5% CO_2. Cells were cultured in DMEM supplemented with 10% FBS, 100 unit/mL of penicillin and 100 μg/mL of streptomycin. Sub-confluent cells were treated with different concentrations of FL118 or with an equivalent amount of solvent DMSO according to the experiments.

2.3. MTT Assay

In vitro inhibitory effects of FL118 on bladder cancer cell growth was performed using MTT assay. The human bladder cancer HT1376, UMUC-3 and T24 cells were plated in 96-well plates at a density of 5000 cells/well and allowed to adhere overnight. The next day, cells were treated with a medium containing DMSO as a vehicle or with 0.5–200 nM FL118 for 24, 48 and 72 hrs. Cell viability was determined at the end of each treatment time by 3-(4,5-dimethylthiazol-2-yl)-2,5-diphenyltetrazolium bromide (MTT) assay, as previously described [17,18]. For this, the cells were incubated with 50 μL of 0.5 mg/mL MTT solution for 4 h, followed by incubation with 150 μL of DMSO for another 30 min at 37 °C. The absorbance was measured at 570 nm in a microtiter plate reader. A blank reading was subtracted from experimental readings for final calculations.

2.4. Immunoblotting

Immunoblotting was performed as previously described [19,20]. Briefly, the cells were lysed in a RIPA lysis buffer containing a protease inhibitor cocktail (Sigma-Aldrich, St. Louis, MO, USA) and supernatants were collected by centrifugation at 13,000 rpm for 15 min at 4 °C. Protein quantification in each sample was performed using a BCA™ protein assay kit (Pierce, Rockford, IL, USA) with bovine serum albumin (BSA) as a standard. Equal amounts of proteins were denatured and fractionated by SDS–PAGE, and the proteins were transferred onto nitrocellulose membranes. Nonspecific binding sites were blocked by incubating the membranes in 5% nonfat milk in TBS containing 0.1% Tween-20. The membranes were probed with appropriate primary antibodies overnight at 4 °C followed by appropriate horseradish peroxidase (HRP) conjugated secondary antibody for 1 h at room temperature. Protein expression was detected by enhanced Western Lightning Plus-ECL, enhanced chemiluminescence substrate (PerkinElmer, Shelton, CT, USA). Images were acquired on a Bio-Rad ChemiDoc system by using Image lab software. Expression of GAPDH was used as an internal control for total protein-loading.

2.5. Lentiviral shRNA-Mediated Knockdown of Kras and Puromycin Selection

Lentiviral vectors encoding scramble control shRNA and Kras-specific shRNA, respectively, were obtained from our Institute's shRNA Core Resource, which owns various shRNA libraries in collaboration with Open Biosystems. Lentiviral shRNA constructs were packaged in pseudo-type viral particles, as described in our previous studies [16]. Subconfluent UMUC-3 cells in 6-well plates were infected with 100 μL/well of lentiviral stock in the presence of 4 μg/mL polybrene. The control scramble shRNA or the previously identified Kras-specific shRNA [21] infected cells in the plate were grown for 24 h, and the media was replaced with fresh growth media. Cells in individual wells were then split, followed by selection with puromycin (5 μg/mL) for 3–7 days. The remaining puromycin selected cell populations specific for Kras shRNA or Control shRNA were used for the experiments.

2.6. Overexpression of $Kras^{G12V}$ in HT1376 Bladder Cancer Cells

HT-1376 cells were transfected with $Kras^{G12V}$ or control vector using Lipofectamine 2000 as per the manufacturer's instructions. Briefly, subconfluent populations of cells were transfected with 1.5 μg of plasmid DNA in one well of the 6 well plates in Opti-MEM for 24 h, followed by recovery in serum-containing medium. After 48 h of transfection, cells were treated with either DMSO or 100 nM FL118 for an additional 48 h. The lysates were prepared using RIPA lysis buffers and used for Western blot analysis.

2.7. Reactive Oxygen Species (ROS) Assay

Cellular reactive oxygen species (ROS) production in the presence of FL118 was measured using a ROS kit from Abcam. The bladder cancer cell lines HT1376, T24 and UMUC-3 were seeded in a black 96-well microplate with clear bottom (20,000 cells per well) and allowed to attach overnight. The next day, the cells were treated with either DMSO as a vehicle or 100 nM FL118 in phenol red-free DMEM for different time points. At the end of treatment, cells were incubated with cell-permeant reagent 2′,7′-dichlorofluorescin diacetate (DCFDA) for 45 min at 37 °C in the dark. DCFDA is a fluorogenic dye that measures hydroxyl, peroxyl and other ROS activity within the cell. After diffusion into the cell, DCFDA is deacetylated by cellular esterases to a non-fluorescent compound, which is later oxidized by ROS into a highly fluorescent compound 2′,7′–dichlorofluorescein (DCF). Plates were read at the end of 45 min incubation on a fluorescent plate reader with excitation wavelength at 485 nm and emission wavelength at 535 nm. Blank readings were subtracted from experimental readings for final calculations.

2.8. *Proteomics Analysis of HT1376 versus UMUC3 Cells after FL118 Treatment*

HT1376 and UMUC3 bladder cancer cells were treated with and without FL118 at 20 nM for 24 h and 48 h in parallel triplicate. The obtained samples were analyzed using the Qu Lab-developed robust IonStar/MS1-based proteomics technology [22]. Briefly, through a process of protein extraction, reduction, alkylation and organic solvent precipitation and digestion of the obtained protein pellets with trypsin, 4 μg peptide samples in 4 μL from each time point sample were gone through the process of Nano LC/UHF-Orbitrap LUMOS MS analyses, as described [22].

A stringent set of criteria were employed for protein identification. The IonStar processing pipeline was used for MS1 quantification of the identified proteins from individual samples. Gene ontology (GO) annotation (quantified proteins) were analyzed using online tools of DAVID Bioinformatics Resources v6.7 (http://david.abcc.ncifcrf.gov/)[23] and/or Ingenuity Pathway Analysis (IPA, Ingenuity Systems). For GO enrichment analysis, all quantified proteins were used as background. Protein function, upstream regulator, and pathway analysis were carried out using IPA for a Core analysis. Biological and functional annotations assigned by the software were manually examined and regrouped into respective categories. Hierarchical cluster analysis (uncentered Pearson correlation distance and centroid-linkage) was analyzed using Cluster 3.0 [24] and displayed by TreeView, supporting tree-based and image-based browsing of hierarchical trees (http://www.eisenlab.org), when needed. In addition to the use of IPA for pathway analyses, we have also analyzed the changes of protein network pathways in FL118-treated and untreated HT1376 cells versus UMUC3 cells using GSEA analysis tools [25,26].

2.9. *Human Bladder Cancer Xenograft Tumor Mouse Model for FL118 Efficacy Testing*

Human subjects were not applicable to this study. All in vivo experimental studies were approved by the Institutional Animal Care and Use Committee (IACUC) and performed following the IACUC-approved mouse protocol at Roswell Park Comprehensive Cancer Center. The animal work followed our previous protocols [16]. Briefly, human bladder cancer xenograft tumors were first generated through implanting 2×10^6 bladder cancer cells at the flank area of severe combined immunodeficiency (SCID) mice. After the tumors grew to 800–1200 mm^3, they were isolated and individual experimental mice were subcutaneously implanted with 30–50 mg of non-necrotic tumor masses at the flank area of individual mice. Seven to 14 days after tumor transplantation, the implanted bladder xenograft tumors were grown to 100–150 mm^3 (defined as day 0), and mice were randomly divided into the required groups (5 mice per group) for treatment via oral administration of FL118 or vehicle. The schedule for FL118 or vehicle treatment was weekly for 4 times (weekly × 4). The FL118 in the current study used a basic oral formulation recipe, which contained FL118 (0.5 mg/mL), hydroxypropyl-β-cyclodextrin (0.5%, *w/v*), propylene glycol (1%) and hydroxypropyl methylcellulose (2% *w/v*, viscosity 40–60 cps) in saline. The formulation process was described in detail in the published patent (PCT/US2015/0022095) [27]. The vehicle solution contained hydroxypropyl-β-cyclodextrin (0.5%, *w/v*), propylene glycol (1%) and hydroxypropyl methylcellulose (2% *w/v*, viscosity 40–60 cps) in saline without FL118. Tumor length (L) and width (W) were measured using digital vernier calipers two times per week until the end of the experimental studies. The tumor volume (v) was calculated using the formula: $v = 0.5\ (L \times W^2)$. Then, the tumor size was divided by the day 0 tumor size, as percentage tumor size versus day 0. The mean tumor volume ± standard deviation (SD) at each time point was derived from 5 mice in each group. The tumor curves were made using Microsoft Excel.

2.10. Statistical Analysis

The experimental data were analyzed using Microsoft Excel and expressed as the mean ± SD. The statistical significance of differences was determined by Student's t-test in two groups and one-way analysis of variance among multiple groups, with a p-value of 0.05 or less considered as significant. * p-value < 0.05, ** p-value < 0.01, *** p-value < 0.001. Protein band relative intensities from various Western blot results were quantified using ImageJ software and normalized against loading controls.

3. Results

3.1. Differential Inhibitory Effects of FL118 on Viability and Growth of Bladder Cancer Cells with Distinct Ras Statuses

The high-grade bladder cancer cell lines HT1376, T24 and UMUC-3 had different oncogenic Ras statuses. While HT1376 cells had wild-type Ras, T24 and UMUC-3 cells containing mutated Hras (G12V) and mutant Kras (G12C), respectively. All of the three cell lines had mutant p53. To evaluate bladder cancer cell growth inhibition by FL118 treatment, HT-1376, T24 and UMUC-3 cells were exposed to 0.5 to 200 nM FL118 for 24–72 h; cell viability was measured using MTT assay. As shown in Figure 1, T24 with Hras G12V and UMUC-3 cells with Kras G12C mutations displayed much higher sensitivity to FL118 than the Ras wild-type HT1376 cells. While maximum cell viability inhibition obtained in the HT1376 cell line was about 40% with 200 nM concentration of FL118 (72 h, Figure 1A), the same concentration of FL118 inhibited 88% of cell viability in T24 (Figure 1B) and 98.8% of cell viability in UMUC-3 cells (Figure 1C). Significantly, the FL118 highly resistant HT1376 cell line and the FL118 highly sensitive UMUC3 cell line-established xenograft tumors were also tested in animal models and support the in vitro result (see below). Additionally, we tested additional human bladder cancer cells with wild-type Ras genes (RT112, 253J B-V, TCCSUP) and found that these cell lines without Kras/Hras/Nras mutation were always relatively resistant to FL118 treatment (Figure S1, Table 1). Kras mutation in bladder cancer was low (8%) [28]. Due to various reasons, we were unable to obtain additional bladder cell lines with Kras mutation. In contrast, the mutation rate of Kras in colorectal cancer (CRC) was at a range of 40–44.7% [29,30]. Therefore, using MTT, we determined cell sensitivity to FL118 in a couple of CRC cell lines with mutant Kras. We found that CRC cell lines with mutant Kras exhibit higher sensitivity to FL118-induced cell growth inhibition (Figure S1D,E). Since the bladder cancer cell lines HT1376, T24 and UMUC3 were commonly used in research, we therefore mainly used these representative three cell lines for the molecular level studies elucidated in this paper.

Table 1. Relative IC50 comparison among the bladder cancer cell lines used in the studies.

Cell Line	Kras/Hras/Nras Status	IC_{50} *
HT1376	Wild type	>200 nM
T-24	Hras mutation	~13 nM
UMUC3	Kras mutation	~3 nM
RT112	Wild type	>160 nM
253 J B-V	Wild type	>110 nM
TCCSUP (HTB-5)	Wild type	>160 nM
SNU-C2B (CRC)	Kras mutation	~2.7 nM
HCT116 (CRC).	Kras mutation	~0.51 nM

* IC_{50} is the 72 h FL118 treatment.

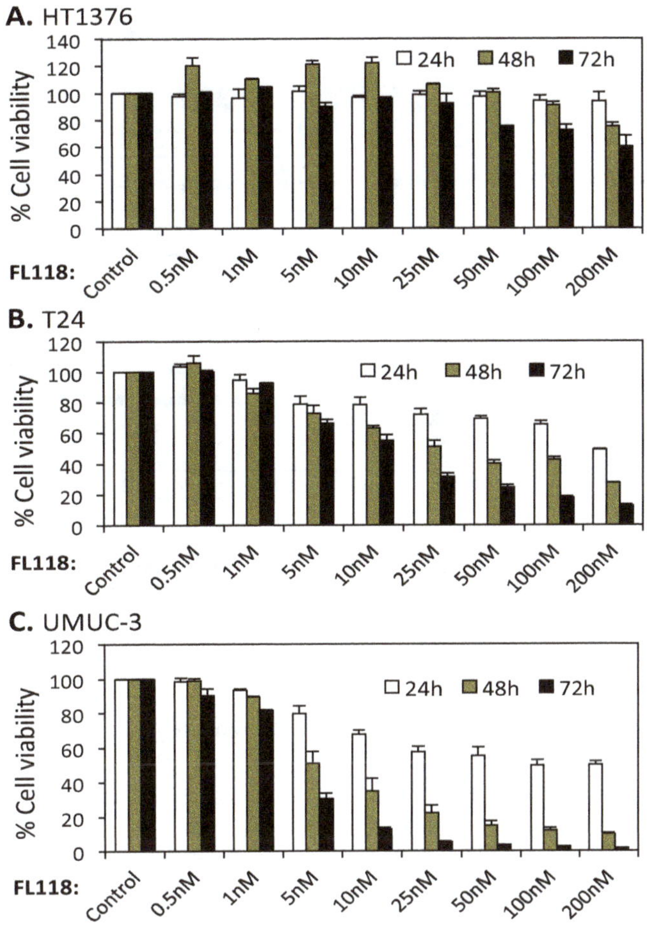

Figure 1. Differential inhibition of human bladder cancer cell growth by FL118. Subconfluent bladder cancer cells HT1376 (wild-type Ras), T24 (Hras G12V mutant) and UMUC-3 (Kras G12C mutant) in 96-well plates were treated with either DMSO (control) or a series of FL118 concentrations for 24 h–72 h followed by MTT assay to determine cell viability. (**A**) HT-1376 cells with wild-type Ras were insensitive to FL118 treatment compared to other cell lines (T24, UMUC-3). (**B**,**C**) Ras mutant T24 and UMUC-3 cells are highly sensitive to FL118 treatment. Each bar in the histogram shown in (**A**–**C**) is the mean ± SD from three independent assays.

3.2. Human Bladder Cancer Cells with Different Ras Statuses Exhibit Differential Sensitivity to FL118-Induced Apoptosis

We anticipated that the differential cell growth and viability inhibition by FL118 in bladder cancer cells would be associated with a differential induction of cell apoptosis. In order to determine the effect of FL118 treatment on the apoptotic potential of bladder cancer cells, we examined PARP cleavage as a hallmark of apoptosis by Western blot analyses. We found that 10–100 nM of FL118 induced strong PARP cleavage in T24 (Figure 2B, Figure S2B) and UMUC-3 (Figure 2C, Figure S2C) bladder cancer cells. In contrast, there was no PARP cleavage difference in HT1376 bladder cancer cells (Figure 2A, Figure S2A). This result is fully consistent with the MTT assay resulted indicating that bladder cancer cells with different Ras statuses exhibited differential sensitivity to FL118 cell growth and viability inhibition (Figure 1, Table 1, Figure S1).

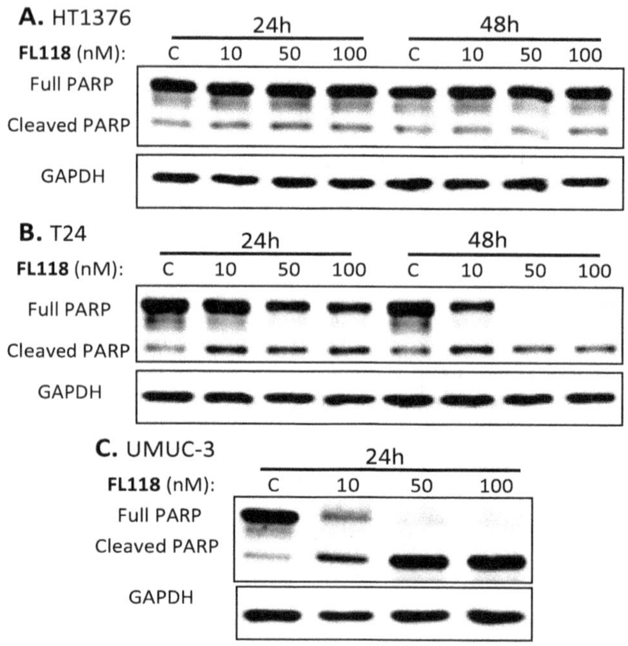

Figure 2. Induction of differential poly (ADP-ribose) polymerase (PARP) cleavage in bladder cancer cells by FL118. Subconfluent bladder cancer cells in 60 mm plates were treated with DMSO (as a vehicle) or with 10, 50 and 100 nM FL118 for 24 h and/or 48 h, as shown, followed by Western blot analyses to determine PARP cleavage. (**A**) HT-1376 cells with wild-type Ras show no significant PARP cleavage after 24 or 48 h FL118 treatment. (**B**) T24 cells with Hras G12V mutation showed the cleavage of PARP with all concentrations of FL118 treatment. (**C**) mutant Kras (UMUC-3) cells with Kras G12C mutation showed the maximum PARP cleavage with the disappearance of total PARP bands after 24 h FL118 treatment. GAPDH (glyceraldehyde 3-phosphate dehydrogenase) shown in A, B and C were used as internal controls of total protein-loading.

3.3. Differential Inhibition of the IAP and Bcl-2 Family Proteins by FL118 Is Associated with FL118 Sensitivity to Bladder Cancer Cells with Different Genetic Backgrounds

Our previous studies in colorectal and head-&-neck cancer cells indicated that FL118 selectively inhibits the expression of survivin, Mcl-1, XIAP and/or cIAP2, which were demonstrated to play important roles in FL118-induced cell growth inhibition and apoptosis induction tested through genetic silencing or overexpression of these genes [16,31]. We then reasoned that the differential effect of FL118 on bladder cancer cell growth inhibition and apoptosis induction might be associated with the differential inhibition of one or more of these anti-apoptotic proteins. Therefore, we determined the expression changes in the members of the IAP and the Bcl-2 family after FL118 treatment in bladder cancer cells through Western blot analyses. We found that FL118 treatment induced different levels of downregulation of the IAP and Bcl-2 family proteins. Specifically, while cIAP2 did not show significant inhibition by FL118 in any of these three cell lines (HT1376, T24, UMUC3), FL118 treatment strongly inhibited the expression of survivin, XIAP and Mcl-1 in UMUC3 cells (Figure 3C, Figure S3C), and inhibited survivin and XIAP in T24 bladder cancer cells (Figure 3B, Figure S3B). However, FL118 failed to inhibit these proteins in HT1376 cells (Figure 3A, Figure S3A). This result is consistent with the ability of FL118 in bladder cancer cell growth inhibition and apoptosis induction shown in Figures 1 and 2. Together, HT1376 cells were resistant to FL118 treatment, while UMUC-3 and T24 cells were sensitive to FL118 treatment, with UMUC-3 being the most sensitive to FL118.

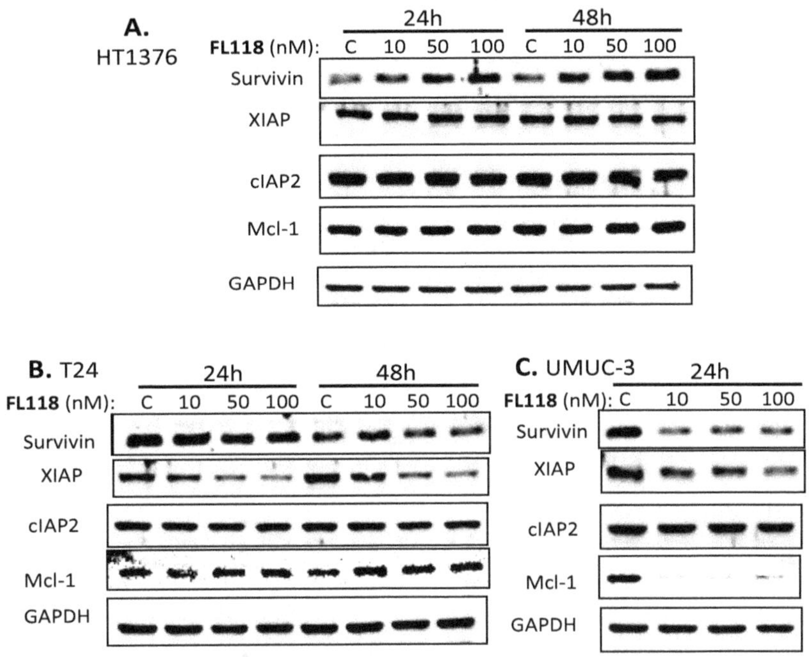

Figure 3. Inhibition of survivin, Mcl-1 and/or XIAP by FL118 in bladder cancer cell lines by FL118. Cells were treated with DMSO or 10–100 nM FL118 for 24 h and/or 48 h, as shown, followed by Western blot analyses to determine the expression of survivin, Mcl-1, XIAP and cIAP2. (**A**) In HT1376 cells, FL118 treatment did not inhibit any of these anti-apoptotic proteins. (**B**) T24 cells showed inhibition of XIAP and survivin after FL118 treatment. (**C**) FL118 treatment showed strong inhibition of Mcl-1, survivin and XIAP in UMUC-3 cells after FL118 treatment. GAPDH shown in A, B and C is the internal control of total protein-loading.

3.4. AKT and ERK1/2 Signaling Pathways May Not Play a Major Role in FL118 Differential Sensitivity in Bladder Cancer Cells

Previous studies have indicated that the activated AKT and MAPK signaling can upregulate the expression of survivin through the AKT [32–36] and/or MAPK signaling transduction pathways [34,36–38]. It is also well known that activated Ras–MAPK and PI3K–Akt pathways promotes cancer cell survival and inhibits apoptosis through upregulation of anti-apoptotic proteins [8]. It is possible that the inhibition of survivin, XIAP and/or Mcl-1 by FL118 were due to the inhibition of AKT and/or MAPK activation by FL118. In other words, it is possible that there are high constitutively active AKT (high phosphorylation of AKT ser473) and/or ERK1/2 (high phosphorylation of Thr202/Tyr204 for human ERK1 and Thr185/Tyr187 for human ERK2) to maintain the high expression of survivin, XIAP and Mcl-1 for bladder cancer cell survival and proliferation. Therefore, we determined the effect of FL118 on the inhibition of the active/phosphorylated AKT and ERK1/2 in these bladder cancer cells. Our studies indicated that there is a high constitutively active AKT (high p-AKT) and ERK1/2 (high p-ERK1/2) in all the three bladder cancer cell lines (Figure 4, Figure S4). This is somehow inconsistent with the fact that these three cell lines exhibited differential sensitivity to FL118 treatment (Figures 1–3, Table 1, Figures S1–S3). This suggests that AKT and ERK1/2 pathways may not play a determinant role in FL118 sensitivity. Consistent with this notion, our studies indicated that FL118 treatment induced inconsistent modulation of total ERK and p-ERK and AKT and p-AKT in the three cell lines (Figure 4, Figure S4). For example, FL118 inhibited p-Akt in both HT1376 and UMUC3 cells at 24 h and 48 h time points (Figure 4A,C). However, HT1376 is resistant to FL118, while UMUC3 is highly sensitive to FL118. In contrast, FL118 significantly induced p-AKT (survival signaling) and p-ERK1/2 (growth signaling) in T24 cells (Figure 4B, Figure S4B). However, T24 cells still exhibited a high sensitivity to FL118 treatment (Figures 1 and 2, Table 1, Figures S2 and S3). Nevertheless, while the current studies could not rule out the possibility that FL118-mediated inhibition of p-AKT and p-ERK1/2, as well as total AKT and total ERK1/2 by FL118, may play a role in FL118 anticancer efficacy, these signaling pathways may not play the critical determinant role in FL118-mediated inhibition of bladder cancer cell viability and the induction of apoptosis. Thus, additional mechanisms appear to be involved in FL118-mediated bladder cancer cell viability inhibition and apoptosis induction.

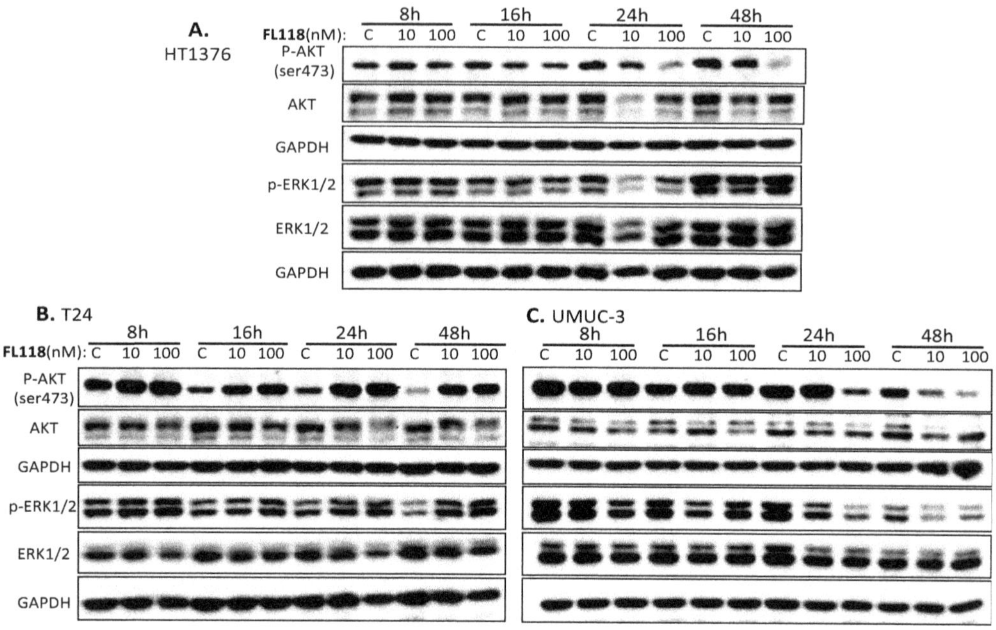

Figure 4. Effect of FL118 on AKT and ERK1/2 expression and phosphorylation/activation in bladder cancer cells. Subconfluent bladder cancer cells were treated with (10, 100 nM) and without (C, control/vehicle) FL118 for 8 h, 16 h, 24 h and 48 h, as shown, followed by Western blot analyses to determine the expression of AKT and ERK1/2 as well as the phospho-AKT (ser473) and phospho-p44/42 MAPK (ERK1/2) (Thr202/Tyr204). (**A**) Treatment of HT1376 cells with FL118 does not significantly modulate the expression and phosphorylation of Erk1/2. At the same time, FL118 reduces the expression of pAKT (ser473). (**B**) Treatment of T24 cells with FL118 enhances the phosphorylation of Akt and Erk1/2. (**C**) Treatment of UMUC-3 cells with FL118 downregulated the expression of active AKT and ERK1/2. GAPDH presented in (**A–C**) is internal controls for total protein-loading.

3.5. Inhibition of Top1 Expression Is Independent of FL118 Sensitivity or Resistance in Bladder Cancer Cells

It has been documented that downregulation of the expression of topoisomerase I (Top1) protein by CPTs is a CPT resistance factor [39–42]. One reason for this is that Top1 inhibition by CPTs is usually associated with a topoisomerase II (Top2) activity increase [41,43]. Thus, Top2 may partially perform the Top1 work in cancer cells, which could not be controlled by CPTs. In fact, the intensity of CPT-induced downregulation of Top1 expression is positively associated with the intensity of cell resistance to CPTs. For example, CPT effectively inhibits Top1 expression in the CPT-resistant breast cancer cell line BT474, while CPT is unable to inhibit Top1 expression in the CPT-sensitive breast cancer cell line ZR75–1 [44]. Consistent with these observations, it has been reported that reduced Top1 expression and/or Top1 catalytic activity in cancer cells is associated with increased resistance to CPTs [45,46], while increased Top1 expression in cancer cells sensitizes CPTs [47–49]. In contrast to these findings for CPTs, the FL118-sensitive bladder cancer cell lines (T24, UMUC-3) resulted in the least Top1 expression after FL118 treatment (Figure 5B,C, Figure S5), while the FL118-resistant HT1376 cell line still had a substantial level of Top1 expression after FL118 treatment (Figure 5A). This observation is consistent with our recent finding that FL118 antitumor efficacy in colorectal cancer cells is irrelevant of Top1 expression status (regardless of Top1 either negative, low or high) [50]. Human xenograft tumors with high Top1 expression may not be sensitive to FL118 treatment, while tumors with low/negative Top1 expression can be highly sensitive to FL118 treatment [50]. Thus, our current data further demonstrated that the differential effect of FL118 on the three bladder cancer cell lines is irrelevant to Top1 expression.

In other words, this Top1 molecular change cannot explain the differential sensitivity of HT1376, T24 and UMUC3 to FL118 treatment.

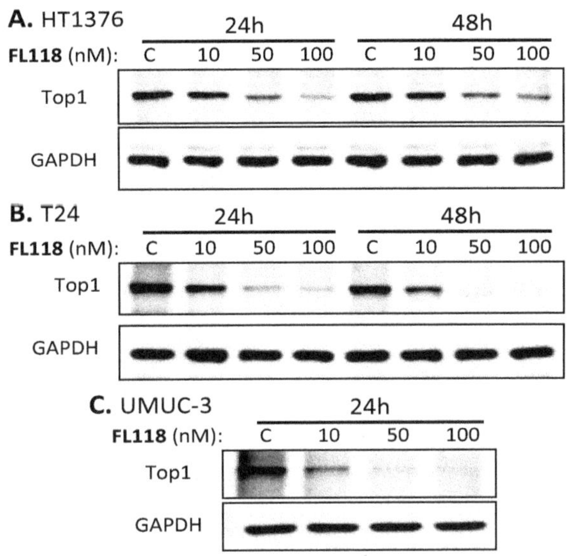

Figure 5. Sensitivity of bladder cancer cells to FL118 is irrelevant to Top1 level after FL118 treatment. Subconfluent bladder cancer cells in 6-well plates were treated with (10, 50, 100 nM) and without (C, vehicle control) FL118 for 24 h and/or 48 h, as shown, followed by Western blot analyses to determine the expression of Top1. (**A**) Treatment of HT1376 cells with FL118 resulted in the least inhibition of Top 1 expression after FL118 treatment. (**B**) Treatment of T24 cells with FL118 resulted in the inhibition of Top 1 expression after FL118 treatment. (**C**) Treatment of UMUC3 cells with FL118 resulted in the most inhibition of Top 1 expression after FL118 treatment. GAPDH presented in (**A**–**C**) is the internal control for total protein-loading.

3.6. Mutant Kras in Bladder Cancer Cells Plays an Important Role in the Increase of FL118 Anticancer Cell Activity

As mentioned before, HT1376 has wild-type Ras, while T24 has mutant Hras and UMUC-3 has mutant Kras. Thus, based on the fact that HT1376 is resistant, but T24 and UMUC-3 are sensitive to FL118 treatment, it is possible that the mutation-activated Ras (mutant Ras) is one factor that contributes to FL118 high sensitivity. To determine whether mutant Ras plays a role in FL118 treatment sensitivity, we employed FL118's most sensitive bladder cancer cell line UMUC-3 and FL118's most resistant bladder cancer cell line HT1376 as our study model system. We first checked the PARP cleavage and the expression of XIAP, Mcl-1 and survivin as the indicators of the apoptotic potential and anti-apoptotic status after FL118 treatment of UMUC-3 cells with no transfection, with control scramble shRNA (CshRNA) transfection and with our previously identified Kras-specific shRNA (KrasshRNA [21]) transfection to silence the activated mutant Kras, respectively. We found that UMUC-3 cells became more resistant to FL118 treatment-induced apoptosis (PARP cleavage) after the silencing of mutant Kras (Figure 6A, Figure S6A). Furthermore, silencing of mutant Kras made FL118 lose or partially lose the ability to inhibit the expression of XIAP, Mcl-1 and survivin (Figure 6A, Figure S6A). We were able to further determine the effect of mutant Kras silencing on FL118-inhibited UMUC-3 cell viability. Consistently, the silencing of mutant Kras decreased FL118's ability to inhibit UMUC-3 cell viability (Figure 6B). This suggests that mutant Kras play an important role in increasing FL118 anticancer efficacy.

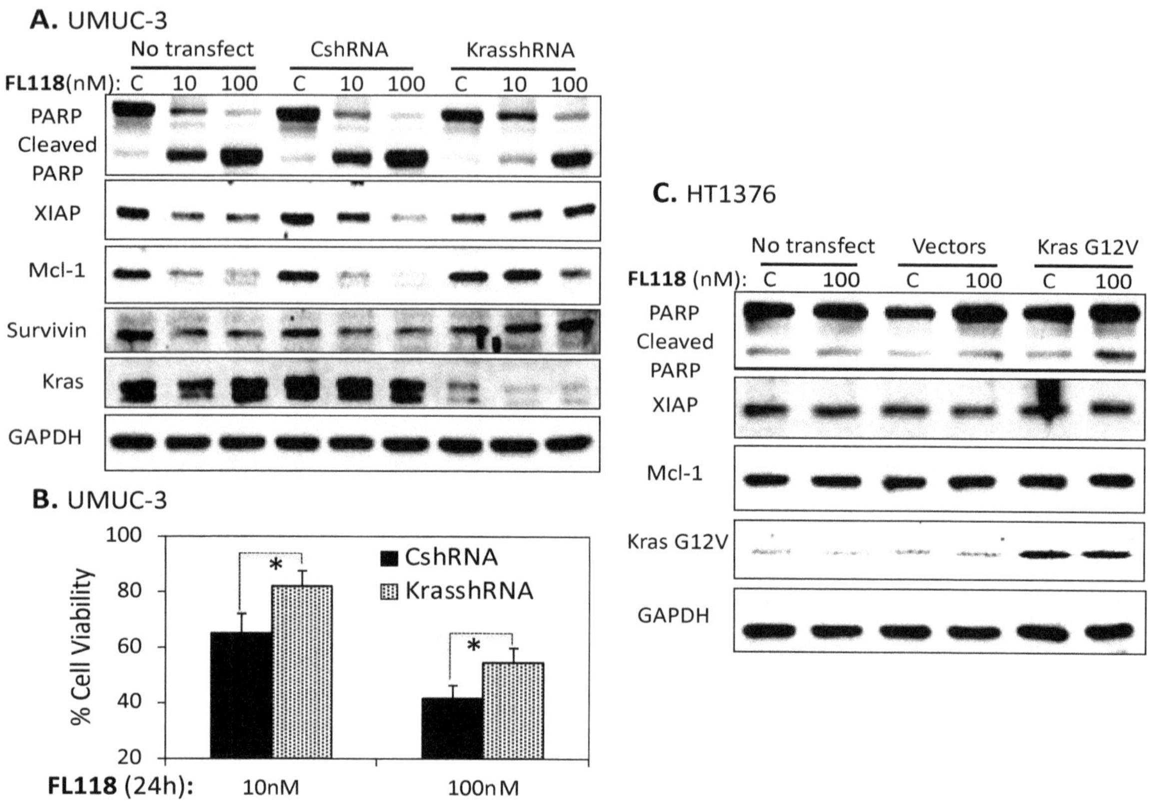

Figure 6. Role of mutant Kras in FL118-mediated apoptosis and inhibition of anti-apoptotic protein expression and cell viability. (**A**) Silencing of Kras G12C via Kras-specific shRNA in UMUC-3 cells increases cell resistance to FL118-induced apoptosis (less PARP cleavage). UMUC-3 cells were infected with Kras-specific lentiviral shRNA identified in our previous studies [21] or control shRNA followed by treatment with DMSO or FL118 (10 and 100 nM) for 24 h. At the end of treatment, Western blot analysis was performed to check PARP cleavage and the expression of anti-apoptotic proteins (XIAP, Mcl-1, survivin). GAPDH was used as an internal control. (**B**) 3-(4,5-dimethylthiazol-2-yl)-2,5-diphenyltetrazolium bromide (MTT) assay was performed to determine cell viability with 10 nM and 100 nM FL118 treatment in UMUC-3 cells infected with control scramble shRNA and Kras-specific shRNA. Each bar in the histogram data is the mean ± SD from three independent assays. (**C**) Effect of forced expression of Kras G12V in HT1376 cells. HT1376 cells were transfected with Kras G12V or control vectors followed by treatment with DMSO or 100 nM FL118 for 48 h. At the end of treatment, Western blot analysis was performed to check the expression of apoptosis-related proteins. GAPDH was used as an internal control of total protein-loading. * p-value < 0.05.

Next, we performed the alternative experiment to determine the effect of overexpression of mutant Kras G12V in FL118-induced apoptosis level in the FL118-resistant HT1376 cells. We found that after forced expression of the constitutive active Kras G12V in HT1376 cells, FL118 treatment showed an increase in PARP cleavage levels (Figure 6C, Figure S6C). However, we repeated this experiment a couple of times, and the result is not very strong. This could be due to multiple reasons, including transfection efficiency and/or endogenous wild-type Kras interferences, etc. Additionally, for this overexpression of the Kras G12V experiment, we were unable to find FL118-mediated inhibition of anti-apoptotic proteins, such as XIAP and Mcl-1 (Figure 6C, Figure S6C).

3.7. FL118 Treatment Increases the Generation of Reactive Oxygen Species (ROS) in Ras-Mutated Bladder Cancer Cells

Previous studies reported that mutant Kras^{G12V} (K-ras V12) promotes the reactive oxygen species (ROS) production in colorectal cancer cells through activation of the p38-PDPK1-PKCδ/p47^{phox}-NOX1 cascade [51], which promotes malignant transformation [51,52]. Therefore, it is possible that FL118 takes advantage of this pathway to promote ROS overproduction to kill cancer cells. Based on this rationale, we measured whether FL118 treatment increases ROS production in bladder cancer cells. In order to measure the effect of FL118 on ROS generation in bladder cancer cells, we used a cell-permeable reagent 2′,7′-dichlorofluorescin diacetate (DCFDA), a fluorogenic dye that measures hydroxyl, peroxyl and other ROS activity within the cell. After diffusion into the cell, DCFDA is deacetylated by cellular esterases to a non-fluorescent compound, which is later oxidized by ROS into 2′,7′-dichlorofluorescein (DCF), giving out fluorescence. Our studies revealed that FL118 did not increase ROS production in the FL118-resistant HT1376 cells (Figure 7A, left panel). In contrast, FL118 significantly increased ROS production in the two FL118-sensitive T24 and UMUC-3 bladder cancer cells (Figure 7A, middle and right panels). Furthermore, the silencing of mutant Kras significantly abrogated FL118-mediated ROS production (Figure 7B). Specifically, we used the UMUC-3 cells as a model system to knock down mutant Kras using Kras-specific shRNA. We found that silencing of mutant Kras significantly reduces ROS production induced by FL118 treatment (Figure 7B). Together, based on the result shown in Figure 7A,B, we conclude that FL118 takes advantage of mutant Kras-mediated ROS generation to further increase ROS overproduction as one-way to kill cancer cells.

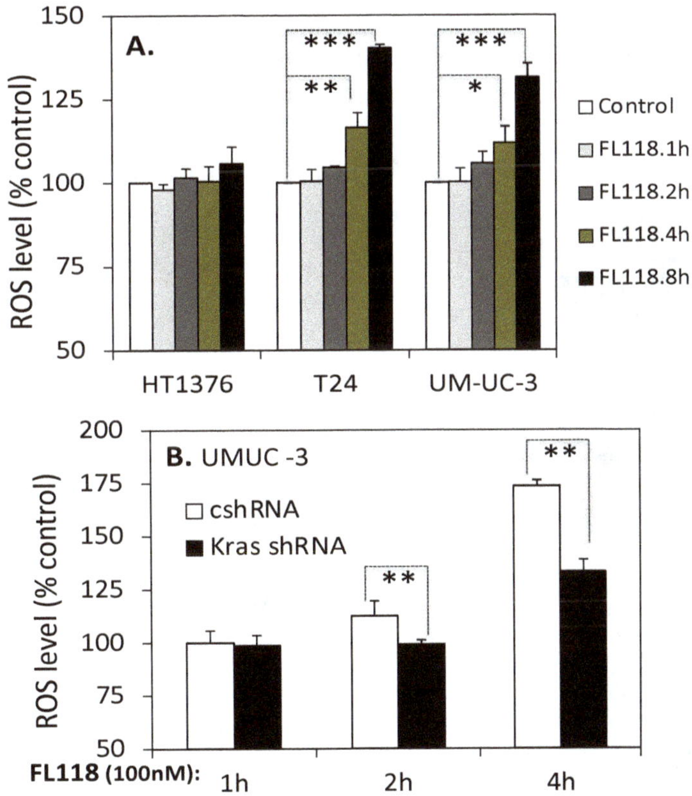

Figure 7. Determination of reactive oxygen species (ROS) production in bladder cancer cells. (**A**) FL118-induced ROS production in bladder cancer cell lines. HT1376, T24 and UMUC-3 cells in 96-well plates were treated with DMSO or 100 nM FL118 for different time points as indicated. At the end of treatment, ROS production was measured using Abcam's 2′,7′-dichlorofluorescin diacetate (DCFDA) cellular reactive oxygen species detection kit, as described in the Materials and Methods section. Values were shown as mean ± SD derived from three experiments. (**B**) Silencing Kras G12C via Kras-specific shRNA in UMUC-3 cells decreases ROS production after FL118 treatment. UMUC-3 cells were infected with Kras-specific lentiviral shRNA or control shRNA followed by treatment with DMSO or 100 nM FL118 for different time periods. At the end of treatment, ROS production was measured as described in the previous experiment. Values were shown as mean ± SD derived from three experiments. * p-value < 0.05, ** p-value < 0.01, *** p-value < 0.001

3.8. Proteomics Analysis Indicates That FL118 Treatment Induced a Profound and Opposed Kras-Relevant Protein Signaling Changes in UMUC3 Cells versus in HT1376 Cells

We hypothesized that if the mutant Kras plays an important role in the FL118 antitumor activity, we should find a differential Kras signaling-relevant downstream protein change in UMUC3 cells versus in HT1376 cells after FL118 treatment. In this regard, we performed a state-of-the-art proteomics analysis of global protein changes after FL118 treatment for 24 h and 48 h in UMUC3 cells versus in HT1376 cells. The proteomics analysis has identified a total of 5902 proteins (Table S1). From the 5902 proteins, we further sorted and identified the proteins that are relevant to the Kras signaling pathway (Table S2). Through analyses of all the 615 Kras signaling pathway-associated proteins (Table S2), we identified 70 proteins that exhibited a significant decrease (p value < 0.05) in FL118-treated UMUC3 cells, while these proteins in HT1376 cells either increased or had no significant change after FL118 treatment (Table S3). In parallel, we also identified 67 proteins that exhibited significant increase (p value < 0.05) in FL118-treated UMUC3 cells, while these proteins in HT1376 cells either decrease or have no significant change after FL118 treatment (Table S4). Based on the function of the total 137 (70 + 67) Kras signaling pathway-relevant proteins (Tables S3 and S4), we further classified them into different classes (Tables S5 and S6). In order to quickly observe the expression behavior difference of these proteins in each class, the data sets were presented in heatmap and histogram in Figure 8 and Figure S7, respectively. These studies revealed that FL118 treatment induced a profound and opposing Kras signaling pathway-relevant signaling protein change in UMUC3 cells versus in HT1376 cells.

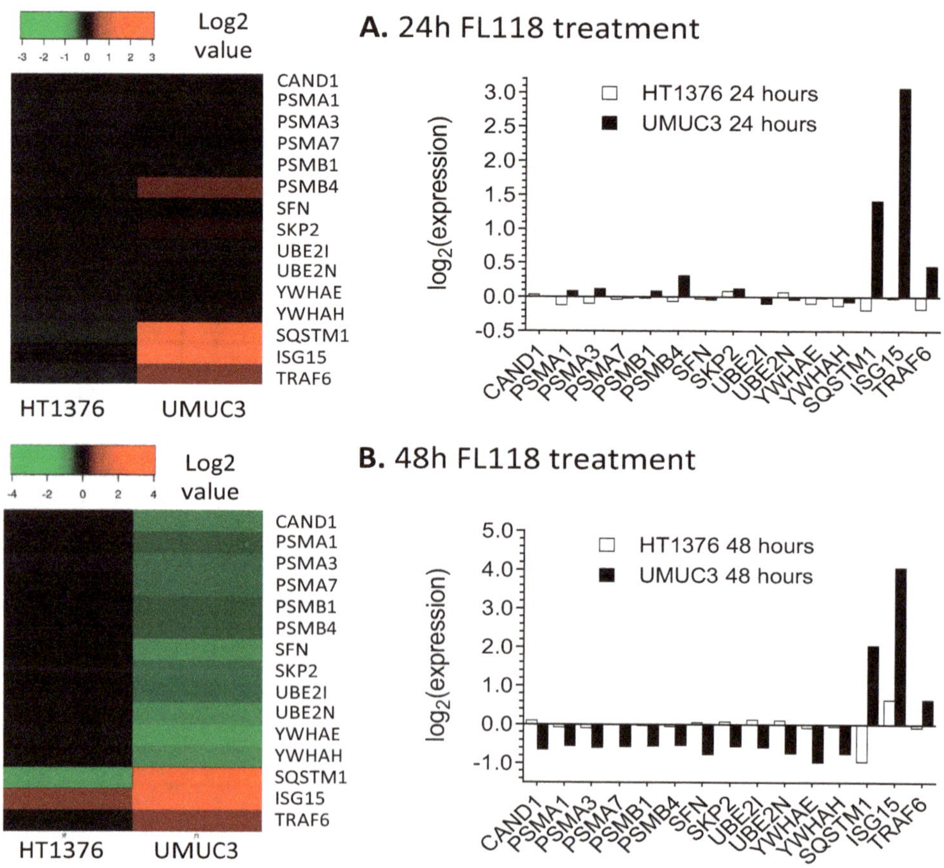

Figure 8. Effects of FL118 on Kras pathway-associated ubiquitination (Ub), de-Ub and proteasome-related proteins. HT1376 and UMUC3 cells were treated with FL118 (20 nM) for 24 h and 48 h. Proteomics analyses were then performed as described in the Method section. The data shown here is the effect of FL118 on the Kras pathway-associated Ub, de-Ub and proteasome-related proteins for 24 h (**A**) and 48 h (**B**). All data in proteomics analyses are in triple replicates in parallel with triple vehicle controls (refer to Table S1).

3.9. UMUC3, but Not HT1376 Bladder Cancer Cell-Derived Xenograft Tumor Exhibits High Sensitivity to FL118 Treatment in Animal Models

Our in vitro experimental data demonstrated that HT1376 bladder cancer cells are highly resistant to FL118 treatment, while UMUC-3 bladder cancer cells are highly sensitive to FL118 treatment in terms of (1) cell growth/viability inhibition (Figure 1, Figure S1), (2) apoptosis induction (Figure 2, Figure S2), (3) anti-apoptotic protein inhibition (Figure 3, Figure S3), (4) the role of Kras status (Figure 6, Figure S6) and (5) ROS production (Figure 7). Consistently, our proteomics data also indicated a profound and opposing modulation of mutant Kras signaling pathway-relevant proteins (Figure 8, Figure S7, Tables S2 and S3). Therefore, it is very important to determine whether the in vitro experimental outcome from FL118 treatment could be mimicked and be consistent with the in vivo outcomes from the HT1376 and UMUC3 bladder cancer cell-derived xenograft tumor in SCID mice. In this regard, we first established HT1376 and UMUC3 bladder cancer xenograft tumors in SCID mice; then, we used these tumor models and determined the FL118 efficacy to inhibit the bladder cancer xenograft tumor growth. As shown, consistent with the in vitro experimental results, UMUC-3 tumors grown in SCID mice exhibited high sensitivity to FL118 treatment (Figure 9A); that is, FL118 can eliminate UMUC3 tumors after three-time treatment (Figure 9A). In contrast, HT1376 tumors grown in SCID mice exhibited high resistance to FL118 treatment (Figure 9B); that is, FL118 was basically unable to inhibit HT1376 tumor growth (Figure 9B). Furthermore, FL118 was less effective in inhibiting the UMUC3 tumors with the partial silencing of mutant Kras (Figure 9E). Together, the in vivo data related to the FL118 efficacy is fully consistent with the in vitro molecular and cell cultural studies with FL118.

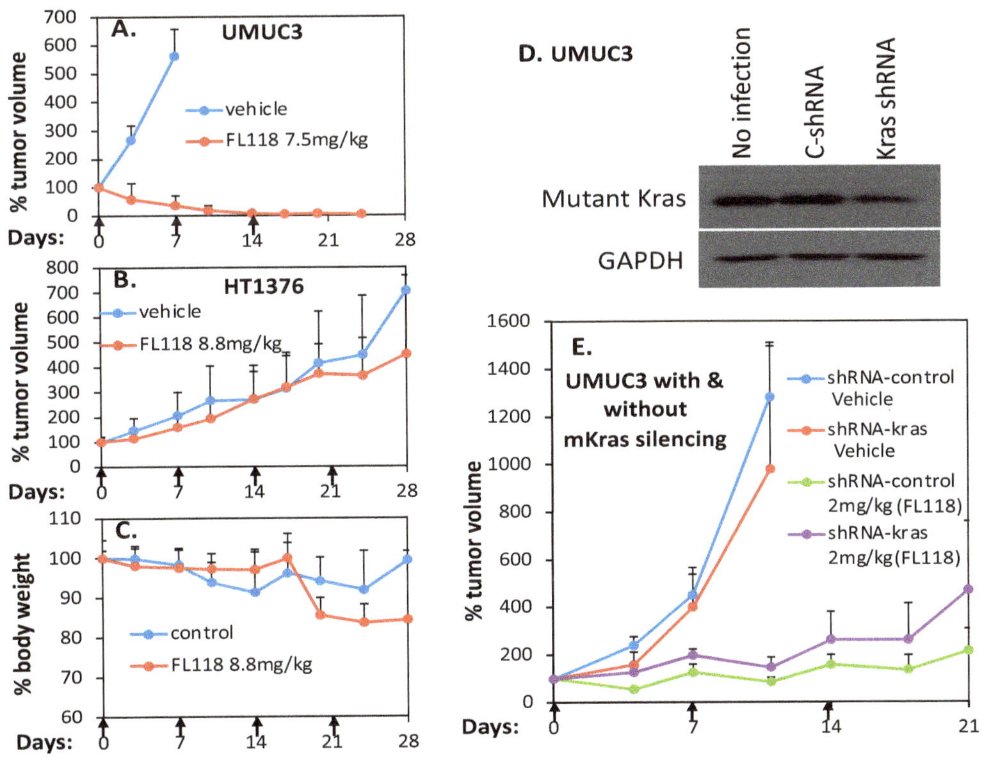

Figure 9. Antitumor efficacy of FL118 in severe combined immunodeficiency (SCID) mice bearing human bladder cancer xenograft tumors. The human bladder cancer xenograft tumors were first generated

through implanting bladder cancer cells at the flank area of SCID mice. Then, the tumors were isolated, and individual experimental mice were subcutaneously implanted with 30–50 mg nonnecrotic tumor masses at the flank area of individual mice. Seven to 14 days after tumor transplantation at which the implanted bladder xenograft tumors were grown to 100–150 mm^3 (defined as day 0), mice were randomly divided into the required groups (5 mice per group) for treatment vial oral administration of FL118 at the doses as shown or vehicles with a schedule of weekly × 3 or 4 (arrowed) as described in the "Materials and Methods" section. (**A**) FL118 efficacy against UMUC-3 bladder cancer cell-established xenograft tumors in SCID mice. (**B**) FL118 efficacy against HT1376 bladder cancer cell-established xenograft tumors in SCID mice. The tumor growth curves shown in A and B are the mean ± SD derived from 5 mice. (**C**) SCID mouse body weight changes after treatment with vehicle or with FL118. The mouse body weight curves shown in C are the mean ± SD derived from 5 mice. (**D**) Western blots validate the expression of mutant Kras in UMUC3 cells in the condition of no infection, with control shRNA lentiviral particle transfection or with Kras shRNA lentiviral particle transfection (Of note, this is the stably infected multiple-infectant mixture, which usually had the issue with some endogenous mutant Kras, due to some unclear reasons). GAPDH is the internal control. (**E**) FL118 exhibited was less effective in inhibiting UMUC3 tumors with a partial silencing of mutant Kras using Kras shRNA. The tumor growth curves shown in E are the mean ± SD derived from 5 mice.

4. Discussion

In order to facilitate a better discussion of the studies reported in this paper, we must first briefly introduce the discovery and the previous findings on FL118. We have generated the survivin promoter-driven luciferase reporter-stably expressed cancer cell models from the colon (HCT116), lung (A549), breast (MCF-7), prostate (PC-3) and ovary (2008) cancer cells [53]. Using these genetically engineered cancer cell models through high throughput screening (HTS) of compound libraries, followed by hit-to-lead in vitro and in vivo testing, we identified the novel small molecule anticancer drug FL118 [16]. We found that FL118 inhibits multiple anti-apoptotic proteins in the inhibitor of apoptosis (IAP) and Bcl-2 families (survivin, Mcl-1, XIAP, cIAP2) [16] as well as other oncogenic proteins such as MdmX/Mdm4 in the p53 signaling pathway [54]. Furthermore, while irinotecan/SN-38 (the active metabolite of irinotecan) and topotecan are substrates of the drug efflux pump proteins ABCG2/BCRP [55–60] and P-gp/MDR1 [61–66], FL118 is not a substrate of ABCG2 and P-gp, and can overcome treatment resistance resulting from the expression of ABCG2 [67] or P-gp [68]. This might be one of the reasons that FL118 can effectively overcome irinotecan and topotecan resistance [68] and can be orally available. Recent studies also revealed that FL118 targets drug-resistant pancreatic cancer cells, cancer stem cells and exhibits exceptional efficacy for the inhibition of pancreatic cancer patient-derived xenograft (PDX) tumors in animal models [69]. Additionally, in terms of the feature of FL118 acting as a non-efflux pump protein substrate, the use of non-efflux pump (e.g., ABCG2) substrate drugs, instead of combination with an efflux pump protein inhibitor, is a new trend in the field for anticancer drug development [70]. In this regard, FL118 is a small molecule drug that is well matched to this trend.

The current targeted agents for human bladder cancer treatment have shown limited efficacy with substantial side effects. Mutations of key genes downstream of the drug target is a key resistance mechanism and a major obstacle to the development of efficacious targeted therapies [8]. In this study, we report the differential sensitivity of high-grade human bladder cancer cell lines with mutant Hras (T24) or with mutant Kras (UMUC-3) versus wild-type Ras (HT1376) to FL118. Intriguingly, our studies revealed that the UMUC-3 and T24 bladder cancer cells with Kras and Hras mutations were highly sensitive to FL118 treatment; in contrast, HT1376 cells without Ras mutation showed resistance to FL118 in the cancer cell viability assay after FL118 treatment (Figure 1). Additional bladder cancer cell lines with wild-type Ras also exhibited much less sensitivity to FL118 treatment in comparison with bladder cancer or CRC cells with mutant Ras (Table 1, Figure S1). Such intriguing observation provides a possibility that mutation of Ras (Hras or Kras in this study) may represent a favorable predictive biomarker for FL118-targeted precision medicine. In order to validate this innovative concept, we performed a series of additional experiments to gain insight into the molecular events and mechanism of action for FL118 using the FL118-sensitive T24 and UMUC-3 bladder cancer cells versus the FL118-insensitive HT1376 bladder cancer cells. Consistent with the effect of FL118 on bladder cancer cell viability (Figure 1), FL118 was able to strongly induce PARP cleavage in both T24 and UMUC-3 cells but failed to induce PARP cleavage in HT1376 cells (Figure 2). Furthermore, the differential effect of FL118 on apoptosis induction in UMUC-3 and T24 cells versus in HT1376 cells were supported by our additional studies that FL118 was able to inhibit the expression of multiple anti-apoptotic proteins in T24 cells (survivin, XIAP) and UMUC-3 (survivin, XIAP, Mcl-1), while FL118 failed to inhibit any of these proteins in HT1376 cells (Figure 3). This is consistent with the previous findings that the inhibition of survivin, Mcl-1, XIAP and cIAP2 by FL118 plays a role in FL118 antitumor efficacy [16,31].

Previous studies demonstrated that activation of the AKT [71–73] and ERK [73–75] signaling is involved in mediating drug resistance and also linked to the upregulation of anti-apoptotic proteins such as XIAP [76]. We previously also found that paclitaxel-induced survivin expression is through activation of the PI3K-AKT and MEK-ERK1/2 pathways as the paclitaxel-resistant factor, and the inhibition of these two pathways by their specific inhibitors decreased survivin expression and sensitized paclitaxel efficacy in breast cancer cells [20]. Therefore, we investigated the effect of FL118 on the modulation of the total and phosphorylated AKT and ERK1/2 over time. We found that all of the three bladder cancer cell lines (HT1376, T24, UMUC-3) have the high constitutive expression and phosphorylation (activation) of AKT (p-Akt on ser473) and ERK1/2 (p-ERK1 on Thr202/Tyr204 and p-ERK2 on Thr185/Tyr187) (Figure 4, Figure S4). However, modulation of the total AKT and p-Akt, as well as the total ERK1/2 and p-ERK1/2 by FL118 treatment (Figure 4, Figure S4), is not fully consistent with the data obtained in the rest of our studies shown in Figure 1 (FL118 effects on cell viability), Figure 2 (FL118 effects on cell apoptosis) and Figure 3 (FL118 effects on anti-apoptotic protein expression), while the data from Figures 1–3 are highly consistent with each other as discussed early. Therefore, we hypothesized that alternative mechanisms of action and signaling pathways for FL118's antitumor activity should exist in bladder cancer cells.

FL118 is structurally similar to topotecan and irinotecan, which are FDA-approved camptothecin (CPT) analogs for cancer treatment. However, the high efficacy of FL118 antitumor ability is irrelevant to CPTs' therapeutic target, Top1 as FL118 can exhibit high antitumor efficacy to tumors that have low or negative Top1 expression [50]. As mentioned earlier, this is in contrast to the reported finding that reduced Top1 expression and/or Top1 catalytic activity in cancer cells is associated with increased resistance to CPTs [45,46] and that the increased Top1 expression in cancer cells sensitizes CPTs [47–49]. Studies have demonstrated that downregulation of Top1 protein by CPT is a CPT resistance mechanism [39–42] and that the intensity of CPT-induced downregulation of Top1 expression is positively associated with the intensity of cell resistance to CPTs [44]. In opposition to these previously documented findings for CPTs, our studies with bladder cancer cells as presented in this report revealed that FL118 has the least ability to inhibit Top1 expression in the resistant cell line HT1376 (Figure 5A), while FL118 has a better ability to inhibit Top1 expression in the FL118-sensitive T24 and UMUC-3 cells (Figure 5B,C). Thus, downregulation of Top1 expression is not a resistant factor to FL118, and Top1 could not be used as a biomarker to predict treatment resistance and sensitivity for FL118. Actually, it should be noted that growing evidence has revealed that CPT and CPT analogs can also have Top1-independent activity to inhibit cancer cells [77] or neutralize HIV-1 [78]. More examples of Top1-independent cases were recently reviewed [79].

Identification of a biomarker for predicting the response to FL118 treatment is important for personalized treatment decisions. We next used UMUC-3 cells as a model system to test whether mutant Kras plays a positive role in FL118 antitumor activity. Our studies revealed that silencing mutant Kras in UMUC-3 cells decreases FL118's ability to induce apoptosis (PARP cleavage) and at least partially abrogates FL118-mediated inhibition of the expression of XIAP, Mcl-1 and survivin (Figure 6A). However, genetic overexpression of Kras G12V in HT1367 cells resulted in no expression changes of XIAP and Mcl-1 while slightly increasing FL118-induced PARP cleavage (Figure 6C). One simple explanation for the minimal effect of forced expression of Kras G12V on FL118 function could be due to low transfection efficiency and/or alternatively, additional protein factors in the HT1376 cells may be involved in FL118-mediated inhibition of multiple anti-apoptotic proteins. This remains to be investigated in the future.

Consistent with the result derived from in vitro studies, UMUC3-established xenograft tumors exhibited high sensitivity to FL118 (Figure 9A), while HT1376-established xenograft tumors exhibited high resistance to FL118 (Figure 9B). Furthermore, Kras shRNA silencing of mutant Kras in the UMUC3 cell-generated xenograft tumor showed less sensitivity to FL118 treatment in comparison with the UMUC3 tumors manipulated with control shRNA (Figure 9E). We noticed that the effective difference is relatively small. This likely contributes to the stably mutant Kras-silencing UMUC3 cells only exhibiting a moderate decrease of mutant Kras expression (i.e., a moderate expression of mutant Kras was still there) in the studies (Figure 9D). Nevertheless, these observations indicate that mutant Kras plays a favorable role in FL118 anti-bladder cancer cell activity and could be used as a biomarker for bladder cancer patient selection for FL118 precision medicine. This finding is highly innovative and significant since Ras mutation, such as Kras mutation, is a well-known major treatment-resistant factor in many types of cancer, especially in pancreatic and colorectal cancers. However, we noticed that in the case of $Kras^{G12D}$ in the pancreatic cancer HPAF-II cell line, the silencing of $Kras^{G12D}$ using Kras shRNA could increase FL118-induced apoptosis [21], suggesting that $Kras^{G12D}$ in HPAF-II cells is somewhat of a resistant factor for FL118. This inconsistency could result from genetic differences in other genes in the background and may not be cancer type-specific or Kras mutation-specific.

Previous studies indicated that the histone deacetylase inhibitor FR901228 selectively induces ROS production in Hras-expressing J82 bladder cancer cells versus the parental cells [80]; ROS induction can render both mutant and wild-type Kras pancreatic cancer cells susceptible to Ad.mda-7/IL-24-induced apoptosis [81]. It was also reported that Kras G12V (K-ras V12) promotes ROS production in colorectal cancer cells through activation of the p38-PDPK1-PKCδ/$p47^{phox}$-NOX1 cascade [51], which promotes malignant transformation [52]. Additionally, ROS-mediated targeted therapies represent a new area of study for the treatment of bladder cancer [82]. In order to have a better understanding of the functional relationship of mutant Kras and mutant Hras with favorable FL118 efficacy, we first determined whether there is a differential ROS induction by FL118 treatment in the three bladder cancer cells (HT1376, T24, UMUC-3). We theorized that FL118 might take advantage of mutant Kras and mutant Hras to stimulate ROS production. As expected, FL118 treatment rapidly increased ROS production in both T24 and UMUC-3 cells, but not in HT1376 cells (Figure 7A), which is consistent with our previous observation that the plant-isolated compound AMR-MeOAc in combination with a low concentration of FL118 increases ROS production in the pancreatic cancer HPAF-II cell line [21]. We then explored the potential signaling pathway of FL118-mediated induction of ROS production through mutant Kras using the bladder cancer UMUC-3 cells as a model system. Our studies revealed that the silencing of mutant Kras by Kras-specific shRNA significantly decreased FL118-induced ROS production (Figure 7B). Thus, our studies at least partially explain why mutant Kras (G12V, G12C) can be used as a favorable biomarker for FL118 efficacy prediction.

Given the other in vitro data obtained, we next investigated the possibility that after FL118 treatment, Kras signaling pathway-relevant proteins may have expression level changes in the FL118-sensitive UMUC3 cells (mutant Kras) distinct from those in the FL118-insensitive HT1376 cells with wild-type Kras. We performed proteomic analyses of UMUC3 cells versus HT1376 cells after FL118 treatment (Tables S1–S6). Our data indicated that many proteins associated with mutant Kras signaling pathways exhibit opposing modulations in UMUC3 versus HT1376 cells after FL118 treatment (Figure 8, Figure S7). These findings are fully consistent with our conclusion that mutant Kras is an important potential biomarker to predict cancer cell sensitivity to FL118 treatment. However, although UMUC3 cells were in an apoptotic state after FL118 treatment, while HT1376 were not, we noted a certain inconsistency between the data from Western blots and the data from proteomics.

For example, for the data shown in Figure S7I, at the time point of FL118 treatment for 24 h, survivin (BIRC5) decreased in UMUC3 cells and increased in HT1376 cells, which is consistent with the results obtained in the Western blots (Figure 3A,C). In contrast, for the data shown in Figure S7I, at the time point of FL118 treatment for 48 h, survivin (BIRC5) increased in both UMUC3 and HT1376 cells, which is unexpected for the UMUC3 cells. We thought that since at the time point of 48 h, only a portion of the UMUC3 cells were attached, the attached UMUC3 cells used in proteomics analyses at the 48 h likely triggered a survival feedback mechanism and induced the expression of certain survival factors like survivin. Consistent with this notion, we determined the expression of survivin after 48 h FL118 treatment using the detached cells and found that the detached UMUC3 cells showed survivin decrease (Figure S3C top panel). Nevertheless, as shown in Figure S7I, Bax (a Bcl-2 family apoptotic protein) increased the UMUC3 cells in both FL118 treatments for 24 and 48 h time points, indicating that UMUC3 cells were in an apoptotic status, while HT1376 cells did not show increased Bax expression in both time points. It is important to note that the dynamic regulation of certain cancer cell survival factors like survivin in a dynamic manner has indicated cancer cell heterogeneity against various treatments, and this has also indicated a complicated network for cancer cell survival factors through various cell survival feedback regulations, especially in the case of survivin as a therapeutic target [83]. This situation may have well explained one interesting observation in our proteomics data shown in Figure S7A–W. The expression modulation of certain proteins by FL118 is in a time course-dependent manner. That is, certain proteins could be upregulated by FL118 treatment at the 24 h time point and then went into another manner to be downregulated by FL118 treatment at the 48 h time point and vice versa (Figure 8 and Figure S7A–W). Such dynamic regulation by a drug is very interesting and may include novel mechanisms that could be further explored for cancer therapeutics.

5. Conclusions

In this report, we have identified the FL118 differential modulation of apoptosis and the expression of anti-apoptotic proteins (survivin, XIAP, Mcl-1) in FL118-sensitive versus FL118-insensitive bladder cancer cells. We have further identified that the mutation-activated Kras (mutant Kras) is positively associated with FL118 efficacy and mechanistically acts as a mediator through which FL118 induces ROS production. Consistently, proteomics studies indicated that FL118 treatment induces a profound and opposing modulation of mutation-activated Kras signaling pathway-relevant proteins in UMUC3 cells versus in HT1376 cells. Significantly, our in vivo studies are fully consistent with the obtained molecular and cell biology data. Thus, our studies suggest that mutant Kras is a favorable biomarker for the prediction of FL118 sensitivity in bladder cancer. This finding will not only benefit a subset of bladder cancer patients with mutant Kras in their tumor but also benefit patients with other types of Kras-mutated cancers. For example, CRC and pancreatic cancers have high Kras mutation rates, and our studies indicated that FL118 has high efficacy to treat CRC cell xenograft tumors [50] and pancreatic cancer patient-derived xenograft (PDX) tumors [69]. Therefore, FL118 will first use CRC and pancreatic cancers in upcoming clinical trials. The significance of the finding in this report is that the use of mutant Kras as a biomarker for patient selection would increase patient response rates to FL118 treatment while avoiding unnecessary treatment. This would decrease costs while increasing the quality of life of these patients.

Supplementary Materials:
Figure S1: FL118 inhibition of bladder cancer cell growth/viability in a series of FL118 concentration for 72 h treatment, Figure S2: FL118-mediated induction of differential PARP cleavage in bladder cancer cells, Figure S3: FL118-mediated inhibition of survivin, Mcl-1 and/or XIAP in bladder cancer cell lines, Figure S4: Effect of FL118 on AKT and ERK1/2 expression and phosphorylation (activation) in bladder cancer cells, Figure S5: Sensitivity of bladder cancer cells to FL118 is irrelevant to Top1 expression level after FL118 treatment, Figure S6: Role of mutant Kras in FL118-mediated apoptosis and inhibition of antiapoptotic protein expression, Figure S7A: Cytokine and growth factor signaling related proteins, Figure S7B: Immunotherapy related proteins and/or antigens, Figure S7C: Membrane receptor signaling related proteins, Figure S7D: Cellular (non-membrane) signaling proteins, Figure S7E: DNA and chromatin remodeling related proteins, Figure S7F: Transcription factor or co-factor related proteins, Figure S7G: Gene expression and DNA damage related proteins, Figure S7H: mRNA regulation related proteins,

Figure S7I: Cell growth, proliferation and apoptosis related proteins, Figure S7J: Metabolism signaling related proteins, Figure S7K: Blood metabolism related proteins, Figure S7L: DNA metabolism and Damage repair related proteins, Figure S7M: Transporter related proteins, Figure S7N: Cell membrane, skeletal and golgi related proteins, Figure S7O: Tissue structure and adhesion related proteins, Figure S7P: Cell migration related proteins, Figure S7Q: Cell vesicle traffic/formation signaling related proteins, Figure S7R: Neuroscience-nerve system regulation signaling-related proteins, Figure S7S: Virus function related proteins, Figure S7T: Cardiovascular and heart function related protein, Figure S7U: Eyes function related proteins, Figure S7V: Protein folding correction relevant chaperonin family proteins, Figure S7W: Nuclear pore complex (NPC) related proteins, Table S1: The original data (results) set derived from the Proteomics analysis of HT1376 versus UMUC3 with and with FL118 treatment for 24 h and 48 h, Table S2: All Kras signaling transduction network-relevant protein molecules resulted from the Proteomics analysis of HT1376 versus UMUC3 with and with FL118 treatment for 24 h and/or 48 h, Table S3: Kras network-relevant proteins that were downregulated in UMUC3 cells but were upregulated or have no changes in HT1376 cells after FL118 treatment for 24 h and/or 48 h, Table S4: Kras network-relevant proteins that were upregulated in UMUC3 cells but were downregulated or roughly have no changes in HT1376 cells after FL118 treatment for 24 h and/or 48 h, Table S5. Kras signaling pathway-relevant proteins (I), Table S6. Kras signaling pathway-relevant proteins (II).

Author Contributions: Conceptualization, X.L. and F.L.; data curation, S.S., X.L., I.A.M.A., S.S.R., X.W. and J.L.; formal analysis, S.S., X.L., I.A.M.A., S.S.R., X.W. and J.L.; funding acquisition, F.L.; investigation, S.S., X.L., I.A.M.A., S.S.R., X.W. and J.L.; methodology, S.S., X.L., I.A.M.A., S.S.R., X.W. and J.L.; project administration, F.L.; resources, J.W., C.F., Q.L., J.Q. and F.L.; software, J.Q.; supervision, Q.L. and F.L.; validation, S.S., X.L., I.A.M.A. and J.L.; visualization, J.W., C.F. and J.Q.; writing–original draft, S.S. and F.L.; writing–review and editing, S.S., X.L., I.A.M.A., S.S.R., X.W., J.L., J.W., C.F., Q.L., J.Q. and F.L. All authors have read and agreed to the published version of the manuscript.

Acknowledgments: We sincerely thank Youcef M. Rustum for his discussion with the corresponding author Li for the significance of the development of anti-bladder cancer drugs. We also thank our colleagues, Yuesheng Zhang and Candace Johnson, for providing the bladder cancer cell lines (HT1376, T24, UMUC-3, RT112, 253J B-V, TCCSUP). Additionally, we thank other members in the Li Lab and/or in Canget BioTekpharma for helpful discussion, suggestion and/or some technical help during the process of this study. Finally, we thank Amanda Hess for editorial proofreading of the manuscript before submission.

References

1. Kamat, A.M.; Hahn, N.M.; Efstathiou, J.A.; Lerner, S.P.; Malmstrom, P.U.; Choi, W.; Guo, C.C.; Lotan, Y.; Kassouf, W. Bladder cancer. *Lancet* **2016**, *388*, 2796–2810. [CrossRef]
2. Knowles, M.A.; Hurst, C.D. Molecular biology of bladder cancer: New insights into pathogenesis and clinical diversity. *Nat. Rev. Cancer* **2015**, *15*, 25–41. [CrossRef] [PubMed]
3. Anastasiadis, A.; de Reijke, T.M. Best practice in the treatment of nonmuscle invasive bladder cancer. *Ther. Adv. Urol.* **2012**, *4*, 13–32. [CrossRef] [PubMed]
4. Ghosh, M.; Brancato, S.J.; Agarwal, P.K.; Apolo, A.B. Targeted therapies in urothelial carcinoma. *Curr. Opin. Oncol.* **2014**, *26*, 305–320. [CrossRef]
5. Bellmunt, J.; Petrylak, D.P. New therapeutic challenges in advanced bladder cancer. *Semin. Oncol.* **2012**, *39*, 598–607. [CrossRef]
6. Wong, Y.N.; Litwin, S.; Vaughn, D.; Cohen, S.; Plimack, E.R.; Lee, J.; Song, W.; Dabrow, M.; Brody, M.; Tuttle, H.; et al. Phase II trial of cetuximab with or without paclitaxel in patients with advanced urothelial tract carcinoma. *J. Clin. Oncol.* **2012**, *30*, 3545–3551. [CrossRef]
7. Pruthi, R.S.; Nielsen, M.; Heathcote, S.; Wallen, E.M.; Rathmell, W.K.; Godley, P.; Whang, Y.; Fielding, J.; Schultz, H.; Grigson, G.; et al. A phase II trial of neoadjuvant erlotinib in patients with muscle-invasive bladder cancer undergoing radical cystectomy: Clinical and pathological results. *BJU Int.* **2010**, *106*, 349–354. [CrossRef]
8. van Kessel, K.E.; Zuiverloon, T.C.; Alberts, A.R.; Boormans, J.L.; Zwarthoff, E.C. Targeted therapies in bladder cancer: An overview of in vivo research. *Nat. Rev. Urol.* **2015**, *12*, 681–694. [CrossRef]

9. Soloway, M.S. Bladder cancer: Lack of progress in bladder cancer—What are the obstacles? *Nat. Rev. Urol.* **2013**, *10*, 5–6. [CrossRef]
10. von der Maase, H.; Sengelov, L.; Roberts, J.T.; Ricci, S.; Dogliotti, L.; Oliver, T.; Moore, M.J.; Zimmermann, A.; Arning, M. Long-term survival results of a randomized trial comparing gemcitabine plus cisplatin, with methotrexate, vinblastine, doxorubicin, plus cisplatin in patients with bladder cancer. *J. Clin. Oncol.* **2005**, *23*, 4602–4608. [CrossRef]
11. Montazeri, K.; Bellmunt, J. Erdafitinib for the treatment of metastatic bladder cancer. *Expert Rev. Clin. Pharmacol.* **2019**, 1–6. [CrossRef]
12. Ewald, J.A.; Downs, T.M.; Cetnar, J.P.; Ricke, W.A. Expression microarray meta-analysis identifies genes associated with Ras/MAPK and related pathways in progression of muscle-invasive bladder transition cell carcinoma. *PLoS ONE* **2013**, *8*, e55414. [CrossRef]
13. McConkey, D.J.; Lee, S.; Choi, W.; Tran, M.; Majewski, T.; Lee, S.; Siefker-Radtke, A.; Dinney, C.; Czerniak, B. Molecular genetics of bladder cancer: Emerging mechanisms of tumor initiation and progression. *Urol. Oncol.* **2010**, *28*, 429–440. [CrossRef]
14. Wu, X.R. Urothelial tumorigenesis: A tale of divergent pathways. *Nat. Rev. Cancer* **2005**, *5*, 713–725. [CrossRef]
15. Jebar, A.H.; Hurst, C.D.; Tomlinson, D.C.; Johnston, C.; Taylor, C.F.; Knowles, M.A. FGFR3 and Ras gene mutations are mutually exclusive genetic events in urothelial cell carcinoma. *Oncogene* **2005**, *24*, 5218–5225. [CrossRef]
16. Ling, X.; Cao, S.; Cheng, Q.; Keefe, J.T.; Rustum, Y.M.; Li, F. A Novel Small Molecule FL118 That Selectively Inhibits Survivin, Mcl-1, XIAP and cIAP2 in a p53-Independent Manner, Shows Superior Antitumor Activity. *PLoS ONE* **2012**, *7*, e45571. [CrossRef]
17. Santha, S.; Viswakarma, N.; Das, S.; Rana, A.; Rana, B. Tumor Necrosis Factor-related Apoptosis-inducing Ligand (TRAIL)-Troglitazone-induced Apoptosis in Prostate Cancer Cells Involve AMP-activated Protein Kinase. *J. Biol. Chem.* **2015**, *290*, 21865–21875. [CrossRef]
18. Ling, X.; Calinski, D.; Chanan-Khan, A.A.; Zhou, M.; Li, F. Cancer cell sensitivity to bortezomib is associated with survivin expression and p53 status but not cancer cell types. *J. Exp. Clin. Cancer Res.* **2010**, *29*, 8. [CrossRef]
19. Santha, S.; Bommareddy, A.; Rule, B.; Guillermo, R.; Kaushik, R.S.; Young, A.; Dwivedi, C. Antineoplastic effects of alpha-santalol on estrogen receptor-positive and estrogen receptor-negative breast cancer cells through cell cycle arrest at G2/M phase and induction of apoptosis. *PLoS ONE* **2013**, *8*, e56982. [CrossRef]
20. Ling, X.; Bernacki, R.J.; Brattain, M.G.; Li, F. Induction of survivin expression by taxol (paclitaxel) is an early event which is independent on taxol-mediated G2/M arrest. *J. Biol. Chem.* **2004**, *279*, 15196–15203. [CrossRef]
21. Rabi, T.; Li, F. Multiple mechanisms involved in a low concentration of FL118 enhancement of AMR-MeOAc to induce pancreatic cancer cell apoptosis and growth inhibition. *Am. J. Cancer Res.* **2018**, *8*, 2267–2283. [PubMed]
22. Shen, X.; Shen, S.; Li, J.; Hu, Q.; Nie, L.; Tu, C.; Wang, X.; Orsburn, B.; Wang, J.; Qu, J. An IonStar Experimental Strategy for MS1 Ion Current-Based Quantification Using Ultrahigh-Field Orbitrap: Reproducible, In-Depth, and Accurate Protein Measurement in Large Cohorts. *J. Proteome Res.* **2017**, *16*, 2445–2456. [CrossRef] [PubMed]
23. Huang da, W.; Sherman, B.T.; Lempicki, R.A. Systematic and integrative analysis of large gene lists using DAVID bioinformatics resources. *Nat. Protoc.* **2009**, *4*, 44–57. [CrossRef] [PubMed]
24. de Hoon, M.J.; Imoto, S.; Nolan, J.; Miyano, S. Open source clustering software. *Bioinformatics* **2004**, *20*, 1453–1454. [CrossRef] [PubMed]
25. Subramanian, A.; Tamayo, P.; Mootha, V.K.; Mukherjee, S.; Ebert, B.L.; Gillette, M.A.; Paulovich, A.; Pomeroy, S.L.; Golub, T.R.; Lander, E.S.; et al. Gene set enrichment analysis: A knowledge-based approach for interpreting genome-wide expression profiles. *Proc. Natl. Acad. Sci. USA* **2005**, *102*, 15545–15550. [CrossRef] [PubMed]
26. Mootha, V.K.; Lindgren, C.M.; Eriksson, K.F.; Subramanian, A.; Sihag, S.; Lehar, J.; Puigserver, P.; Carlsson, E.; Ridderstrale, M.; Laurila, E.; et al. PGC-1alpha-responsive genes involved in oxidative phosphorylation are coordinately downregulated in human diabetes. *Nat. Genet.* **2003**, *34*, 267–273. [CrossRef] [PubMed]

27. Ling, X.; Li, F. Use of the FL118 Core Chemical Structure Platform to Generate FL118 Derivatives for Treatment of Human Disease (PCT/US2015/022095). 2015. Available online: https://patentswarm.com/patents/US10344037B2 as well as https://patentscope.wipo.int/search/en/detail.jsf?docId=WO2015148415 (accessed on 18 November 2020).
28. Earl, J.; Rico, D.; Carrillo-de-Santa-Pau, E.; Rodriguez-Santiago, B.; Mendez-Pertuz, M.; Auer, H.; Gomez, G.; Grossman, H.B.; Pisano, D.G.; Schulz, W.A.; et al. The UBC-40 Urothelial Bladder Cancer cell line index: A genomic resource for functional studies. *BMC Genom.* **2015**, *16*, 403. [CrossRef]
29. Fearon, E.R. Molecular genetics of colorectal cancer. *Annu. Rev. Pathol.* **2011**, *6*, 479–507. [CrossRef]
30. Cox, A.D.; Fesik, S.W.; Kimmelman, A.C.; Luo, J.; Der, C.J. Drugging the undruggable RAS: Mission possible? *Nat. Rev. Drug Discov.* **2014**, *13*, 828–851. [CrossRef]
31. Zhao, J.; Ling, X.; Cao, S.; Liu, X.; Wan, S.; Jiang, T.; Li, F. Antitumor activity of FL118, a survivin, Mcl-1, XIAP, cIAP2 selective inhibitor, is highly dependent on its primary structure and steric configuration. *Mol. Pharm.* **2014**, *11*, 457–467. [CrossRef]
32. Asanuma, H.; Torigoe, T.; Kamiguchi, K.; Hirohashi, Y.; Ohmura, T.; Hirata, K.; Sato, M.; Sato, N. Survivin expression is regulated by coexpression of human epidermal growth factor receptor 2 and epidermal growth factor receptor via phosphatidylinositol 3-kinase/AKT signaling pathway in breast cancer cells. *Cancer Res.* **2005**, *65*, 11018–11025. [CrossRef] [PubMed]
33. Xing, H.; Weng, D.; Chen, G.; Tao, W.; Zhu, T.; Yang, X.; Meng, L.; Wang, S.; Lu, Y.; Ma, D. Activation of fibronectin/PI-3K/Akt2 leads to chemoresistance to docetaxel by regulating survivin protein expression in ovarian and breast cancer cells. *Cancer Lett.* **2008**, *261*, 108–119. [CrossRef] [PubMed]
34. Ye, Q.; Cai, W.; Zheng, Y.; Evers, B.M.; She, Q.B. ERK and AKT signaling cooperate to translationally regulate survivin expression for metastatic progression of colorectal cancer. *Oncogene* **2014**, *33*, 1828–1839. [CrossRef] [PubMed]
35. Sun, L.; Zhao, Y.; Shi, H.; Ma, C.; Wei, L. LMP-1 induces survivin expression to inhibit cell apoptosis through the NF-kappaB and PI3K/Akt signaling pathways in nasal NK/T-cell lymphoma. *Oncol. Rep.* **2015**, *33*, 2253–2260. [CrossRef] [PubMed]
36. Tsubaki, M.; Takeda, T.; Ogawa, N.; Sakamoto, K.; Shimaoka, H.; Fujita, A.; Itoh, T.; Imano, M.; Ishizaka, T.; Satou, T.; et al. Overexpression of survivin via activation of ERK1/2, Akt, and NF-kappaB plays a central role in vincristine resistance in multiple myeloma cells. *Leuk. Res.* **2015**, *39*, 445–452. [CrossRef] [PubMed]
37. Carter, B.Z.; Mak, D.; Schober, W.D.; Cabreira-Hansen, M.; Beran, M.; McQueen, T.; Chen, W.; Andreeff, M. Regulation of survivin expression through Bcr-Abl/MAPK cascade: Targeting survivin overcomes Imatinib resistance and increases Imatinib sensitivity in Imatinib responsive CML cells. *Blood* **2006**, *107*, 1555–1563. [CrossRef] [PubMed]
38. Zhang, Y.; Chen, H.X.; Zhou, S.Y.; Wang, S.X.; Zheng, K.; Xu, D.D.; Liu, Y.T.; Wang, X.Y.; Wang, X.; Yan, H.Z.; et al. Sp1 and c-Myc modulate drug resistance of leukemia stem cells by regulating survivin expression through the ERK-MSK MAPK signaling pathway. *Mol. Cancer* **2015**, *14*, 56. [CrossRef] [PubMed]
39. Sugimoto, Y.; Tsukahara, S.; Oh-hara, T.; Isoe, T.; Tsuruo, T. Decreased expression of DNA topoisomerase I in camptothecin-resistant tumor cell lines as determined by a monoclonal antibody. *Cancer Res.* **1990**, *50*, 6925–6930.
40. Kanzawa, F.; Sugimoto, Y.; Minato, K.; Kasahara, K.; Bungo, M.; Nakagawa, K.; Fujiwara, Y.; Liu, L.F.; Saijo, N. Establishment of a camptothecin analogue (CPT-11)-resistant cell line of human non-small cell lung cancer: Characterization and mechanism of resistance. *Cancer Res.* **1990**, *50*, 5919–5924.
41. Woessner, R.D.; Eng, W.K.; Hofmann, G.A.; Rieman, D.J.; McCabe, F.L.; Hertzberg, R.P.; Mattern, M.R.; Tan, K.B.; Johnson, R.K. Camptothecin hyper-resistant P388 cells: Drug-dependent reduction in topoisomerase I content. *Oncol. Res.* **1992**, *4*, 481–488.
42. Ando, K.; Shah, A.K.; Sachdev, V.; Kleinstiver, B.P.; Taylor-Parker, J.; Welch, M.M.; Hu, Y.; Salgia, R.; White, F.M.; Parvin, J.D.; et al. Camptothecin resistance is determined by the regulation of topoisomerase I degradation mediated by ubiquitin proteasome pathway. *Oncotarget* **2017**, *8*, 43733–43751. [CrossRef] [PubMed]
43. Sugimoto, Y.; Tsukahara, S.; Oh-hara, T.; Liu, L.F.; Tsuruo, T. Elevated expression of DNA topoisomerase II in camptothecin-resistant human tumor cell lines. *Cancer Res.* **1990**, *50*, 7962–7965. [PubMed]

44. Desai, S.D.; Li, T.K.; Rodriguez-Bauman, A.; Rubin, E.H.; Liu, L.F. Ubiquitin/26S proteasome-mediated degradation of topoisomerase I as a resistance mechanism to camptothecin in tumor cells. *Cancer Res.* **2001**, *61*, 5926–5932. [PubMed]
45. Kapoor, R.; Slade, D.L.; Fujimori, A.; Pommier, Y.; Harker, W.G. Altered topoisomerase I expression in two subclones of human CEM leukemia selected for resistance to camptothecin. *Oncol. Res.* **1995**, *7*, 83–95.
46. Liao, Z.; Robey, R.W.; Guirouilh-Barbat, J.; To, K.K.; Polgar, O.; Bates, S.E.; Pommier, Y. Reduced expression of DNA topoisomerase I in SF295 human glioblastoma cells selected for resistance to homocamptothecin and diflomotecan. *Mol. Pharmacol.* **2008**, *73*, 490–497. [CrossRef] [PubMed]
47. Kotoh, S.; Naito, S.; Yokomizo, A.; Kumazawa, J.; Asakuno, K.; Kohno, K.; Kuwano, M. Increased expression of DNA topoisomerase I gene and collateral sensitivity to camptothecin in human cisplatin-resistant bladder cancer cells. *Cancer Res.* **1994**, *54*, 3248–3252.
48. Sakai, A.; Kasahara, K.; Ohmori, T.; Kimura, H.; Sone, T.; Fujimura, M.; Nakao, S. MET increases the sensitivity of gefitinib-resistant cells to SN-38, an active metabolite of irinotecan, by up-regulating the topoisomerase I activity. *J. Thorac. Oncol.* **2012**, *7*, 1337–1344. [CrossRef]
49. Smith, P.J.; Makinson, T.A.; Watson, J.V. Enhanced sensitivity to camptothecin in ataxia-telangiectasia cells and its relationship with the expression of DNA topoisomerase I. *Int. J. Radiat. Biol.* **1989**, *55*, 217–231. [CrossRef]
50. Li, F.; Ling, X.; Harris, D.L.; Liao, J.; Wang, Y.; Westover, D.; Jiang, G.; Xu, B.; Boland, P.M.; Jin, C. Topoisomerase I (Top1): A major target of FL118 for its antitumor efficacy or mainly involved in its side effects of hematopoietic toxicity? *Am. J. Cancer Res.* **2017**, *7*, 370–382.
51. Park, M.T.; Kim, M.J.; Suh, Y.; Kim, R.K.; Kim, H.; Lim, E.J.; Yoo, K.C.; Lee, G.H.; Kim, Y.H.; Hwang, S.G.; et al. Novel signaling axis for ROS generation during K-Ras-induced cellular transformation. *Cell Death Differ.* **2014**, *21*, 1185–1197. [CrossRef]
52. Suh, Y.; Lee, S.J. KRAS-driven ROS promote malignant transformation. *Mol. Cell Oncol.* **2015**, *2*, e968059. [CrossRef] [PubMed]
53. Li, F. Compositions and Methods for Identifying Agents that Alter Expression of Survivin. US Patent 7,569,221 B2, 4 August 2009.
54. Ling, X.; Xu, C.; Fan, C.; Zhong, K.; Li, F.; Wang, X. FL118 Induces p53-Dependent Senescence in Colorectal Cancer Cells by Promoting Degradation of MdmX. *Cancer Res.* **2014**, *74*, 7487–7497. [CrossRef] [PubMed]
55. Houghton, P.J.; Germain, G.S.; Harwood, F.C.; Schuetz, J.D.; Stewart, C.F.; Buchdunger, E.; Traxler, P. Imatinib mesylate is a potent inhibitor of the ABCG2 (BCRP) transporter and reverses resistance to topotecan and SN-38 in vitro. *Cancer Res.* **2004**, *64*, 2333–2337. [CrossRef] [PubMed]
56. Su, Y.; Hu, P.; Lee, S.H.; Sinko, P.J. Using novobiocin as a specific inhibitor of breast cancer resistant protein (BCRP/ABCG2) to assess the role of transporter in the absorption and disposition of topotecan. *J. Pharm. Pharm. Sci.* **2007**, *10*, 519–536. [CrossRef]
57. Su, Y.; Lee, S.H.; Sinko, P.J. Inhibition of efflux transporter ABCG2/BCRP does not restore mitoxantrone sensitivity in irinotecan-selected human leukemia CPT-K5 cells: Evidence for multifactorial multidrug resistance. *Eur. J. Pharm. Sci. Off. J. Eur. Fed. Pharm. Sci.* **2006**, *29*, 102–110. [CrossRef]
58. Yoshikawa, M.; Ikegami, Y.; Sano, K.; Yoshida, H.; Mitomo, H.; Sawada, S.; Ishikawa, T. Transport of SN-38 by the wild type of human ABC transporter ABCG2 and its inhibition by quercetin, a natural flavonoid. *J. Exp. Ther. Oncol.* **2004**, *4*, 25–35.
59. Shishido, Y.; Ueno, S.; Yamazaki, R.; Nagaoka, M.; Matsuzaki, T. ABCG2 inhibitor YHO-13351 sensitizes cancer stem/initiating-like side population cells to irinotecan. *Anticancer Res.* **2013**, *33*, 1379–1386.
60. Maliepaard, M.; van Gastelen, M.A.; de Jong, L.A.; Pluim, D.; van Waardenburg, R.C.; Ruevekamp-Helmers, M.C.; Floot, B.G.; Schellens, J.H. Overexpression of the BCRP/MXR/ABCP gene in a topotecan-selected ovarian tumor cell line. *Cancer Res.* **1999**, *59*, 4559–4563.
61. Kruijtzer, C.M.; Beijnen, J.H.; Rosing, H.; ten Bokkel Huinink, W.W.; Schot, M.; Jewell, R.C.; Paul, E.M.; Schellens, J.H. Increased oral bioavailability of topotecan in combination with the breast cancer resistance protein and P-glycoprotein (Pgp) inhibitor GF120918. *J. Clin. Oncol. Off. J. Am. Soc. Clin. Oncol.* **2002**, *20*, 2943–2950. [CrossRef]
62. de Vries, N.A.; Zhao, J.; Kroon, E.; Buckle, T.; Beijnen, J.H.; van Tellingen, O. P-glycoprotein (Pgp) and breast cancer resistance protein (BCRP): Two dominant transporters working together in limiting the brain penetration of topotecan. *Clin. Cancer Res. Off. J. Am. Assoc. Cancer Res.* **2007**, *13*, 6440–6449. [CrossRef]

63. Takeba, Y.; Sekine, S.; Kumai, T.; Matsumoto, N.; Nakaya, S.; Tsuzuki, Y.; Yanagida, Y.; Nakano, H.; Asakura, T.; Ohtsubo, T.; et al. Irinotecan-induced apoptosis is inhibited by increased P-glycoprotein expression and decreased p53 in human hepatocellular carcinoma cells. *Biol. Pharm. Bull.* **2007**, *30*, 1400–1406. [CrossRef] [PubMed]
64. Tagen, M.; Zhuang, Y.; Zhang, F.; Harstead, K.E.; Shen, J.; Schaiquevich, P.; Fraga, C.H.; Panetta, J.C.; Waters, C.M.; Stewart, C.F. P-glycoprotein, but not multidrug resistance protein 4, plays a role in the systemic clearance of irinotecan and SN-38 in mice. *Drug Metab. Lett.* **2010**, *4*, 195–201. [CrossRef] [PubMed]
65. Filipski, E.; Berland, E.; Ozturk, N.; Guettier, C.; van der Horst, G.T.; Levi, F.; Okyar, A. Optimization of irinotecan chronotherapy with P-glycoprotein inhibition. *Toxicol. Appl. Pharmacol.* **2014**, *274*, 471–479. [CrossRef] [PubMed]
66. Hendricks, C.B.; Rowinsky, E.K.; Grochow, L.B.; Donehower, R.C.; Kaufmann, S.H. Effect of P-glycoprotein expression on the accumulation and cytotoxicity of topotecan (SK&F 104864), a new camptothecin analogue. *Cancer Res.* **1992**, *52*, 2268–2278. [PubMed]
67. Westover, D.; Ling, X.; Lam, H.; Welch, J.; Jin, C.; Gongora, C.; Del Rio, M.; Wani, M.; Li, F. FL118, a novel camptothecin derivative, is insensitive to ABCG2 expression and shows improved efficacy in comparison with irinotecan in colon and lung cancer models with ABCG2-induced resistance. *Mol. Cancer* **2015**, *14*, 92. [CrossRef] [PubMed]
68. Ling, X.; Liu, X.J.; Zhong, K.; Smith, N.; Prey, J.; Li, F. FL118, a novel camptothecin analogue, overcomes irinotecan and topotecan resistance in human tumor xenograft models. *Am. J. Transl. Res.* **2015**, *7*, 1765–1781.
69. Ling, X.; Wu, W.; Fan, C.; Xu, C.; Liao, J.; Rich, L.J.; Huang, R.Y.; Repasky, E.A.; Wang, X.; Li, F. An ABCG2 non-substrate anticancer agent FL118 targets drug-resistant cancer stem-like cells and overcomes treatment resistance of human pancreatic cancer. *J. Exp. Clin. Cancer Res.* **2018**, *37*, 240. [CrossRef]
70. Westover, D.; Li, F. New trends for overcoming ABCG2/BCRP-mediated resistance to cancer therapies. *J. Exp. Clin. Cancer Res.* **2015**, *34*, 159. [CrossRef]
71. Szanto, A.; Bognar, Z.; Szigeti, A.; Szabo, A.; Farkas, L.; Gallyas, F., Jr. Critical role of bad phosphorylation by Akt in cytostatic resistance of human bladder cancer cells. *Anticancer Res.* **2009**, *29*, 159–164.
72. Yuge, K.; Kikuchi, E.; Hagiwara, M.; Yasumizu, Y.; Tanaka, N.; Kosaka, T.; Miyajima, A.; Oya, M. Nicotine Induces Tumor Growth and Chemoresistance through Activation of the PI3K/Akt/mTOR Pathway in Bladder Cancer. *Mol. Cancer Ther.* **2015**, *14*, 2112–2120. [CrossRef]
73. Dong, Q.; Fu, L.; Zhao, Y.; Tan, S.; Wang, E. Derlin-1 overexpression confers poor prognosis in muscle invasive bladder cancer and contributes to chemoresistance and invasion through PI3K/AKT and ERK/MMP signaling. *Oncotarget* **2017**, *8*, 17059–17069. [CrossRef] [PubMed]
74. Takeuchi, A.; Eto, M.; Shiota, M.; Tatsugami, K.; Yokomizo, A.; Kuroiwa, K.; Itsumi, M.; Naito, S. Sunitinib enhances antitumor effects against chemotherapy-resistant bladder cancer through suppression of ERK1/2 phosphorylation. *Int J. Oncol.* **2012**, *40*, 1691–1696. [CrossRef] [PubMed]
75. Huang, L.; Luan, T.; Chen, Y.; Bao, X.; Huang, Y.; Fu, S.; Wang, H.; Wang, J. LASS2 regulates invasion and chemoresistance via ERK/Drp1 modulated mitochondrial dynamics in bladder cancer cells. *J. Cancer* **2018**, *9*, 1017–1024. [CrossRef] [PubMed]
76. Shrader, M.; Pino, M.S.; Lashinger, L.; Bar-Eli, M.; Adam, L.; Dinney, C.P.; McConkey, D.J. Gefitinib reverses TRAIL resistance in human bladder cancer cell lines via inhibition of AKT-mediated X-linked inhibitor of apoptosis protein expression. *Cancer Res.* **2007**, *67*, 1430–1435. [CrossRef] [PubMed]
77. Wolff, D.; Lee, M.H.; Jothi, M.; Mal, M.; Li, F.; Mal, A.K. Camptothecin exhibits topoisomerase1-independent KMT1A suppression and myogenic differentiation in alveolar rhabdomyosarcoma cells. *Oncotarget* **2018**, *9*, 25796–25807. [CrossRef] [PubMed]
78. Bennett, R.P.; Stewart, R.A.; Hogan, P.A.; Ptak, R.G.; Mankowski, M.K.; Hartman, T.L.; Buckheit, R.W., Jr.; Snyder, B.A.; Salter, J.D.; Morales, G.A.; et al. An analog of camptothecin inactive against Topoisomerase I is broadly neutralizing of HIV-1 through inhibition of Vif-dependent APOBEC3G degradation. *Antiviral Res.* **2016**, *136*, 51–59. [CrossRef] [PubMed]
79. Li, F.; Jiang, T.; Li, Q.; Ling, X. Camptothecin (CPT) and its derivatives are known to target topoisomerase I (Top1) as their mechanism of action: Did we miss something in CPT analogue molecular targets for treating human disease such as cancer? *Am. J. Cancer Res.* **2017**, *7*, 2350–2394.

80. Choudhary, S.; Wang, H.C. Role of reactive oxygen species in proapoptotic ability of oncogenic H-Ras to increase human bladder cancer cell susceptibility to histone deacetylase inhibitor for caspase induction. *J. Cancer Res. Clin. Oncol.* **2009**, *135*, 1601–1613. [CrossRef]
81. Lebedeva, I.V.; Su, Z.Z.; Sarkar, D.; Gopalkrishnan, R.V.; Waxman, S.; Yacoub, A.; Dent, P.; Fisher, P.B. Induction of reactive oxygen species renders mutant and wild-type K-ras pancreatic carcinoma cells susceptible to Ad.mda-7-induced apoptosis. *Oncogene* **2005**, *24*, 585–596. [CrossRef]
82. Wang, H.C.; Choudhary, S. Reactive oxygen species-mediated therapeutic control of bladder cancer. *Nat. Rev. Urol.* **2011**, *8*, 608–616. [CrossRef]
83. Li, F.; Aljahdali, I.; Ling, X. Cancer therapeutics using survivin BIRC5 as a target: What can we do after over two decades of study? *J. Exp. Clin. Cancer Res.* **2019**, *38*, 368. [CrossRef] [PubMed]

2

Malignancy Grade-Dependent Mapping of Metabolic Landscapes in Human Urothelial Bladder Cancer: Identification of Novel, Diagnostic and Druggable Biomarkers

Aikaterini Iliou [1,†], Aristeidis Panagiotakis [1,†], Aikaterini F. Giannopoulou [2,†], Dimitra Benaki [1], Mariangela Kosmopoulou [1], Athanassios D. Velentzas [2], Ourania E. Tsitsilonis [3], Issidora S. Papassideri [2], Gerassimos E. Voutsinas [4], Eumorphia G. Konstantakou [5], Evagelos Gikas [1,*,‡], Emmanuel Mikros [1,*,‡] and Dimitrios J. Stravopodis [2,*,‡]

1 Section of Pharmaceutical Chemistry, Department of Pharmacy, School of Health Sciences, National and Kapodistrian University of Athens (NKUA), 15701 Athens, Greece; katerinail@pharm.uoa.gr (A.I.); arispan@pharm.uoa.gr (A.P.); dbenaki@pharm.uoa.gr (D.B.); mrgkosm@gmail.com (M.K.)

2 Section of Cell Biology and Biophysics, Department of Biology, School of Science, National and Kapodistrian University of Athens (NKUA), 15701 Athens, Greece; aigiann@biol.uoa.gr (A.F.G.); tveletz@biol.uoa.gr (A.D.V.); ipapasid@biol.uoa.gr (I.S.P.)

3 Section of Animal and Human Physiology, Department of Biology, School of Science, National and Kapodistrian University of Athens (NKUA), 15701 Athens, Greece; rtsitsil@biol.uoa.gr

4 Laboratory of Molecular Carcinogenesis and Rare Disease Genetics, Institute of Biosciences and Applications, National Center for Scientific Research (NCSR) "Demokritos", 15701 Athens, Greece; mvoutsin@bio.demokritos.gr

5 Harvard Medical School, Massachusetts General Hospital Cancer Center (MGHCC), Charlestown, MA 021004, USA; ekonstantakou@mgh.harvard.edu

* Correspondence: vgikas@pharm.uoa.gr (E.G.); mikros@pharm.uoa.gr (E.M.); dstravop@biol.uoa.gr (D.J.S.)

† These authors contributed equally to this work.

‡ These authors contributed equally to this work.

Abstract: Background: Urothelial bladder cancer (UBC) is one of the cancers with the highest mortality rate and prevalence worldwide; however, the clinical management of the disease remains challenging. Metabolomics has emerged as a powerful tool with beneficial applications in cancer biology and thus can provide new insights on the underlying mechanisms of UBC progression and/or reveal novel diagnostic and therapeutic schemes. Methods: A collection of four human UBC cell lines that critically reflect the different malignancy grades of UBC was employed; RT4 (grade I), RT112 (grade II), T24 (grade III), and TCCSUP (grade IV). They were examined using Nuclear Magnetic Resonance, Mass Spectrometry, and advanced statistical approaches, with the goal of creating new metabolic profiles that are mechanistically associated with UBC progression toward metastasis. Results: Distinct metabolic profiles were observed for each cell line group, with T24 (grade III) cells exhibiting the most abundant metabolite contents. AMP and creatine phosphate were highly increased in the T24 cell line compared to the RT4 (grade I) cell line, indicating the major energetic transformation to which UBC cells are being subjected during metastasis. Thymosin $\beta4$ and $\beta10$ were also profiled with grade-specific patterns of expression, strongly suggesting the importance of actin-cytoskeleton dynamics for UBC advancement to metastatic and drug-tolerant forms. Conclusions: The present study unveils a novel and putatively druggable metabolic signature that holds strong promise for early diagnosis and the successful chemotherapy of UBC disease.

Keywords: biomarker; bladder; cancer; grade; metabolomics; MS; NMR

1. Introduction

Urothelial bladder cancer (UBC) exhibits the highest mortality rate worldwide, being categorized as the second most common genitourinary disease in the USA [1]. UBC still remains a major clinical challenge and its treatment mainly depends on early diagnosis [2]. It can be generally classified as a low-grade (I and II) non-muscle-invasive and a high-grade (III and IV) muscle-invasive disease that is prone to metastasis, based on histological differentiations from normal bladder cells [3]. One third of non-muscle-invasive UBCs progress to high(er) grades or stages of malignancy [4], which, along with the symptom-to-treatment delay for affected patients [5], compromise the therapeutic effectiveness and success of clinically applied regimens. UBC is characterized by high recurrence rates, with the continuous monitoring of patients being a medical practice of great importance [6]. Notably, despite their initial chemosensitivity, UBC patients will eventually develop chemoresistance due to tumors' mutational heterogeneity, leading to a median survival expectancy of 13–19 months [7,8]. Thereby, novel, early diagnosis, and druggable biomarkers for UBC need to be promptly discovered.

Metabolomics, according to Professor J. Nicolson's definition, is "the quantitative measurement of the dynamic and multi-parametric metabolic response of living systems to pathophysiological stimuli or genetic modifications" [9], with its great potential and promise in cancer research being continuously proved. The reprogramming of cellular metabolism seems to act as a strong force in tumorigenesis [10]. Malignant hallmarks, such as cell survival under stress conditions, as well as tumors' ability to utilize nutrients and successfully encounter high-energy demands, are tightly correlated with metabolic alterations, thus indicating the major roles of metabolic landscapes in Cancer Biology [11–14]. Metabolic activities may significantly differ among distinct subtypes or malignancy grades/stages of the same type of cancer, leading to different metabolic networks and metabolomes [15,16]. Metabolomics has gained great value, power, and importance for cancer research, not only as a multifaceted tool in early diagnosis, but also as a valuable platform for the discovery of novel mechanisms controlling tumorigenesis, thus paving the way to new treatment strategies and therapies. Research on several cancers has significantly profited from the engagement of metabolomics technology. However, its application to early detection, progression, and the chemotherapeutic management of human malignancies and especially UBC remains still limited, and it needs to be further expanded [15–20].

Most metabolomics studies in UBC cell lines have focused on differentiating between normal bladder and UBC cells, and they have shown the importance of several metabolites involved in pathways related to energy production, such as fatty acids, amino acids, and organic acids. [21,22]. The effect of the oncometabolome on progression of the disease has recently emerged as a new field in UBC research [23–26]. Few studies used two cell lines, for low and high-grade UBC, in order to find distinct metabolic profiles between the two grades [27,28]. They observed that pyruvate consumption, as well as alanine and lactate levels, might be related to UBC aggressiveness, and they also suggested the role of fatty acid biosynthesis and amino acid metabolism in disease progression.

To further expand these studies, we herein engaged a collection of four human UBC cell lines that critically reflect the distinct de-differentiation stage, malignancy grade (I, II, III, and IV), mutational signature, genetic heterogeneity, metastatic capacity, and chemotherapeutic tolerance of UBC to thoroughly investigate the metabolic alterations to which UBC cells are being subjected during disease progression. Our findings are expected to shed light into mechanisms regulating the transition of normal to the oncogenic and, finally, metastatic cell phase. Employment of the two state-of-the-art analytical platforms, Nuclear Magnetic Resonance (NMR) and Mass Spectrometry (MS), which are complementary, allows the more comprehensive metabolic profiling of UBC, with the grade-specific metabolic signatures revealed essentially contributing to the significant advancement in the success, efficacy, and safety of conducted research. High-scale UBC cell culturing enabled the high-resolution metabolic landscaping, while the high density of cells upon harvesting portrayed tumor architectural organization in vivo.

2. Results

In this study, a comparative NMR and LC-MS-mediated metabolic profiling was performed in four UBC human cell lines in order to thoroughly examine the effects of oncometabolome composition on progression of the disease.

2.1. NMR Analysis

The ^{1}H 1D NMR spectra of the four UBC cell lines with the respective standard deviations obtained from each group are shown in Figure 1. The observed within-group variability has proved to be very low, thus confirming the precision and high-technical value of the procedure being followed for sample preparation and the subsequent instrumental analysis. In total, 42 metabolites have been identified (Supplementary Table S1), with the annotated and grade-dependent metabolites being described in Figure 2 as boxplot-type graphs.

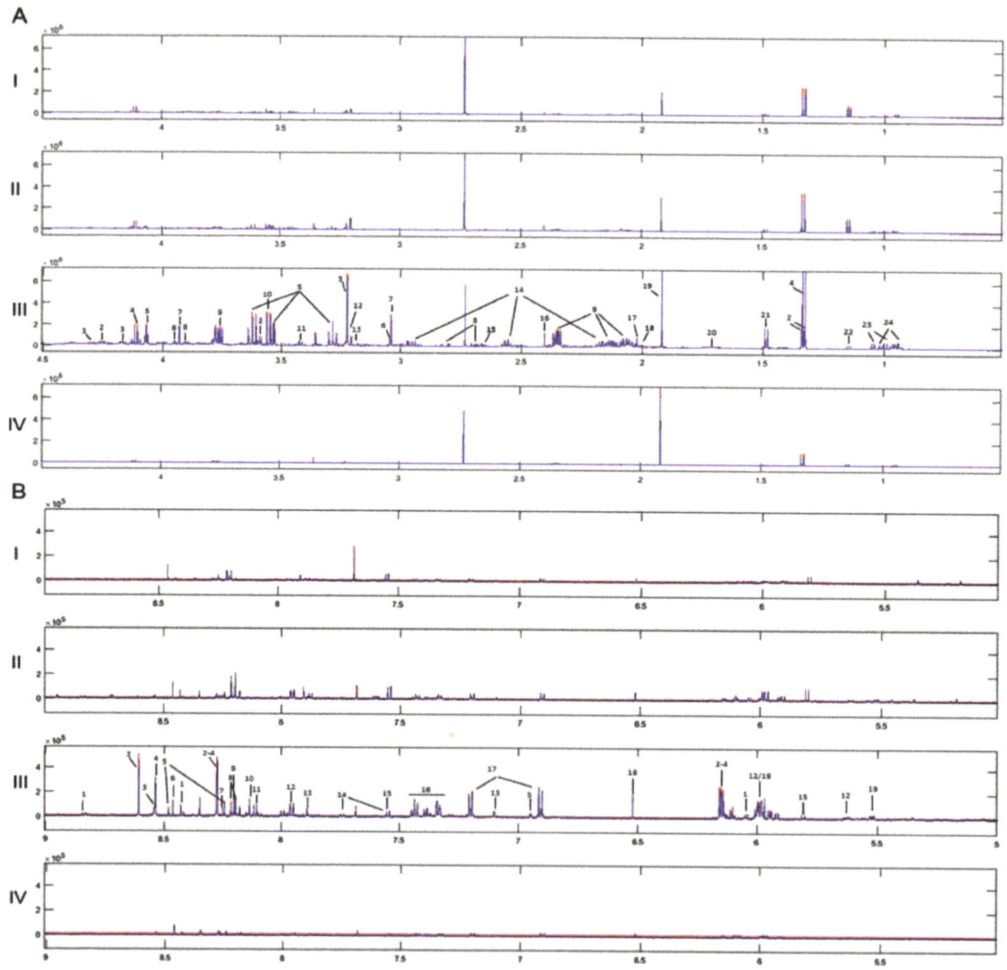

Figure 1. Average ^{1}H NMR spectra of the four groups and their standard deviation, where very low within-group variability is observed. Annotation is shown on the most abundant spectrum of the grade III group. (I. Grade I, II. Grade II, III. Grade III, IV. Grade IV). Red Line: Average + standard deviation, Blue Line: Average–standard deviation. (**A**) Aliphatic region: 1. UDPs, 2. Threonine, 3. Choline phosphate, 4. Lactate, 5. Myo-inositol, 6. Creatine phosphate, 7. Creatine, 8. Aspartate, 9. Glutamate, 10. Glycine, 11. Taurine, 12. Choline, 13. β-Alanine, 14. Glutathione, 15. Malate, 16. Succinate, 17. N-Acetylglutamine, 18. Proline, 19. Acetate, 20. Leucine, 21. Alanine, 22. Propylene glycol, 23. Valine, 24. Isoleucine. (**B**) Aromatic region: 1. NAD+, 2. AMP, 3. ATP, 4. ADP, 5. NADH, 6. Formate, 7. Adenine, 8. Hypoxanthine, 9. Oxypurinol, 10. GTP, 11. UMP, 12. UDPs, 13. Histidine, 14. Tryptophan, 15. Uracil, 16. Phenylalanine, 17. Tyrosine, 18. Fumarate, 19. UDP-GlcNAc.

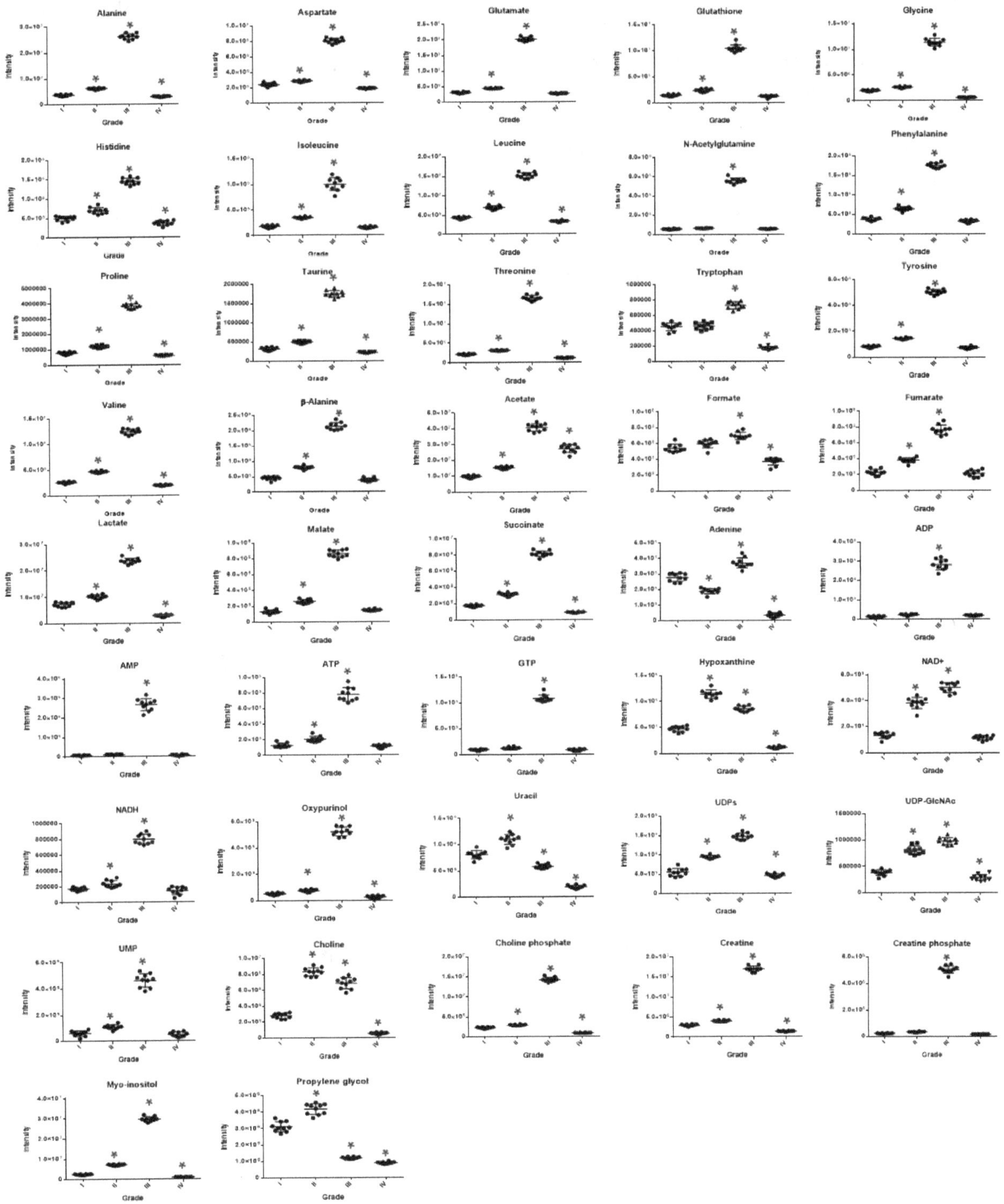

Figure 2. Boxplots of the 42 most significant metabolites, using ANOVA for the four-group urothelial bladder cancer (UBC) member comparisons. Myo-inositol, creatine phosphate, amino acids (e.g., histidine), organic acids (e.g., malate, succinate, and acetate), AXPs (AMP, ADP, and ATP), GTP, UMP, and oxypurinol follow the pattern of "metabolic inversion" that is being typified by their highly elevated contents in grade III (T24) group but reduced (restored) to the cell line-reference-like ones (RT4; grade I) in the grade IV (TCCSUP) UBC cell group. However, some metabolites are not subjected to the same pattern of grade-dependent deregulation (e.g., tryptophan, formate, uracil, adenine, propylene glycol, and choline). Remarkably, uracil and propylene glycol are presented with significant decreases during cellular transition from low to high grades (III and IV) of UBC malignancy.

For the multivariate analysis, Principal Component Analysis (PCA) was first conducted to search for outliers and trends of discrimination. No outliers were detected (Hotteling eclipse, 95% confidence level), and a clear separation of the four UBC groups was observed (Supplementary Figure S1). Partial Least Square-Discriminant Analysis (PLS-DA) confirmed the clear separation of the examined groups, with good quality parameters and prediction power [R2X(cum) = 0.982 and Q2(cum) = 0.977]. Orthogonal Partial Least Square-Discriminant Analysis (OPLS-DA) pairwise comparisons were also performed to search for discriminatory variables for each grade-specific UBC cell line. The S-plot between grade I (RT4) and grade III (T24) UBC cells revealed that the T24 cell line exhibits notably upregulated levels of most metabolites, including, among others, amino acids (glutamate, alanine, threonine), organic acids (acetate, lactate), myo-inositol, creatine, and choline phosphate, while decreased contents of few metabolites (uracil, histidine, and propylene glycol) were observed (Figure 3A).

The S-plot between grade III (T24) and grade IV (TCCSUP) UBC cells unveiled that the grade IV-specific levels of most metabolites were significantly reduced and restored almost to the grade I (RT4) respective levels, indicating a "metabolic inversion" effect during the advanced (late stage) UBC development (Figure 3B). This is observed in the PLS-DA scores plot of UBC groups, with RT4 and TCCSUP showing an inability to be discriminated on the first PC, while grade III (T24) was being proved as the most distant UBC group on the same component (Figure 3C). Validation of the PLS-DA model using permutation testing is shown in Figure 3D. Table 1 summarizes the results of univariate analysis of the identified metabolites, considering grade I (RT4) as the UBC cell line of reference (control) in order to explore malignancy grade-specific metabolic changes occurring during disease progression.

Grade-dependent metabolites were detected and shown to be implicated in diverse metabolic pathways, such as amino acid metabolism, the tricarboxylic acid (TCA) cycle, and energy metabolism, as well as purine and pyrimidine metabolism. In accordance to the multivariate analysis, elevated contents of most metabolites are observed in grade III (T24), whereas they are restored (reduced) to their respective levels of the reference grade I group (RT4) [Fold Change (x) close to 1], or even lower, in the grade IV (TCCSUP) cells. Since the majority of metabolites (40 out of 42) exhibited significant increase in the grade III (T24) group, further investigation was performed in order to take into account dilution effects and metabolic dependencies. For the identified metabolites, all pairwise ratios were examined, and the fold change (x) of each metabolic trait was calculated. A heat map of the fold change (x) values of metabolic ratios between grade III (T24) and grade I (RT4) UBC cell groups is presented in Supplementary Figure S2. Among the 42 metabolites that were found to be significant, the pairwise ratios analysis highlighted the importance of a sub-collection containing 14 of them.

Remarkably, uracil, hypoxanthine, adenine, tryptophan, propylene glycol, formate, UDPs, and choline ratios exhibited the highest decrease in grade III (T24) compared to grade I (RT4), whereas ADP, AMP, GTP, oxypurinol, creatine phosphate, and myo-inositol ratios showed the most significant increase in grade III (T24) [compared to grade I (RT4) reference group] cells. Importantly, the reduced metabolite contents, except for the uracil and propylene glycol ones, were found to be elevated in the analysis of metabolite concentrations only (expressed as signals). On the contrary, most of these metabolite ratios were shown to be decreased, which suggests that the analysis of metabolite concentrations only may lead to erroneous results when such enormous biological differences between compared groups are observed.

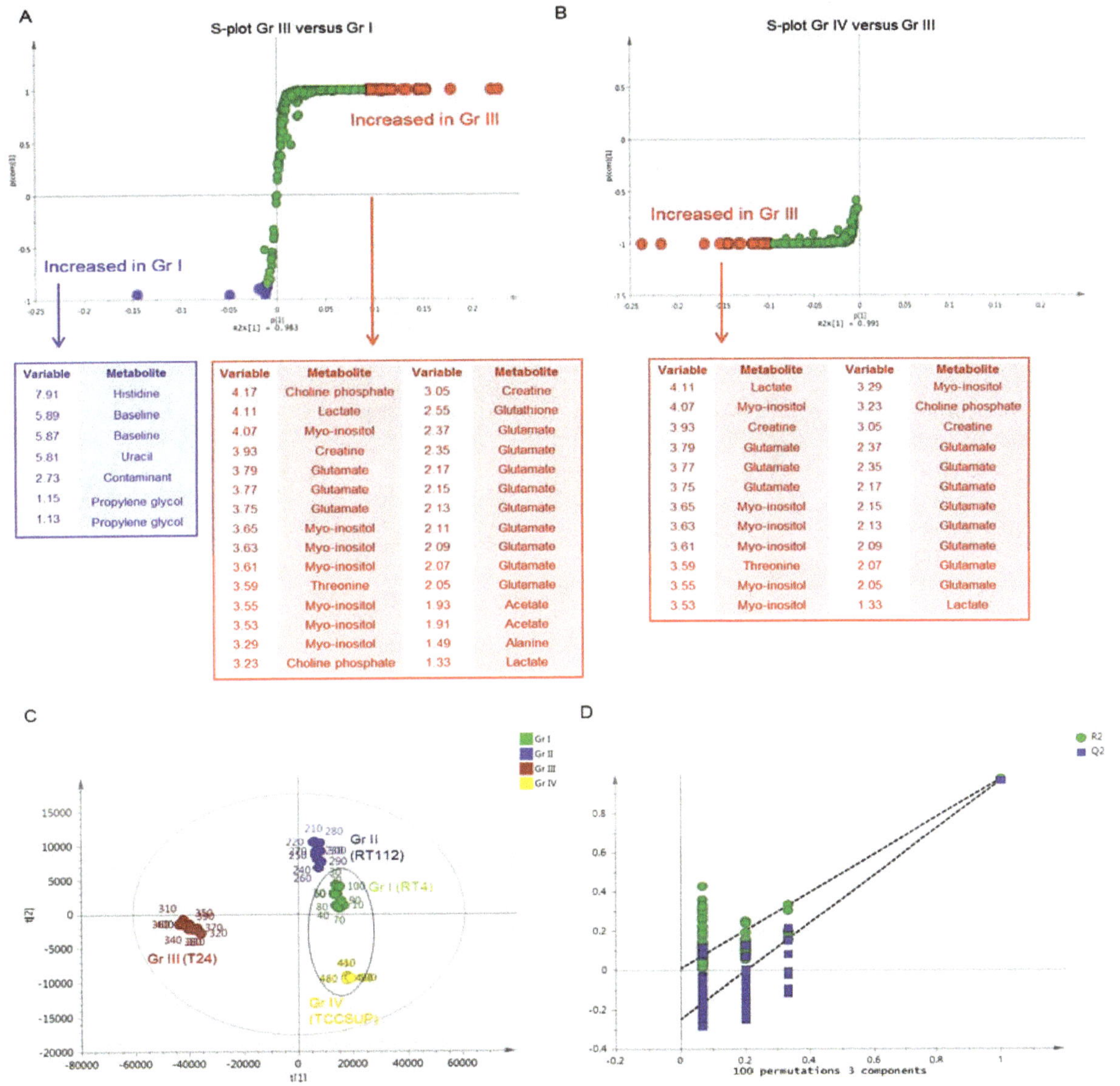

Variable	Metabolite
7.91	Histidine
5.89	Baseline
5.87	Baseline
5.81	Uracil
2.73	Contaminant
1.15	Propylene glycol
1.13	Propylene glycol

Variable	Metabolite	Variable	Metabolite
4.17	Choline phosphate	3.05	Creatine
4.11	Lactate	2.55	Glutathione
4.07	Myo-inositol	2.37	Glutamate
3.93	Creatine	2.35	Glutamate
3.79	Glutamate	2.17	Glutamate
3.77	Glutamate	2.15	Glutamate
3.75	Glutamate	2.13	Glutamate
3.65	Myo-inositol	2.11	Glutamate
3.63	Myo-inositol	2.09	Glutamate
3.61	Myo-inositol	2.07	Glutamate
3.59	Threonine	2.05	Glutamate
3.55	Myo-inositol	1.93	Acetate
3.53	Myo-inositol	1.91	Acetate
3.29	Myo-inositol	1.49	Alanine
3.23	Choline phosphate	1.33	Lactate

Variable	Metabolite	Variable	Metabolite
4.11	Lactate	3.29	Myo-inositol
4.07	Myo-inositol	3.23	Choline phosphate
3.93	Creatine	3.05	Creatine
3.79	Glutamate	2.37	Glutamate
3.77	Glutamate	2.35	Glutamate
3.75	Glutamate	2.17	Glutamate
3.65	Myo-inositol	2.15	Glutamate
3.63	Myo-inositol	2.13	Glutamate
3.61	Myo-inositol	2.09	Glutamate
3.59	Threonine	2.07	Glutamate
3.55	Myo-inositol	2.05	Glutamate
3.53	Myo-inositol	1.33	Lactate

Figure 3. Multivariate analysis of ^{1}H NMR spectra of the four UBC cell lines. (**A**) S-plot of Orthogonal Partial Least Square-Discriminant Analysis (OPLS-DA) model of grade I (RT4) versus grade III (T24) cell line and the respective loadings. Red dots: increased in grade III (T24), Blue dots: increased in grade I (RT4). (**B**) S-plot of OPLS-DA model of grade III (T24) versus grade IV (TCCSUP) cell line and the respective loadings. Red dots: increased in grade III (T24). (**C**) Scores plot of Partial Least Square-Discriminant Analysis (PLS-DA) model of the four UBC cell lines. Grade I (RT4) and grade IV (TCCSUP) groups seem unable to be discriminated, among each other, on the first principal component, while the grade III (T24) group is the most distant from the initial conditions on the same component. (**D**) Permutation test of the PLS-DA model of the four UBC cell lines. Gr: (malignancy) grade.

In order to systemically map and integrate the metabolic hits into their related biological pathways, the statistically significant metabolites were imported into CytoScape 3.7.0, using MetScape for metabolomics data visualization. Extracted pathway and metabolic course analyses are illustrated in Figure 4A. Among others, it seems that purine and pyrimidine metabolism (including the one of uracil) can critically control (positively or negatively) UBC progression to late-malignancy stages (Figure 4B). Importantly, propylene glycol (Kyoto Encyclopedia of Genes and Genomes (KEGG): 1, 2 propanediol), which is implicated in lactaldehyde metabolism, as shown in the constructed network (Figure 4A), may also be notably downregulated during UBC advancement toward metastasis (e.g., T24; grade III).

Figure 4C describes the enzymatic reaction of aldo-keto reductase family 1 member B (AKR1B1), which is the enzyme that catalyzes the NADP-dependent conversion of propylene glycol to lactaldehyde in human (KEGG Reaction R02577, EC 1.1.1.21).

Table 1. The identified metabolites and the calculated fold change (×) during UBC progression, taking grade I (RT4) as the cell group of reference. A three-color gradient is applied, depending on the fold change (×) value. Red denotes the highest value(s). Gr: (malignancy) grade.

Metabolites	Gr II/Gr I	Gr III/Gr I	Gr IV/Gr I
Alanine	1.66	6.99	0.81
Aspartate	1.18	3.33	0.78
Glutamate	1.41	6.44	0.88
Glutathione	1.65	7.18	0.87
Glycine	1.33	5.71	0.32
Histidine	1.41	2.91	0.74
Isoleucine	1.96	5.62	0.86
Leucine	1.61	3.51	0.77
N-Acetylglutamine	1.14	10.17	0.99
Phenylalanine	1.82	5.92	0.86
Proline	1.5	4.77	0.75
Taurine	1.55	5.5	0.67
Threonine	1.42	5.38	0.74
Tryptophan	1.01	1.6	0.37
Tyrosine	1.77	6.25	0.88
Valine	1.79	4.81	0.74
β-Alanine	1.68	4.54	0.82
Acetate	1.56	4.17	2.78
Formate	1.13	1.28	0.68
Fumarate	1.65	3.34	0.92
Lactate	1.39	3.22	0.39
Malate	1.95	6.5	1.12
Succinate	1.79	4.65	0.51
Adenine	0.68	1.33	0.12
ADP	1.76	20.76	1.49
AMP	1.45	34.33	0.79
ATP	1.6	6.1	0.88
GTP	1.29	11.31	0.88
Hypoxanthine	2.41	1.81	0.24
NAD+	2.86	3.76	0.86
NADH	1.36	4.62	0.83
Oxypurinol	1.46	10.16	0.45
Uracil	1.36	0.72	0.23
UDPs	1.71	2.66	0.83
UDP-GlcNAc	2.43	3.25	0.75
UMP	1.82	7.77	0.82
Choline	2.96	2.44	0.19
Choline phosphate	1.27	6.26	0.37
Creatine	1.35	5.73	0.45
Creatine phosphate	1.51	22.99	0.66
Myo-inositol	2.89	12.06	0.37
Propylene glycol	1.34	0.38	0.29

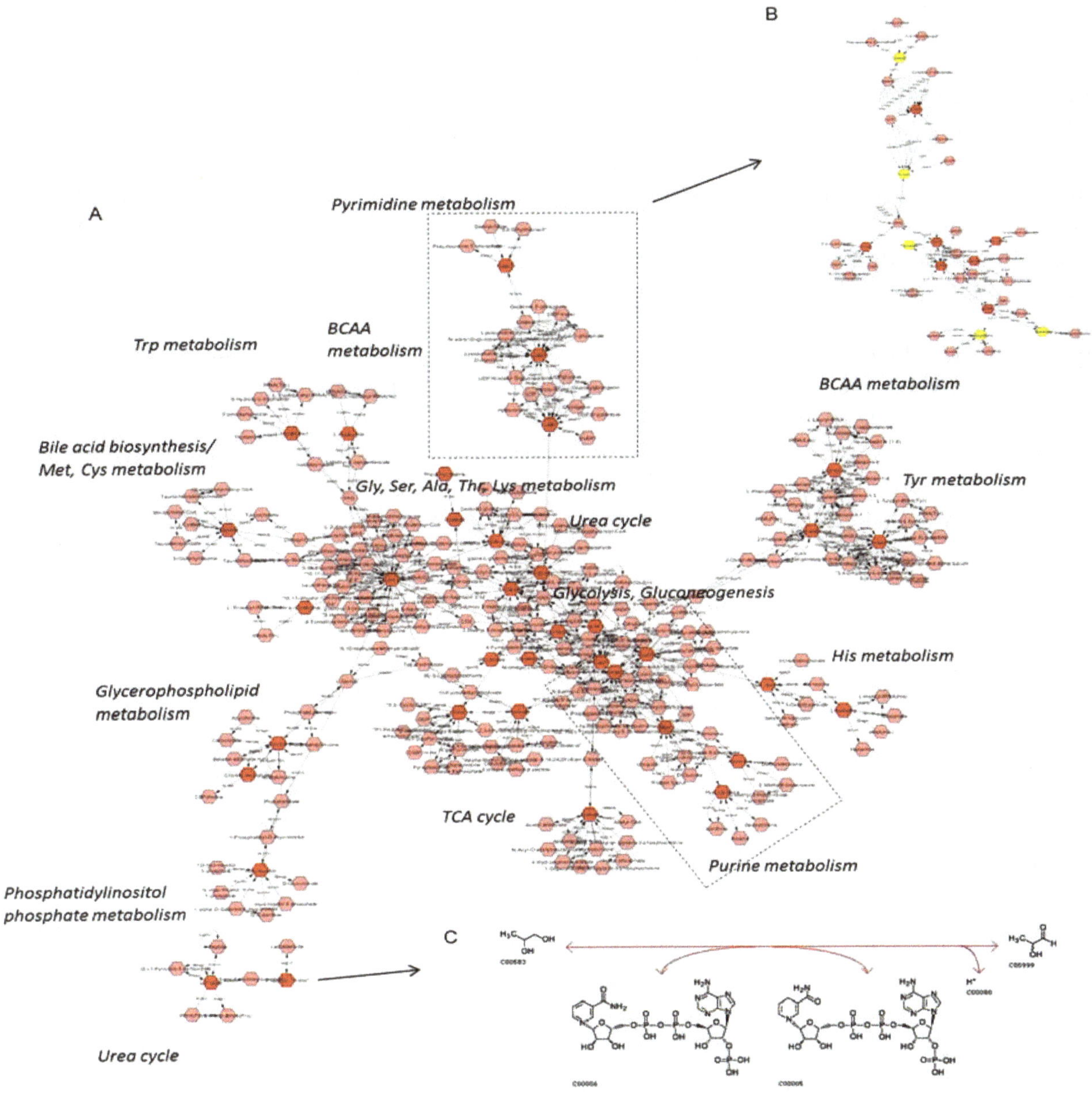

Figure 4. UBC metabolic network construction. (**A**) Hits (red) of the ^{1}H NMR metabolomic analysis inserted into Cytoscape and the related pathways assembled. Purine/pyrimidine metabolism seems to play a crucial role in UBC progression. (**B**) Hits of the purine/pyrimidine metabolism in grade III (T24) versus grade I (RT4) cell group comparison. Red: increased in grade III (T24), Yellow: decreased in grade III (T24). (**C**) Propylene glycol (or propane-1, 2-diol) has emerged as a novel, putative biomarker, with the EC 1.1.1.21 enzyme reaction for propylene glycol having been taken from KEGG.

2.2. *MS Analysis*

Representative LC-MS chromatograms of each one of the four UBC cell lines are shown in Supplementary Figure S3. PCA scores plots, before and after filtering of the features based on the % Relative Standard Deviation in Quality Control samples (QCs) and QC-based Signal-correction Method (QC-RLSC) correction (Supplementary Figure S4A,B, respectively), for instrument drift and signal attenuation, remarkably lead to more consistent clustering of QCs after normalization, therefore improving the repeatability and accuracy of the study.

In order to more deeply investigate for grade-specific variables among the four UBC cell groups that are able to uniquely reflect urothelial bladder-tumor pathologies (e.g., grade, stage, metastatic capacity, mutational load, and genetic heterogeneity), different multivariate approaches were employed, including the PLS-DA (SIMCA-P), KODAMA (R package), and Breiman's Random-Forest (BR-F) (StatTarget) tools. The results obtained from multivariate analyses were evaluated based on their multi-ROC (Receiver Operating Characteristic) values (calculated for every MS feature) and are summarized in Table 2, wherein the features with an Area Under Curve (AUC) > 0.9 and their respective ranking after employing the different methodologies are shown. Loadings and Kruskal–Wallis ranking are the different platforms used by the Knowledge Discovery by Accuracy Maximization Analysis (KODAMA) algorithm for variable selection. The results described in Table 2 strongly suggest that KODAMA loadings and BF-R classification exhibit better performance for the four-group UBC-member comparisons than the classical PLS-DA model. Figure 5 presents the scores plot constructed using the three models. It is observed that the obtained results are in accordance with the ones derived from NMR analysis, with the grade III (T24) UBC cell group showing the highest separation on the first principal component in all three methods used. Detailed results for testing each variable's importance using the different methodologies KODAMA, PLS-DA, and multi-ROC AUC are shown in Supplementary Table S2, while the first 50 ranked variables using BF-R are summarized in Supplementary Table S3.

Table 2. MS features with multi-ROC AUC > 0.9 and their ranking, based on different multivariate approaches. Knowledge Discovery by Accuracy Maximization Analysis (KODAMA) loadings and Breiman's Random-Forest (BF-R) classification exhibit better performance for the four-group UBC-member comparisons than the classical PLS-DA model.

Feature	Multi-ROC AUC	Variable Importance in Projection (VIP) (PLS-DA)	Loadings Ranking	Kruskal Ranking	Random Forest (RF) (p-Value)
993.7033_3.7	0.995	56	11	54	2
828.2532_3.71	0.982	77	6	58	5
129.1015_3.71	0.98	79	4	61	2
993.3025_3.7	0.973	66	5	53	6
348.7831_0.69	0.972	22	3	1	7
993.5029_3.7	0.972	58	13	66	11
828.0866_3.71	0.96	69	9	57	20
136.0611_3.3	0.955	1	66	11	8
827.9193_3.71	0.952	71	14	65	12
828.4207_3.71	0.95	74	7	33	9
696.5591_0.69	0.942	49	52	17	41
823.9269_3.79	0.938	55	12	24	16
824.0938_3.8	0.938	52	32	70	13
120.08_2.03	0.935	99	57	4	15
823.4258_3.79	0.932	51	2	3	16
823.5929_3.8	0.932	41	15	31	5
823.7596_3.8	0.928	53	23	25	18
380.7729_0.69	0.925	86	49	28	38
118.0643_2.01	0.922	39	37	16	28
988.1106_3.8	0.917	54	20	12	1
828.7551_3.7	0.913	67	10	69	18
622.646_0.68	0.912	65	16	8	34
350.7812_0.69	0.91	47	26	20	31
212.8509_0.69	0.908	19	38	36	30
828.5893_3.79	0.908	112	30	55	14
988.7121_3.78	0.907	62	17	47	26
330.7728_0.66	0.902	36	33	13	45
486.713_0.66	0.902	34	28	6	>50
827.7527_3.7	0.9	84	21	79	22

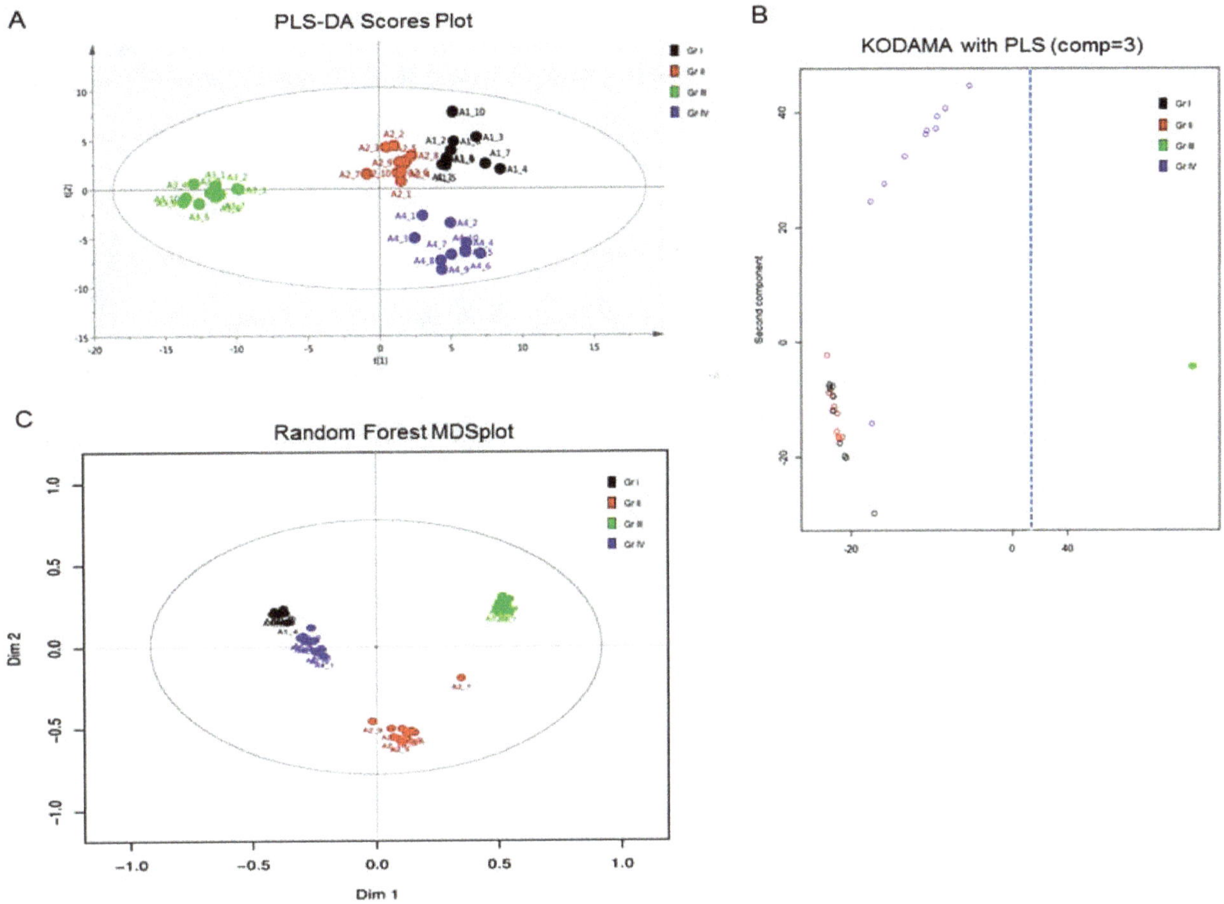

Figure 5. Comparison of the PLS-DA modeling of MS analysis, with KODAMA and Random Forest methods for the four UBC cell lines herein examined. All methods presented the greatest separation for the grade III (T24) group, highlighting T24 as the most suitable cell line to study the metabolic signature of highly malignant and strongly metastatic UBC disease. Black: grade I (RT4), Red: grade II (RT112), Green: grade III (T24), and Blue: grade IV (TCCSUP). (**A**) Principal Component (PC) scores plot from PLS-DA model. (**B**) PC scores plot from the KODAMA-PLS model. Figure is cut on the x-axis (dashed line), as grade III (T24) is far removed from the initial conditions. (**C**) Multidimensional Scaling (MDS) plot from the Random Forest model. Gr: (malignancy) grade.

Among the top ranked variables, peaks corresponding to two peptides have been herein identified, after deconvolution of multiple charged peaks and isotope clusters. Accordingly, for the first peptide, penta- (*m/z* 993.5027), exa- (*m/z* 828.0855), and epta- (*m/z* 709.9307) charged ions of *N*-Acetyl Thymosin β4 (Tβ4) were recognized, while the monoisotopic mass M + H = 4961.4792 was also obtained after deconvolution of the Electro-Spray Ionization (ESI) spectra. For the second peptide, Thymosin β10 (Tβ10), penta- (*m/z* 988.2166), exa- (*m/z* 823.5936), and epta- (*m/z* 705.7941) charged ions were identified, with the deconvoluted mass of 4934.5153 corresponding again to the *N*-Acetyl form of Tβ10 peptide. The previous identification of thymosin-type peptides [29] has revealed that the fragmentation of Tβ4 generates mainly fragments of the b series, while that of Tβ10 generates mainly fragments of the y series. The respective ions were searched in the MS/MS spectra of the penta- and exa-charged ions, using the peptide-fragmentation tool of mMass after noise filtering. The matched ions for Tβ4 and Tβ10 are described in Table 3.

Table 3. Matched ions of b series, with the MS/MS fragmentation profile of the penta- (*m/z* 993.5027) and exa- (*m/z* 828.0855) charged (acetylated) thymosin β4 (Tβ4), and matched ions of the y series, with the MS/MS fragmentation profile of the penta- (*m/z* 988.2166) and exa- (*m/z* 823.5936) charged (acetylated) thymosin β10 (Tβ10).

m/z	Ion	z	Sequence	Error (Da)	Deconvoluted Mass
			Ions of b Series, (Acetylated) Thymosin β4 (Tβ4)		
774.9006	b13	2	.SDKPDMAEIEKFD.k [1xAcetyl]	0.053	1547.696
946.616	b16	2	.SDKPDMAEIEKFDKSK.l [1xAcetyl]	0.157	1890.9178
1067.2304	b18	2	.SDKPDMAEIEKFDKSKLK.k [1xAcetyl]	0.182	2132.097
831.2934	b21	3	.SDKPDMAEIEKFDKSKLKKTE.t [1xAcetyl]	0.197	2490.2895
355.2822	b27	9	.SDKPDMAEIEKFDKSKLKKTETQEKNP.l [1xAcetyl]	0.096	3187.6722
850.3742	b29	4	.SDKPDMAEIEKFDKSKLKKTETQEKNPLP.s [1xAcetyl]	−0.069	3397.7732
936.3339	b32	4	.SDKPDMAEIEKFDKSKLKKTETQEKNPLPSKE.t [1xAcetyl]	−0.152	3741.9428
869.5772	b37	5	.SDKPDMAEIEKFDKSKLKKTETQEKNPLPSKETIEQE.k [1xAcetyl]	0.132	4342.2255
1086.6825	b37	4	.SDKPDMAEIEKFDKSKLKKTETQEKNPLPSKETIEQE.k [1xAcetyl]	0.128	4342.218
1164.2402	b40-NH_3	4	.SDKPDMAEIEKFDKSKLKKTETQEKNPLPSKETIEQEKQA.g [1xAcetyl]	0.145	4669.4134
788.6117	b41	6	.SDKPDMAEIEKFDKSKLKKTETQEKNPLPSKETIEQEKQAG.e [1xAcetyl]	−0.129	4726.4448
1182.801	b41	4	.SDKPDMAEIEKFDKSKLKKTETQEKNPLPSKETIEQEKQAG.e [1xAcetyl]	0.194	4726.4304
971.9887	b42	5	.SDKPDMAEIEKFDKSKLKKTETQEKNPLPSKETIEQEKQAGE.s [1xAcetyl]	−0.107	4855.48
			Ions of y Series, (Acetylated) Thymosin β10 (Tβ10)		
m/z	Ion	z	Sequence	Error (Da)	Deconvoluted Mass
839.5505	y14	2	p.TKETIEQEKRSEIS.	0.1142	1676.8726
592.5017	y15	3	l.PTKETIEwebQEKRSEIS.	0.1909	1773.9327
1775.0578	y15	1	l.PTKETIEQEKRSEIS.	0.1397	1790.9491
944.3809	y16	2	t.LPTKETIEQEKRSEIS.	−0.1239	1887.0094
663.8185	y17	3	n.TLPTKETIEQEKRSEIS.	0.1304	1988.0643
994.9422	y17	2	n.TLPTKETIEQEKRSEIS.	−0.0864	1988.0572
1052.2492	y18	2	k.NTLPTKETIEQEKRSEIS.	0.1992	2119.131
1244.6476	y21	2	t.QEKNTLPTKETIEQEKRSEIS.	−0.0005	2504.3272
863.8784	y22	3	e.TQEKNTLPTKETIEQEKRSEIS.	0.0947	2605.3821
1295.2735	y22	2	e.TQEKNTLPTKETIEQEKRSEIS.	0.1016	2605.3748
983.2832	y25	3	k.KTETQEKNTLPTKETIEQEKRSEIS.	0.1044	2946.5364
1130.0686	y29	3	k.AKLKKTETQEKNTLPTKETIEQEKRSEIS.	0.1194	3403.8786
1172.5977	y30	3	d.KAKLKKTETQEKNTLPTKETIEQEKRSEIS.	−0.0498	3531.9735
630.6308	y32	6	s.FDKAKLKKTETQEKNTLPTKETIEQEKRSEIS.	0.1209	3777.0594
756.3638	y32	5	s.FDKAKLKKTETQEKNTLPTKETIEQEKRSEIS.	−0.0466	3777.0525
945.1581	y32	4	s.FDKAKLKKTETQEKNTLPTKETIEQEKRSEIS.	−0.1031	3777.0452
810.8174	y35	5	e.IASFDKAKLKKTETQEKNTLPTKETIEQEKRSEIS.	0.1763	4048.2055
807.212	y35-NH_3	5	e.IASFDKAKLKKTETQEKNTLPTKETIEQEKRSEIS.	−0.0238	4048.21
1059.3714	y37	4	m.GEIASFDKAKLKKTETQEKNTLPTKETIEQEKRSEIS.	−0.1943	4251.2934
744.6523	y39-H_2O	6	p.DMGEIASFDKAKLKKTETQEKNTLPTKETIEQEKRSEIS.	−0.07	4480.3443
1116.7269	y39-H_2O	4	p.DMGEIASFDKAKLKKTETQEKNTLPTKETIEQEKRSEIS.	0.1471	4479.3502
916.6534	y40	5	k.PDMGEIASFDKAKLKKTETQEKNTLPTKETIEQEKRSEIS.	0.1754	4594.421
965.1255	y42	5	a.DKPDMGEIASFDKAKLKKTETQEKNTLPTKETIEQEKRSEIS.	0.0231	4837.5425
1206.0731	y42	4	a.DKPDMGEIASFDKAKLKKTETQEKNTLPTKETIEQEKRSEIS.	−0.053	4837.5354
801.7036	y42-NH3	6	a.DKPDMGEIASFDKAKLKKTETQEKNTLPTKETIEQEKRSEIS.	0.1215	4820.5236

Pairwise comparisons, using OPLS-DA models and univariate analysis, have also been performed. Hence, T24 (grade III) were compared to RT4 (grade I) that serve as reference cells. Figure 6 presents the pairwise comparison between the lower (I) and higher (III) UBC grade, using both multivariate and univariate approaches.

OPLS-DA analysis of these two UBC cell lines (RT4 and T24) was carried out to unveil important variables for their grade-specific and metabolic signature-dependent discrimination. In the OPLS-DA derived S-plot, features with the highest variation and reliability were selected. Tβ4 and Tβ10 were found to be strikingly elevated in the grade III (T24) UBC cell group. In the univariate analysis of the grade I (RT4) versus grade III (T24) UBC group, comparably similar results were obtained. Tβ10 peaks exhibit a $\log_2$ (FC) < -5, indicating a ca. 40-fold (x) increase in the grade III (T24) UBC cell group, while Tβ4 shows a $\log_2$ (FC) $= -3$, corresponding to a ca. 10-fold (x) increase for T24 cells, again.

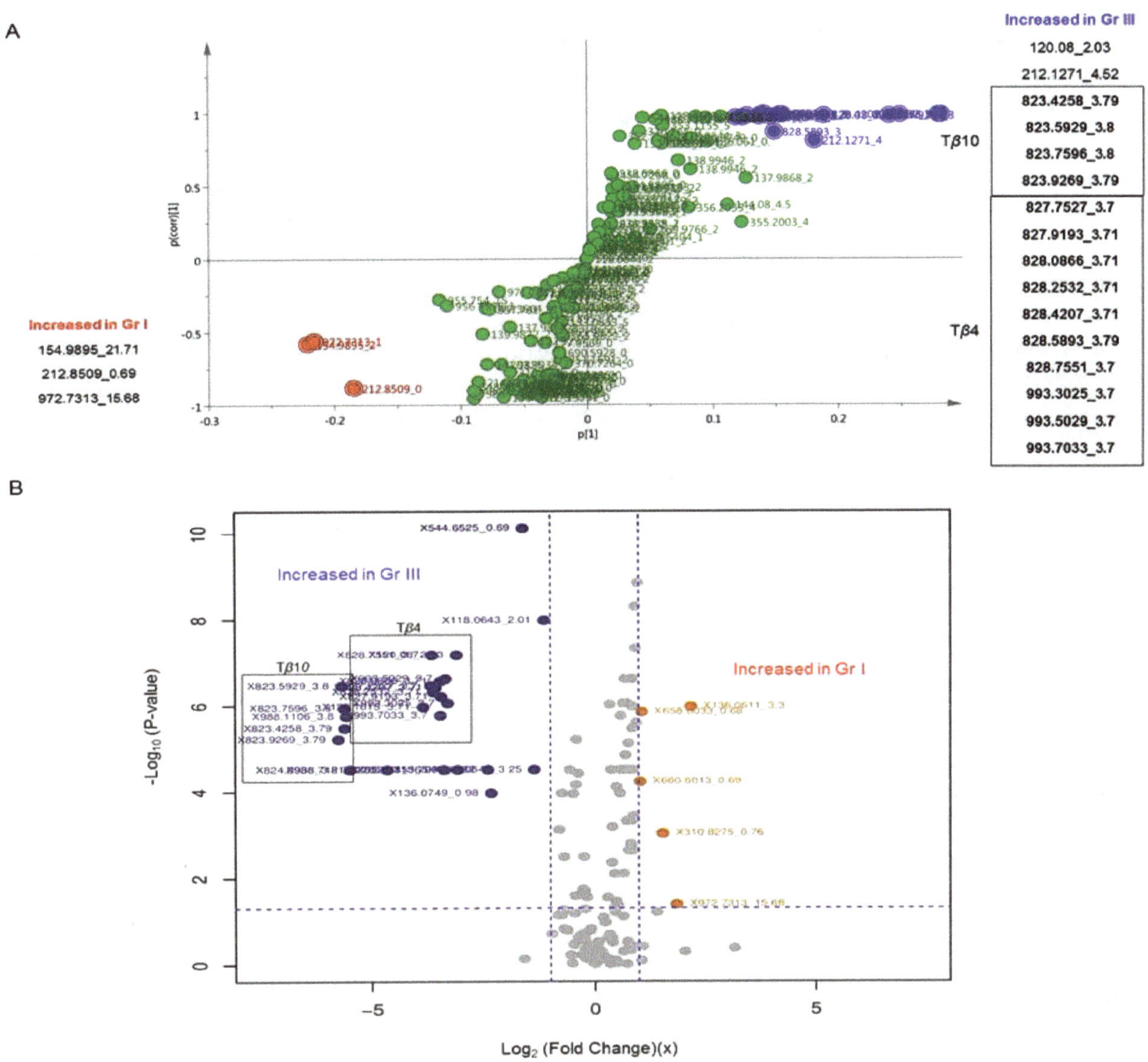

Figure 6. Comparison of the grade I (RT4) versus grade III (T24) cell groups and the significant MS analysis features. Tβ4 and Tβ10 charged peaks, and their respective isotopes, were found to be elevated in the grade III (T24) UBC cell group, using both univariate and multivariate approaches. Blue: increased in grade III (T24), Red: increased in grade I (RT4). (**A**) S-plot from OPLS-DA modeling multivariate approach. (**B**) Volcano plot of $\log_2$ [fold change (FC) (x)] versus p-values, and the selected variables with $p < 0.05$ and FC > 2, or < 0.5 (univariate approach). Gr: (malignancy) grade.

3. Discussion

Cancer research has considerably benefited from cultured-cell metabolomics, which offers a number of advantages, such as minor ethical issues, cost-efficiency merit, and low biological variation, as compared to human biofluids [30,31]. In vitro metabolomics approaches facilitate the more integrated, systemic, and reliable experimental design, and, most importantly, the successful investigation of metabolic alterations that are directly and/or mechanistically linked to the tumorigenic process, and these may not be captured by blood and/or urine classical biochemical examination. However, there are still some challenges to cope with, such as the fast quenching of metabolism and data normalization [32,33]. To successfully encounter these challenges, we have chosen a grade-specific unique collection of UBC human cell lines that are able to largely maintain and thus mimic the pathology of the disease, including both its clinical features and molecular subtypes. Immediate freezing of UBC cultured cells ensured metabolism's fast quenching equally for all the four cell lines examined, with RT4 (grade I) serving as the line of reference (control), due to its lowest malignancy grade among all. Data statistical processing, via the engagement of advanced algorithmic platforms, unearthed the major biological importance of our results to UBC progression toward tissue metastasis and refractory responses to chemotherapies.

To our knowledge, this is the first time all major UBC malignancy-grade cell types, I, II, III, and IV, with different mutational loads and metastatic proficiencies, are being metabolically fingerprinted, combining both NMR and LC-MS state-of-the-art technologies. Powerful and multifaceted statistical processing of the metabolic data ensures their biological validity and highlights the role of metabolomics pathways in UBC progression toward metastasis in vivo. Remarkably, each grade-specific UBC cell line has proved to carry its own unique metabolic signature that diagnostically, mechanistically, and therapeutically typifies each distinct tumorigenic phenotype examined. The question is whether the grade-dependent metabolome governs UBC pathology and aggressiveness, or, vice versa, the advancement to metastatic state(s) compels the acquisition of metabolic aberrations and the generation of derailed UBC metabolomes. It must be the grade-specific molecular signature of each UBC cell type that defines its unique metabolic landscape. However, the four cell lines herein examined carry different mutational profiles, with some mutations being likely unrelated (due to their generation stochasticity) to UBC aggressiveness. Hence, the possibility that these (non-causative for tumor features) mutations could be linked to some of the observed metabolic alterations cannot be excluded. Nevertheless, the major mutation contents of the cell lines used are indeed grade dependent, and they can be classified according to the UBC grade, metastatic capacity, and general disease pathology. In any case, the high grade-specific oncometabolomes (e.g., of T24) seem to contain a number of critical metabolites that can serve as novel and powerful biomarkers for both the diagnosis and drug-mediated clinical management of UBC disease.

In this study, a four-cell-line group of a human UBC model has been in vitro engaged to thoroughly investigate the metabolic alterations that tumor cells likely undergo during UBC advancement, thus highlighting the importance of a malignancy grade, mutational signature, de-differentiation state and metastatic activity to "diagnostic biomarkering" and "targeted therapeutic drugging" of the disease. The four human UBC cell lines that have been analyzed critically reflect the distinct de-differentiation state and malignancy grade (I–IV) of UBC in vivo. Our results clearly indicate that T24 (grade III) can serve as a powerful, informative, and versatile cell-line system that can be successfully exploited to illuminate the role of metabolic reprogramming in UBC progression toward metastasis. It seems that the elevated contents of most metabolites specifically identified in T24 are tightly associated with the highly oncogenic character of the cells. Notably, PCA analysis showed that the grade III-specific T24-cell group exhibits the clearest separation on the first principal component, both in NMR and MS analysis, thus explaining the maximal amount of variation for its discrimination among the four cell groups. These results are strongly supported by biological data interpretations, since T24 cells bear a heavy mutational load and strong tumorigenic capacity. They are characterized by the mutant, oncogenic, form H-RAS^{G12V} and the disruption of stress-induced activation of mutant p53 ($\Delta\Upsilon^{126}$) protein [34]. Hence, the aberrant signaling activity of H-RAS^{G12V}, in a cellular environment that lacks the genome-protecting properties of p53, may render T24 cells susceptible to severe metabolic reprogramming, with grade III-specific metabolites fostering and promoting highly tumorigenic features and pathologies, including genetic instability, clonal heterogeneity, chemoresistance, immune escape, and organ metastasis (tissue invasion). Interestingly, a role of *H-RAS*^{G12V} oncogene (*RAS*) in metabolic reprogramming during early mammary carcinogenesis has been previously reported, with the MCF10A-*RAS* transfected human breast epithelial cells exhibiting enhanced glycolytic activity and lactate production [35], consistently with the cancer hallmark of the classic "Warburg effect" [36,37]. Comparative genomics evidence that indicates that the T24 cell line (https://depmap.org/portal/cell_line/ACH-000018?tab=mutation) reliably reflects the mutational profile of muscle-invasive bladder cancer patients (https://www.cbioportal.org; Bladder Cancer, TCGA Cell 2017, 413 Total Samples) supports and increases the utilization of T24 as a valid, pre-clinical, cell-model system for advanced bladder cancer research in diagnosis and therapy. Remarkably, besides the *H-RAS* and *TP53* (encodes p53) mutated oncogenes, T24 cells share with muscle-invasive UBC patients multiple genes carrying molecular alterations, including (among others) the *KDM6A*, *MAGEF1*, *DIDO1*, and *EP300* ones, with 37%, 31%, 30% and 30% of detection frequency, respectively, in the UBC patient cohort studied (Supplementary Table S4).

Among all UBC–cell pairs, embracing different grades being compared [e.g., II versus I, III versus I, and IV versus I; I (RT4) herein serves as the cell line of reference], only the grade III (T24) versus grade I (RT4) proved to significantly differ in the majority of metabolite contents examined, thus indicating the major role of the T24-specific mutational signature (including H-RAS^{G12V} and p53$^{\Delta Y126}$) in metabolome composition and its oncogenic proficiency. The surprising resemblance between grade I (RT4) and grade IV (TCCSUP) metabolic profiles strongly suggests the engagement of a "metabolic inversion" process that likely favors late-metastasis cells to successfully encounter energetic challenges, nutritional demands, and oxygen deprivations. It is possible that a pre-metastatic UBC cell, after it becomes metastatic and invades other (proximal or/and distal) tissues/organs, will undergo a dramatic metabolic reprogramming to suppress its ability for a second metastasis event. If so, it may always be the primary tumor mass that feeds metastasis, with a metastatic-cell clonal population likely colonizing tissues outside the urinary bladder only once. In accordance, cell dissemination seems to occur during the early stages of tumor evolution, with cells from early and low-density lesions displaying more "stemness" features, migrating more and founding more metastases than cells derived from dense and advanced tumors [38–40].

The majority of previous UBC metabolomics reports have underlined the importance of amino acids to urothelium oncometabolome, with most amino acid levels being upregulated compared to controls; similar differential patterns were described for advanced UBC stage(s) compared to early stage(s). Interestingly, increased contents of glutathione were found in UBC cell lines, while glycine was elevated in the tumorigenic cells as well [21,22]. Alanine was also increased in the TCCSUP (high-grade) cell line compared to the RT4 (low grade) one [28]. An abundance of amino acids is important for the proliferative cancer cells, not only as substrates of protein synthesis, but also for energy generation, cellular redox homeostasis, and nucleotide biosynthesis [41]. Pyruvate consumption and alterations in glycolytic profile have also been related to UBC aggressiveness, as anaerobic conditions in high(er) grade UBC favor the conversion of pyruvate to lactate, or alanine [28]. In our study, and in accordance with previous results, T24 (grade III) exhibited elevated contents of totally 17 amino acids and derivatives, with the highest increase being detected for N-acetylglutamine, glutathione, alanine, and glutamate, together with a 3x increase of lactate. Nucleotides are also involved in biomass build-up observed in cancer cells and in the changes of ATP concentrations that indicate the energetic status (usually crisis) of tumors [42]. In serum samples of UBC patients, the raised levels of hypoxanthine and reduced levels of uracil indicated a perturbed breakdown of purine nucleotides, favoring the purine synthesis pathway (reviewed in ref. [17]). Notably, herein, purine metabolism has emerged as one of the most important networks in our *in silico* analysis (Figure 4), thus highlighting its major contribution to UBC aggressiveness and progression toward metastasis. Increased contents of hypoxanthine and adenosine nucleotides (AMP/ADP/ATP), with up to a 34x striking increase for AMP, were observed in T24 (grade III), but they were surprisingly restored (again) to the initial (RT4-like) levels in TCCSUP (grade IV) cells. In a study of urine samples derived from UBC patients, it has been suggested that the high(er) levels of choline phosphate may reflect increased lipid membrane remodeling, which has also been reported for other cancers [24,42]. Choline phosphate and, to lower extent, choline contents were also increased in our T24 (grade III) cell-line group, with a 6x and 2x rise, respectively. As expected, the elevated contents of these metabolites were reduced in TCCSUP (grade IV) cells, indicating the activation of a "metabolic inversion" effect. Regarding the two major metabolites involved in osmoregulation and volume regulation, taurine and myo-inositol, contradictory results were previously reported, with either upregulated or downregulated levels detected (reviewed in ref. [17,42]), likely implicating the role of cellular micro-environments in metabolome compositions. Interestingly, herein, significantly elevated contents of myo-inositol (12x) and taurine (5x) were observed in T24 (grade III), indicating the high grade-dependent ability of UBC to regulate osmosis and volume, in favor of promoting cell motility and tumor metastasis.

Taking into account that the majority of the identified metabolites (40 out of 42) were increased in the grade III (T24) group, multivariate analysis and the use of pairwise ratios were employed in order to highlight metabolites with major alterations. Notably, multivariate analysis of the obtained NMR data indicated the importance of, among others, glutamate and myo-inositol level deregulations to UBC pathology, while AXPs (AMP, ADP and ATP), GTP, oxypurinol, and creatine phosphate content increases were presented with the strongest statistical significance in the grade III/I cell pair (III/I). The use of pairwise ratios allowed us to account for dilution and signal instability effects and to unveil alterations that are masked by the "metabolic inversion" phenomenon. Increased ratios were found in III/I for metabolites that were also profiled with a "metabolic inversion" effect in IV/I (e.g., AMP, oxypurinol, myo-inositol, and creatine phosphate); thus, they might critically contribute to UBC advancement. On the other hand, decreased ratios were observed in III/I for several metabolites that were also presented with downregulated proportions in IV/I (e.g., uracil and propylene glycol) and, as such, they could presumably function as UBC-specific "oncosuppressing" modulators/inducers. Further discussion will focus on those metabolites that were herein identified as the most important by both (NMR and LC-MS) applied technologies, and especially the ones with the highest fold change (x) in metabolite levels and the highest alterations in all pairwise metabolic ratios.

Regarding the top two metabolites with the highest elevation contents in grade III (T24) versus grade I (RT4) UBC cells, creatine phosphate and AMP, they were remarkably presented with 23x and 34x positive change (upregulation), respectively (Table 1). Strikingly, by taking uracil as the metabolite of reference (since it was downregulated both in III/I and IV/I cell pairs), their respective fold changes (x) were further increased up to 32x and 50x values (Supplementary Table S5). Since colon cancer-derived liver metastases carry higher creatine kinase brain type (CKB) levels compared to primary tumors [43,44], UBC metastatic populations, in order to overcome hypoxia and other metabolic stresses, may also upregulate CKB expression or/and activity. This allows (after CKB secretion) energy to be likely captured from the extracellular ATP-mediated generation of creatine phosphate and its subsequent SLC6A8-dependent import into metastatic cells to regenerate ATP. Similarly to colon cancer cells [45], hypoxic UBC cells, in the absence of functional Hypoxia-Inducible Factor 1-alpha (HIF1α) (a key regulator of hypoxia response) pathway, could adapt their energy metabolism via the upregulation of creatine metabolism (and synthesis), thus opening a new chemotherapeutic window for metastatic UBC targeting and management in the clinic. Most importantly, T24 (grade III) cells contain a mutant version of the EP300 (KAT3B/p300) transcriptional co-activator (Supplementary Table S4) (https://depmap.org/portal/cell_line/ACH-000018?tab=mutation), which, in its wild-type form, is required for the transcriptional activation of HIF1α-target genes [46]. This indicates their competence to survive and grow in adverse hypoxic environments through the engagement of HIF1α-independent, but likely creatine-dependent, metabolic pathways. Given that the calculated fold change (x) in the III/I pair for ADP is 20.76x, which is a value close to the 22.99x of creatine phosphate (Table 1) (an approximately 1:1 molecular stoichiometry), T24 (grade III) cells may utilize intracellular creatine phosphate as a phosphate donor to the available ADP to finally produce ATP.

The remarkably elevated content of AMP in T24 (grade III) versus RT4 (grade I) cells indicates its major value for UBC progression toward chemoresistance and metastasis. High levels of ADP and AMP in a cell undergoing energetic stress/crisis cause significant increase in the AMPK kinase activity [47]. Activated AMPK phosphorylates a number of target substrates to regulate cell growth, metabolism, and autophagy [48]. Interestingly, activated H-RAS (G12V) requires autophagy for the maintenance of tumorigenesis [49]. Therefore, it seems that the major AMP/ADP/ATP (AXPs) metabolic reprogramming specifically observed in grade III (T24) cells may be tightly related to the aberrant signaling of the H-RAS^{G12V} mutant oncoprotein. If so, H-RAS^{G12V}–AMP/ADP–AMPK–autophagy must operate as an indispensable axis for UBC cell survival and growth in unfavorable and adverse (e.g., hypoxic or nutritionally deprived) environments. Since we have previously shown that T24 cells are characterized by constitutively activated basal autophagy [34], the H-RAS^{G12V}-induced intracellular energetic stress, in the form of AMP (and ADP) highly upregulated levels (this study), serves as a valuable and powerful metabolic biomarker, with its implicated enzymes/regulators likely opening a new therapeutic window for UBC metastasis and drug tolerance.

Intriguingly, propylene glycol and uracil herein emerged as metabolites that were downregulated in both III/I and IV/I grade cell pairs. Especially for propylene glycol, a prominent reduction in its intracellular contents was observed for both T24 (grade III) and TCCSUP (grade IV) compared to RT4 (grade I) cells of reference. Propylene glycol is produced by the conversion of pyruvaldehyde to lactaldehyde, which is then converted to propylene glycol via the aldehyde reductase mediation. Aldo-keto reductases family 1 members A1 and B1 (AKR1A1 and AKR1B1) are part of the Aldo-keto reductase superfamily and catalyze the reduction of several aldehydes. Data derived from the TCGA (The Cancer Genome Atlas) platform (https://www.cbioportal.org) strengthen our interpretation for perturbed (compromised) aldehyde reductase activities in advanced metastatic UBC disease, with 16% and 7% of the examined muscle-invasive UBC patients (Bladder Cancer, Cell 2017, z: 1.5) exhibiting deregulated expression/activity of the AKR1A1 and AKR1B1 enzymes, respectively, and 2.67% of them bearing low mRNA levels of the *AKR1A1* gene (https://www.cbioportal.org). Thereby, it seems that T24 may have originated from a patient with a molecular signature of downregulated *AKR1A1* gene expression in the tumor cells.

A major advantage (and novelty) of the present study is the employment of two complementary, state-of-the-art, analytical platforms: Nuclear Magnetic Resonance (NMR) and Mass Spectrometry (MS). Their successful combination offers a comprehensive metabolic characterization that covers a variety of chemical structures and concentrations of profiled metabolites. Strikingly, application of the MS-based metabolomics technology led to the detection and identification of novel molecules that could significantly contribute to UBC progression toward metastasis. Two peptides, Tβ4 and Tβ10, were identified with a high confidence level, and proved to be statistically significant both in the discrimination of the four (I, II, III, and IV) groups and of the low(er) or high(er) malignancy grade pairwise comparisons. Members of the β thymosin family form a (1:1) complex with the monomeric G-Actin protein, acting as its sequestration peptides, thus critically controlling actin cytoskeleton dynamics [50].

Furthermore, in contrast to Tβ4, Tβ10 can also directly bind to RAS, inhibiting its signaling activity, in an endothelial cell environment [51]. Nevertheless, in a T24-specific cellular setting, Tβ10 could no longer interact with the mutant H-RAS^{G12V} form, thus presumably releasing its aberrant signaling function(s) to drive the oncogenic and metastatic phenotypes of grade III UBC cells. Hence, the strikingly elevated contents of Tβ4 (10x) and Tβ10 (40x) in T24 (grade III) compared to RT4 (grade I; reference) cell line strongly suggest their actin cytoskeleton remodeling-dependent role in UBC advancement to metastasis, with oncogenic H-RAS^{G12V} (after its presumable release from Tβ10) also orchestrating UBC aggressiveness and drug/radiation resistance. Accordingly, Tβ10 overexpression correlates with the poor prognosis and progression of UBC disease [52], while Tβ4 expression is associated with clinical outcomes and clinicopathological parameters of UBC patients (it is significantly increased in UBC patients versus normal (control) volunteers) [53]. Most importantly, TCGA-derived data unveiled 6% of muscle-invasive UBC cases (bladder cancer, "amplification" and "mRNA high", Cell 2017, z: 1.5) to be carrying upregulated levels of *TMSB10* gene (encodes Tβ10) expression (https://www.cbioportal.org), thus indicating the in vivo importance of Tβ10 (and Tβ4) to UBC progression toward high-malignancy grades and aggressive metastatic stages that are characterized by resistance to (chemo/radio)therapy, shorter survival of patients, and, generally, poor prognosis.

4. Materials and Methods

4.1. Chemicals and Reagents

The detailed information for chemicals and reagents is listed in Supplementary Materials.

4.2. Cell Lines and Culture Conditions

The UBC human cell lines RT4, RT112, T24, and TCCSUP were used in the present study. RT4 was obtained from ECACC-Sigma-Aldrich (Munich, Germany). RT112 was kindly provided by Professor J.R. Masters (London, England, UK). T24 and TCCSUP were purchased from ATCC-LGC Standards GmbH (Wesel, Germany). All cell lines were derived from urothelial cell carcinomas of human urinary bladder, with RT4 being classified as malignancy grade I, RT112 as grade I–II (II), T24 as grade III, and TCCSUP as grade IV. All four UBC cell lines were authenticated mainly using in-house established technologies. Cell authentication was based on several combinational criteria, such as the cell-specific morphology, growth rate, nutritional requirement, mitotic index, immunofluorescence pattern (e.g., Epithelial–Mesenchymal Transition (EMT) phenotype), mutational load (e.g., *H-RAS* and *TP53*), signaling activity (e.g., Akt and p44/42 MAPK {ERK1/2}), protein content, gene-expression profiling, drug response, motility (e.g., wound-healing assay) and tumorigenicity (e.g., xenograft in Severe Combined ImmunoDeficient (SCID) mouse). All four UBC human cell lines were being tested periodically, but, most importantly, they were thoroughly examined just before the commencement of their large-scale growth for the herein implemented metabolomics analysis. The detailed culture conditions are described in the Supplementary Materials.

4.3. Cell Collection and Storage

The analytical protocols of cell collection and storage are described in the Supplementary Materials.

4.4. Metabolomics Experiments

The detailed protocols of metabolomics experiments (e.g., metabolite extraction, sample preparation, NMR, and MS analysis) are described in the Supplementary Materials.

4.5. Data Preprocessing

The binning of NMR spectra was conducted (0.001/0.02 ppm) using the AMIX software. Regions of water and contaminations being observed at the blank solutions were removed from the analysis. Pairwise ratios of the metabolites identified in NMR analysis were also calculated ($42 \times 42 = 1.764$ metabolic traits). In MS analysis, data preprocessing was performed using the XCMS online. Peak-based normalization was applied in order to correct data within the batch experiment. Specifically, a QC-based signal-correction method (QC-RLSC), engaging the non-linear local polynomial regression (LOESS), was performed using the MetaX R package [54]. KNN (*K*-Nearest Neighbor) imputation for missing values and filtering of features based on the % Relative Standard Deviation (RSD) in QCs were applied.

4.6. Metabolite/Pathway Identification

The Chenomx NMR suite (Chenomx Inc., Alberta, Canada) was utilized for the NMR-mediated metabolite identification. For the recognition of peptides, the mMass peptide tool v. 5.5.0 was suitably employed [55]. The Cytoscape platform was engaged for visualizing molecular networks of significant metabolites derived from the NMR analysis [56,57].

4.7. Statistical Analysis

Principal Component Analysis (PCA), Partial Least Square-Discriminant Analysis (PLS-DA), and Orthogonal Partial Least Square-Discriminant Analysis (OPLS-DA), using SIMCA-P 14.0 (Umetrics, Umea, Sweden), were suitably applied. The quality of obtained models was assessed via R2X (variance explained by X Matrix) and Q2 (Goodness of prediction) obtained by 7x cross-validation, parameters, and permutation test results (100 random permutations for the PLS-DA and OPLS-DA models). The Knowledge Discovery by Accuracy Maximization Analysis (KODAMA) R package [58] was performed for the unsupervised extraction of variables in the MS analysis. The selected classifier was PLS-DA, and the procedure was repeated 100 times. Two methods implemented in the same package were used for the ranking of variables' importance; Kruskal–Wallis test and the model's loadings. Breiman's Random-Forest (BR-F) algorithm was also evaluated using the StatTarget tool [59]. A number of 500 grown trees and 20 permutations were imported as model parameters. Multi-ROC AUC was used for the evaluation of methods performance using the multi-ROC R package [60].

5. Conclusions

In the present study, the metabolic landscapes of grade I, II, III, and IV UBC human cell lines were extensively mapped. Obtained results indicated a prominently perturbed amino acid and purine/pyrimidine metabolism with a remarkable increase of most metabolites being identified in grade III (T24) UBC cells, using RT4 (grade I) as the line of reference. Surprisingly, insignificant changes were observed for grade IV (TCCSUP) cells, thus implying the activation of a "metabolic inversion" process. T24 (grade III) has proved the most powerful and versatile cell line, which is able to accurately and reliably unveil the metabolic signature of highly malignant and strongly metastatic UBC pathology. "Metabolic inversion" has to be mechanistically investigated, in order to open new chemotherapeutic windows for UBC advancement to drug-resistant metastasis. Analysis of NMR-derived metabolite contents and ratios showed significant perturbations in purine and pyrimidine metabolism, while MS analysis demonstrated the importance of Tβ4 and Tβ10 peptides to UBC progression toward metastasis. AMP (and ADP) highly upregulated levels indicate the H-RAS^{G12V}-induced intracellular energetic stress/crisis, and they can serve as valuable metabolic biomarkers, while the remarkably elevated contents of Tβ4 and Tβ10 in the T24 (grade III) compared to RT4 (grade I) cell line strongly suggest their actin cytoskeleton remodeling-dependent role in UBC advancement to metastasis and drug tolerance. Furthermore, decreased levels of propylene glycol are indicative of dysregulated *AKR1A1* gene expression in the tumor cells of urinary bladder, thus rendering it (propylene glycol) as a potentially significant biomarker.

Our work also made use of novel statistical approaches for metabolomics data analysis. Metabolic ratios are strongly suggested to account for the size effect present in the data and to highlight novel metabolic pathways. Hence, their combined employment and biological interpretation are crucial in order to avoid erroneous results. A common bottleneck in the untargeted MS analysis is the selection of important variables. We herein compared the typical PLS-DA method used in metabolomics analyses with other statistical tools carrying different merits and drawbacks (e.g., KODAMA and BF-R). Our results underline the importance of either pairwise comparisons or the implementation of more sophisticated multivariate approaches, such as the Random Forest models, which may exhibit better performances.

Most importantly, the integration of high-resolution metabolic maps with high-scale proteomic profiles containing enzymes/regulators that are able to control the homeostasis of grade-dependent UBC intracellular metabolites will shed light on mechanisms of urothelial bladder tumorigenesis, and they will benefit our tools in terms of the safe, efficient, and generally successful (including reduced medical costs) diagnostic and therapeutic management of the advanced UBC disease in the clinic.

Author Contributions: Conceptualization, D.J.S.; methodology, A.I., A.P., A.F.G., D.B., E.G., E.M. and D.J.S.; software, A.I., A.P., D.B., M.K., E.G. and E.M.; validation, A.I., A.P., A.F.G., D.B., M.K., A.D.V., O.E.T., I.S.P., G.E.V., E.G.K., E.G., E.M. and D.J.S.; resources, E.M. and D.J.S.; writing—original draft preparation, A.I., E.G., E.M. and D.J.S.; writing—review and editing, E.M. and D.J.S.; supervision, D.B., E.M. and D.J.S.; project administration, D.B., E.G., E.M. and D.J.S.; funding acquisition, A.I., E.M. and D.J.S. All authors have read and agreed to the published version of the manuscript.

Acknowledgments: Dimitrios J. Stravopodis (DJS) at NKUA devotes the present article to the memory of his beloved mother who suddenly passed away in October 2015.

Abbreviations

AKR1A1/AKR1B1	Aldo-keto Reductases Family 1 Member(s) A1/B1
AUC-ROC	Area Under the Receiver Operating Characteristic Curve
BR-F	Breiman's Random-Forest
KEGG	Kyoto Encyclopedia of Genes and Genomes
KODAMA	Knowledge Discovery by Accuracy Maximization Analysis
OPLS-DA	Orthogonal Partial Least Squares-Discriminant Analysis
PCA	Principal Component Analysis
PLS-DA	Partial Least Squares-Discriminant Analysis
QC-RLSC	QC-based Signal-correction Method
QCs	Quality Control Samples
UBC	Urothelial Bladder Cancer
VIP	Variable Importance in Projection

References

1. Burger, M.; Catto, J.W.; Dalbagni, G.; Grossman, H.B.; Herr, H.; Karakiewicz, P.; Kassouf, W.; Kiemeney, L.A.; La Vecchia, C.; Shariat, S.; et al. Epidemiology and risk factors of urothelial bladder cancer. *Eur. Urol.* **2013**, *63*, 234–241. [CrossRef]
2. Huang, Z.; Lin, L.; Gao, Y.; Chen, Y.; Yan, X.; Xing, J.; Hang, W. Bladder cancer determination via two urinary metabolites: A biomarker pattern approach. *Mol. Cell. Proteom.* **2011**, 10. [CrossRef] [PubMed]
3. Montironi, R.; Cheng, L.; Scarpelli, M.; Lopez-Beltran, A. Pathology and genetics: Tumours of the urinary system and male genital system: Clinical implications of the 4th edition of the who classification and beyond. *Eur. Urol.* **2016**, *70*, 120–123. [CrossRef] [PubMed]
4. Hurle, R.; Losa, A.; Manzetti, A.; Lembo, A. Upper urinary tract tumors developing after treatment of superficial bladder cancer: 7-year follow-up of 591 consecutive patients. *Urology* **1999**, *53*, 1144–1148. [CrossRef]
5. Hansen, R.P.; Vedsted, P.; Sokolowski, I.; Søndergaard, J.; Olesen, F. Time intervals from first symptom to treatment of cancer: A cohort study of 2,212 newly diagnosed cancer patients. *BMC Health Serv. Res.* **2011**, *11*, 284. [CrossRef] [PubMed]
6. James, A.C.; Gore, J.L. The costs of non-muscle invasive bladder cancer. *Urol. Clin. N. Am.* **2013**, *40*, 261–269. [CrossRef]
7. Vlachostergios, P.J.; Faltas, B.M. Treatment resistance in urothelial carcinoma: An evolutionary perspective. *Nat. Rev. Clin. Oncol.* **2018**, *15*, 495–509. [CrossRef] [PubMed]
8. Giannopoulou, A.F.; Velentzas, A.D.; Konstantakou, E.G.; Avgeris, M.; Katarachia, S.A.; Papandreou, N.; Kalavros, N.; Mpakou, V.E.; Iconomidou, V.A.; Anastasiadou, E.; et al. Revisiting histone deacetylases in human tumorigenesis: The paradigm of urothelial bladder cancer. *Int. J. Mol. Sci.* **2019**, *20*, 1291. [CrossRef]
9. Nicholson, J.K.; Lindon, J.C.; Holmes, E. Metabonomics: Understanding the metabolic responses of living systems to pathophysiological stimuli via multivariate statistical analysis of biological nmr spectroscopic data. *Xenobiotica* **1999**, *29*, 1181–1189. [CrossRef]
10. Locasale, J.W.; Cantley, L.C.; Heiden, M.G.V. Cancer's insatiable appetite. *Nat. Biotechnol.* **2009**, *27*, 916–917. [CrossRef]
11. Hanahan, D.; Weinberg, R.A. Hallmarks of cancer: The next generation. *Cell* **2011**, *144*, 646–674. [CrossRef] [PubMed]

12. Aboud, O.A.; Weiss, R.H. New opportunities from the cancer metabolome. *Clin. Chem.* **2013**, *59*, 138–146. [CrossRef] [PubMed]
13. DeBerardinis, R.J.; Chandel, N.S. Fundamentals of cancer metabolism. *Sci. Adv.* **2016**, *2*, e1600200. [CrossRef] [PubMed]
14. Boroughs, L.K.; DeBerardinis, R.J. Metabolic pathways promoting cancer cell survival and growth. *Nat. Cell Biol.* **2015**, *17*, 351–359. [CrossRef] [PubMed]
15. Sahu, D.; Lotan, Y.; Wittmann, B.; Neri, B.; Hansel, D.E. Metabolomics analysis reveals distinct profiles of nonmuscle-invasive and muscle-invasive bladder cancer. *Cancer Med.* **2017**, *6*, 2106–2120. [CrossRef] [PubMed]
16. Denkert, C.; Budczies, J.; Kind, T.; Weichert, W.; Tablack, P.; Sehouli, J.; Darb-Esfahani, S.; Könsgen, D.; Dietel, M.; Fiehn, O. Mass spectrometry-based metabolic profiling reveals different metabolite patterns in invasive ovarian carcinomas and ovarian borderline tumors. *Cancer Res.* **2006**, *66*, 10795–10804. [CrossRef]
17. Rodrigues, D.; Jerónimo, C.; Henrique, R.; Belo, L.; Bastos, M.D.L.; De Pinho, P.G.; Carvalho, M. Biomarkers in bladder cancer: A metabolomic approach using in vitro and ex vivo model systems. *Int. J. Cancer* **2016**, *139*, 256–268. [CrossRef]
18. Catchpole, G.; Platzer, A.; Weikert, C.; Kempkensteffen, C.; Johannsen, M.; Krause, H.; Jung, K.; Miller, K.; Willmitzer, L.; Selbig, J.; et al. Metabolic profiling reveals key metabolic features of renal cell carcinoma. *J. Cell. Mol. Med.* **2011**, *15*, 109–118. [CrossRef]
19. Cheng, Y.; Xie, G.; Chen, T.; Qiu, Y.; Zou, X.; Zheng, M.; Tan, B.; Feng, B.; Dong, T.; He, P.; et al. Distinct urinary metabolic profile of human colorectal cancer. *J. Proteom. Res.* **2012**, *11*, 1354–1363. [CrossRef]
20. Huang, Q.; Tan, Y.; Yin, P.; Ye, G.; Gao, P.; Lu, X.; Wang, H.; Xu, G. Metabolic characterization of hepatocellular carcinoma using nontargeted tissue metabolomics. *Cancer Res.* **2013**, *73*, 4992–5002. [CrossRef]
21. Pendyala, L.; Velagapudi, S.; Toth, K.; Zdanowicz, J.; Glaves, D.; Slocum, H.; Perez, R.; Huben, R.; Creaven, P.J.; Raghavan, D. Translational studies of glutathione in bladder cancer cell lines and human specimens. *Clin. Cancer Res.* **1997**, *3*, 793–798.
22. Pasikanti, K.K.; Norasmara, J.; Cai, S.; Mahendran, R.; Esuvaranathan, K.; Ho, P.C.; Chan, E.C.Y. Metabolic footprinting of tumorigenic and nontumorigenic uroepithelial cells using two-dimensional gas chromatography time-of-flight mass spectrometry. *Anal. Bioanal. Chem.* **2010**, *398*, 1285–1293. [CrossRef] [PubMed]
23. Bansal, N.; Gupta, A.; Mitash, N.; Shakya, P.S.; Mandhani, A.; Mahdi, A.A.; Sankhwar, S.N.; Mandal, S.K. Low- and high-grade bladder cancer determination via human serum-based metabolomics approach. *J. Proteom. Res.* **2013**, *12*, 5839–5850. [CrossRef] [PubMed]
24. Wittmann, B.M.; Stirdivant, S.M.; Mitchell, M.; Wulff, J.E.; McDunn, J.E.; Li, Z.; Dennis-Barrie, A.; Neri, B.P.; Milburn, M.V.; Lotan, Y.; et al. Bladder cancer biomarker discovery using global metabolomic profiling of urine. *PLoS ONE* **2014**, *9*, e115870. [CrossRef] [PubMed]
25. Tan, G.; Wang, H.; Yuan, J.; Qin, W.; Dong, X.; Wu, H.; Meng, P. Three serum metabolite signatures for diagnosing low-grade and high-grade bladder cancer. *Sci. Rep.* **2017**, *7*, 46176. [CrossRef]
26. Kouznetsova, V.L.; Kim, E.; Romm, E.L.; Zhu, A.; Tsigelny, I. Recognition of early and late stages of bladder cancer using metabolites and machine learning. *Metabolomics* **2019**, *15*, 94. [CrossRef]
27. Rodrigues, D.; Pinto, J.; Araujo, A.M.; Jerónimo, C.; Henrique, R.; Bastos, M.D.L.; De Pinho, P.G.; Carvalho, M. Gc-ms metabolomics reveals distinct profiles of low- and high-grade bladder cancer cultured cells. *Metabolites* **2019**, *9*, 18. [CrossRef]
28. Conde, V.R.; Oliveira, P.F.; Nunes, A.R.; Rocha, C.S.; Ramalhosa, E.; Pereira, J.A.; Alves, M.G.; Silva, B.M. The progression from a lower to a higher invasive stage of bladder cancer is associated with severe alterations in glucose and pyruvate metabolism. *Exp. Cell Res.* **2015**, *335*, 91–98. [CrossRef]
29. Inzitari, R.; Cabras, T.; Pisano, E.; Fanali, C.; Manconi, B.; Scarano, E.; Faa, G. Hplc-esi-ms analysis of oral human fluids reveals that gingival crevicular fluid is the main source of oral thymosins β4 and β10. *J. Sep. Sci.* **2009**, *32*, 57–63. [CrossRef]
30. León, Z.; García-Cañaveras, J.C.; Donato, M.T.; Lahoz, A. Mammalian cell metabolomics: Experimental design and sample preparation. *Electrophoresis* **2013**, *34*, 2762–2775. [CrossRef]
31. Kalluri, U.; Naiker, M.; Myers, M.A. Cell culture metabolomics in the diagnosis of lung cancer-the influence of cell culture conditions. *J. Breath Res.* **2014**, *8*, 027109. [CrossRef] [PubMed]

32. Čuperlović-Culf, M.; Barnett, D.; Culf, A.S.; Chute, I. Cell culture metabolomics: Applications and future directions. *Drug Discov. Today* **2010**, *15*, 610–621. [CrossRef] [PubMed]
33. Bi, H.; Krausz, K.W.; Manna, S.K.; Li, F.; Johnson, C.H.; Gonzalez, F.J. Optimization of harvesting, extraction, and analytical protocols for uplc-esi-ms-based metabolomic analysis of adherent mammalian cancer cells. *Anal. Bioanal. Chem.* **2013**, *405*, 5279–5289. [CrossRef] [PubMed]
34. Konstantakou, E.G.; Voutsinas, G.E.; Velentzas, A.D.; Basogianni, A.-S.; Paronis, E.; Balafas, E.; Kostomitsopoulos, N.; Syrigos, K.; Anastasiadou, E.; Stravopodis, D.J. 3-brpa eliminates human bladder cancer cells with highly oncogenic signatures via engagement of specific death programs and perturbation of multiple signaling and metabolic determinants. *Mol. Cancer* **2015**, *14*, 135. [CrossRef] [PubMed]
35. Zheng, W.; Tayyari, F.; Gowda, G.N.; Raftery, D.; McLamore, E.S.; Porterfield, D.M.; Donkin, S.; Bequette, B.; Teegarden, R. Altered glucose metabolism in harvey-ras transformed mcf10a cells. *Mol. Carcinog.* **2015**, *54*, 111–120. [CrossRef] [PubMed]
36. Gatenby, R.A.; Gillies, R.J. Why do cancers have high aerobic glycolysis? *Nat. Rev. Cancer* **2004**, *4*, 891–899. [CrossRef] [PubMed]
37. Koppenol, W.H.; Bounds, P.L.; Dang, C.V. Otto warburg's contributions to current concepts of cancer metabolism. *Nat. Rev. Cancer* **2011**, *11*, 325–337. [CrossRef]
38. Harper, K.L.; Sosa, M.S.; Entenberg, D.; Hosseini, H.; Cheung, J.F.; Nobre, R.; Farias, E.F. Mechanism of early dissemination and metastasis in her^2 mammary cancer. *Nature* **2016**, *540*, 588–592. [CrossRef]
39. Hosseini, H.; Obradović, M.M.S.; Hoffmann, M.; Harper, K.L.; Sosa, M.S.; Werner-Klein, M.; Nanduri, S.L.K.; Werno, C.; Ehrl, C.; Maneck, M.; et al. Early dissemination seeds metastasis in breast cancer. *Nature* **2016**, *540*, 552–558. [CrossRef]
40. Yachida, S.; Jones, S.; Bozic, I.; Antal, T.; Leary, R.; Fu, B.; Kamiyama, M.; Hruban, R.H.; Eshleman, J.R.; Nowak, M.A.; et al. Distant metastasis occurs late during the genetic evolution of pancreatic cancer. *Nature* **2010**, *467*, 1114–1117. [CrossRef]
41. Vettore, L.; Westbrook, R.L.; Tennant, D.A. New aspects of amino acid metabolism in cancer. *Br. J. Cancer* **2020**, *122*, 150–156. [CrossRef] [PubMed]
42. Griffin, J.L.; Shockcor, J.P. Metabolic profiles of cancer cells. *Nat. Rev. Cancer* **2004**, *4*, 551–561. [CrossRef] [PubMed]
43. Loo, J.M.; Scherl, A.; Nguyen, A.; Man, F.Y.; Weinberg, E.; Zeng, Z.; Saltz, L.B.; Paty, P.B.; Tavazoie, S.F. Extracellular metabolic energetics can promote cancer progression. *Cell* **2015**, *160*, 393–406. [CrossRef] [PubMed]
44. Sullivan, W.J.; Christofk, H.R. The metabolic milieu of metastases. *Cell* **2015**, *160*, 363–364. [CrossRef]
45. Valli, A.; Morotti, M.; Zois, C.E.; Albers, P.K.; Soga, T.; Feldinger, K.; Fischer, R.; Frejno, M.; McIntyre, A.; Bridges, E.; et al. Adaptation to hif1α deletion in hypoxic cancer cells by upregulation of glut14 and creatine metabolism. *Mol. Cancer Res.* **2019**, *17*, 1531–1544. [CrossRef]
46. Kung, A.; Zabludoff, S.D.; France, D.S.; Freedman, S.J.; Tanner, E.A.; Vieira, A.; Cornell-Kennon, S.; Lee, J.; Wang, B.; Wang, J.; et al. Small molecule blockade of transcriptional coactivation of the hypoxia-inducible factor pathway. *Cancer Cell* **2004**, *6*, 33–43. [CrossRef]
47. Hardie, D.G.; Ross, F.A.; Hawley, S.A. Ampk: A nutrient and energy sensor that maintains energy homeostasis. *Nat. Rev. Mol. Cell Biol.* **2012**, *13*, 251–262. [CrossRef]
48. Mihaylova, M.M.; Shaw, R.J. The ampk signalling pathway coordinates cell growth, autophagy and metabolism. *Nat. Cell Biol.* **2011**, *13*, 1016–1023. [CrossRef]
49. Guo, J.Y.; Chen, H.-Y.; Mathew, R.; Fan, J.; Strohecker, A.M.; Karsli-Uzunbas, G.; Kamphorst, J.J.; Chen, G.; Lemons, J.M.; Karantza, V.; et al. Activated ras requires autophagy to maintain oxidative metabolism and tumorigenesis. *Genes Dev.* **2011**, *25*, 460–470. [CrossRef]
50. Sribenja, S.; Wongkham, S.; Wongkham, C.; Yao, Q.C.; Chen, C. Roles and mechanisms of β-thymosins in cell migration and cancer metastasis: An update. *Cancer Investig.* **2013**, *31*, 103–110. [CrossRef]
51. Lee, S.H.; Son, M.J.; Oh, S.H.; Rho, S.B.; Park, K.; Kim, Y.J.; Lee, J.H. Thymosin β10 inhibits angiogenesis and tumor growth by interfering with ras function. *Cancer Res.* **2005**, *65*, 137–148. [PubMed]
52. Wang, B.; Wang, Z.; Zhang, T.; Yang, G. Overexpression of thymosin β10 correlates with disease progression and poor prognosis in bladder cancer. *Exp. Ther. Med.* **2019**, *18*, 3759–3766. [CrossRef]

53. Wang, Z.Y.; Zhang, W.; Yang, J.; Song, D.K.; Wei, J.X.; Gao, S. Association of thymosin β4 expression with clinicopathological parameters and clinical outcomes of bladder cancer patients. *Neoplasma* **2016**, *63*, 991–998. [CrossRef]
54. Wen, B.; Mei, Z.; Zeng, C.; Liu, S. Metax: A flexible and comprehensive software for processing metabolomics data. *BMC Bioinform.* **2017**, *18*, 183. [CrossRef] [PubMed]
55. Strohalm, M.; Kavan, D.; Novák, P.; Volny, M.; Havlicek, V. Mmass 3: A cross-platform software environment for precise analysis of mass spectrometric data. *Anal. Chem.* **2010**, *82*, 4648–4651. [CrossRef] [PubMed]
56. Gao, J.; Tarcea, V.G.; Karnovsky, A.; Mirel, B.R.; Weymouth, T.E.; Beecher, C.W.; Cavalcoli, J.D.; Athey, B.; Omenn, G.S.; Burant, C.; et al. Metscape: A cytoscape plug-in for visualizing and interpreting metabolomic data in the context of human metabolic networks. *Bioinformatics* **2010**, *26*, 971–973. [CrossRef] [PubMed]
57. Shannon, P.; Markiel, A.; Ozier, O.; Baliga, N.S.; Wang, J.T.; Ramage, D.; Amin, N.; Schwikowski, B.; Ideker, T. Cytoscape: A software environment for integrated models of biomolecular interaction networks. *Genome Res.* **2003**, *13*, 2498–2504. [CrossRef]
58. Cacciatore, S.; Tenori, L.; Luchinat, C.; Bennett, P.R.; MacIntyre, D.A. Kodama: An r package for knowledge discovery and data mining. *Bioinformatics* **2017**, *33*, 621–623. [CrossRef]
59. Luan, H.; Ji, F.; Chen, Y.; Cai, Z. Stattarget: A streamlined tool for signal drift correction and interpretations of quantitative mass spectrometry-based omics data. *Anal. Chim. Acta* **2018**, *1036*, 66–72. [CrossRef]
60. Robin, X.; Turck, N.; Hainard, A.; Tiberti, N.; Lisacek, F.; Sanchez, J.-C.; Müller, M. Proc: An open-source package for r and s+ to analyze and compare roc curves. *Bmc Bioinform.* **2011**, *12*, 77. [CrossRef]
61. Wu, H.; Southam, A.D.; Hines, A.; Viant, M.R. High-throughput tissue extraction protocol for NMR- and MS-based metabolomics. *Anal. Biochem.* **2008**, *372*, 204–212. [CrossRef] [PubMed]
62. Dunn, W.B.; Broadhurst, D.; Begley, P.; Zelena, E.; Francis-McIntyre, S.; Anderson, N.; Brown, M.; Knowles, J.D.; Halsall, A.; Haselden, J.N.; et al. Procedures for large-scale metabolic profiling of serum and plasma using gas chromatography and liquid chromatography coupled to mass spectrometry. *Nat. Protoc.* **2011**, *6*, 1060–1083. [CrossRef] [PubMed]

3

Moving towards Personalized Medicine in Muscle-Invasive Bladder Cancer: Where are we Now and Where are we Going?

Juan Carlos Pardo [1,2,†], Vicenç Ruiz de Porras [2,3,†], Andrea Plaja [1,2], Cristina Carrato [4], Olatz Etxaniz [1,2], Oscar Buisan [5] and Albert Font [1,2,*]

1 Department of Medical Oncology, Catalan Institute of Oncology, University Hospital Germans Trias i Pujol, Ctra. Can Ruti-Camí de les Escoles s/n, 08916 Badalona, Spain; jcpardor@iconcologia.net (J.C.P.); aplaja@iconcologia.net (A.P.); oetxaniz@iconcologia.net (O.E.)

2 Catalan Institute of Oncology, Badalona Applied Research Group in Oncology (B·ARGO), Ctra. Can Ruti-Camí de les Escoles s/n, 08916 Badalona, Spain; vruiz@igtp.cat

3 Germans Trias i Pujol Research Institute (IGTP), Ctra. Can Ruti-Camí de les Escoles s/n, 08916 Badalona, Spain

4 Pathology Department, Hospital Germans Trias i Pujol, 08916 Badalona, Spain; criscarrato@gmail.com

5 Urology Department, University Hospital Germans Trias i Pujol, 08916 Badalona, Spain; obuisan2903@gmail.com

* Correspondence: afont@iconcologia.net

† These authors contribute equally to this work.

Abstract: Neoadjuvant cisplatin-based chemotherapy followed by radical cystectomy is the recommended treatment, with the highest level of evidence, for patients with muscle-invasive bladder cancer (MIBC). However, only a minority of patients receive this treatment, mainly due to patient comorbidities, the relatively small survival benefit, and the lack of predictive biomarkers to select those patients most likely to benefit from this multimodal approach. In addition, adjuvant chemotherapy has been recommended for patients with high-risk MIBC, although randomized trials have not provided conclusive evidence on the impact of this approach. At present, however, this situation is changing, largely due to our improved knowledge of the molecular biology of bladder cancer, which has enabled us to identify new prognostic and predictive biomarkers that can be used to select the most appropriate treatment for each patient. Moreover, new active treatments, especially immunotherapy, have shown promising results in the neoadjuvant setting. In addition, the gene expression profile of bladder tumors can be used to classify them into different subtypes, which correlate with specific clinical-pathological characteristics and with treatment response or resistance. Therefore, the main objective for the near future is to introduce these translational breakthroughs into routine clinical practice in order to personalize treatment for each patient.

Keywords: muscle-invasive bladder cancer; chemotherapy; immunotherapy; personalized medicine; predictive biomarker

---

1. Neoadjuvant Therapy in Muscle-Invasive Bladder Cancer (MIBC): An Overview

The prognosis of bladder cancer (BC) has not improved significantly over the last 30 years, as few advances have been made in treatment options since the introduction of cisplatin-based chemotherapy in the mid-1980s. While it is true that platinum-based schemes have somewhat improved survival of patients with advanced disease, less than 50% of patients initially respond and most eventually develop resistance. In platinum-resistant patients, second-line chemotherapy provides poor survival expectations [1]. Despite these limitations, chemotherapy has been incorporated into the treatment of muscle-invasive bladder cancer (MIBC) in combination with local treatments, such as cystectomy or radiotherapy. However, the limited survival benefit and the absence of predictive biomarkers have led to some reluctance to incorporate these strategies into the routine management of the disease, especially with regard to the use of neoadjuvant chemotherapy (NAC) in MIBC. Although international clinical guidelines recommend NAC with cisplatin-based schemes with the highest level of evidence [2,3], less than 20% of patients with MIBC receive this treatment in clinical practice [4]. There are two main reasons for this: firstly, cisplatin-based chemotherapy is contraindicated in approximately 50% of patients due to renal failure or other comorbidities [5]; and secondly, there is a lack of clinical and pathological markers to identify patients who will benefit from NAC, while delaying local treatment in those who will not benefit can have a negative impact on prognosis [6].

Fortunately, this discouraging scenario has changed in recent years, mainly due to two advances. Firstly, the molecular characterization of BC has made it possible to identify potential prognostic and predictive biomarkers, as well as new therapeutic targets. Secondly, the recent introduction of new active therapies, especially immunotherapy, has expanded the therapeutic arsenal in BC beyond platinum-based chemotherapy.

Importantly, it is essential to identify biomarkers to select those patients likely to benefit from these novel treatment options, including immunotherapy—either alone or in combination with chemotherapy and/or biological therapies. This would also help to avoid the administration of ineffective treatments that may lead to unnecessary toxicities, delays in the administration of more effective therapies, and lowered cost-effectiveness. Studies with DNA and RNA sequencing have demonstrated the heterogeneity of bladder tumors at the molecular and genetic level and have identified specific profiles—based on differences in the type and frequency of mutations, in gene copy numbers, and in methylation patterns—that can help define patient prognosis and sensitivity to specific treatments [7]. However, despite these advances, only around 40% of bladder tumors present genomic alterations that are potentially treatable with targeted therapies. Moreover, in contrast to other cancers, such as melanoma, gastrointestinal stromal tumors, and breast and lung cancers, in which 20–60% of patients can be treated with therapies selected by the analysis of biomarkers [8], no biomarkers for BC have been approved for use in clinical practice. It is crucial, therefore, to transfer advances in molecular biology as quickly and efficiently as possible into clinical practice if we are to improve the survival of patients.

Here, we describe the potential applications of molecular biology in the diagnosis and treatment of BC, and especially of MIBC, based on the concept of precision medicine.

2. Predictive Biomarkers of Response to Cisplatin-Based Chemotherapy

Cisplatin-based chemotherapy remains the standard treatment for BC both for advanced disease and for the perioperative or conservative treatment of localized BC [2]. The antitumor mechanism of action of cisplatin is based on the formation of adducts that cause DNA damage, which prevents cell replication and induces cell death [9]. Cisplatin induces DNA damage either as single-strand breaks (SSBs), double-strand breaks (DSBs), or interstrand-crosslinks. However, cancer cells have several mechanisms to repair DNA damage. SSBs can be repaired by base excision repair, mismatch repair, or nucleotide excision repair (NER), while DSBs can be repaired by non-homologous end joining or homologous recombination (HR). The analysis of genes involved in the different pathways of DNA damage repair (DDR) may enable us to identify predictive biomarkers of response to cisplatin [10].

The NER pathway, which repairs SSBs, includes the ERCC excision repair 1 (ERCC1) and ERCC excision repair 2 (ERCC2) proteins. High levels of ERCC1 indicate a gain of NER pathway function, leading to greater repair of the DNA damage caused by cisplatin and thus decreased efficacy of the drug [11]. Bellmunt et al. demonstrated that in patients with metastatic BC treated with a cisplatin-based combination, those with high *ERCC1* expression had worse prognosis [12]. Several studies have analyzed the role of *ERCC2* mutations as predictive biomarkers in BC. *ERCC2* mutations are found in 12% of BCs, mostly in the helicase domain of the gene, and have been associated with a loss of NER pathway function in preclinical studies [13]. Interestingly, *ERCC2* mutations confer sensitivity to both cisplatin and carboplatin, but not to treatments with doxorubicin, ionizing radiation or poly (ADP-ribose) polymerase (PARP) inhibitors [13]. Whole exome sequencing of 50 MIBC tumor samples treated with cisplatin-based NAC demonstrated that *ERCC2* mutations were significantly associated with treatment response. Specifically, *ERCC2* mutations were detected in 36% of patients who responded to chemotherapy (<ypT1), while no mutations were detected in non-responders (>ypT2) [14]. These results were confirmed in a subsequent validation study [15]. In the joint analysis of the two series, *ERCC2* mutations were found in 38% (17/45) of responders and in only 6% (3/53) of non-responders [13]. Taken together, these data suggest that ERCC2 may well be a predictive biomarker of response to cisplatin-based chemotherapy. In this line, a recent study by the Memorial Sloan Kettering Cancer Center (MSKCC) compared the genomic profile of primary vs. secondary MIBC patients treated with NAC. They found that not only was the benefit of NAC limited to primary MIBC but also that *ERCC2* mutations were observed more frequently in primary MIBC (12% vs. 1.2%), which could explain the lack of benefit of NAC in secondary MIBC [13]. Other studies have also correlated mutations in the ATM serine/threonine kinase (*ATM*), RB transcriptional corepressor 1 (*RB1*) and FA complementation group C (*FANCC*) repair genes with efficacy of NAC in MIBC. In the study of Plimack et al., 13 of 15 cisplatin-responders (87%) presented mutations in some of these genes, while none of the non-responders harbored these mutations. In their validation study, 64% of responders presented some of these mutations as compared to only 15% of non-responders [16]. In a recent update of this study, a significant improvement in the five-year disease-specific survival was observed in carriers of at least one mutation compared to patients without mutations (90% vs. 49%, $p = 0.0015$) [17]. The presence of mutations in DDR pathways can identify patients likely to respond to NAC, who could be potential candidates for a bladder-sparing approach. The ongoing phase II RETAIN trial in patients treated with NAC aims to identify candidates for bladder preservation among patients who attain a complete response and have mutations in *ATM*, *RB1*, *FANCC*, or *ERCC2* (NCT02710734).

HR is used to repair DSBs. In a molecular profile analysis using the NGS600 testing platform, mutations in HR genes were detected in 17% of 17,566 tumors and in 23% of BCs, which had the third highest frequency of HR-DDR mutations (after endometrial and biliary tract carcinomas). The most frequently mutated genes in BC were AT-rich interaction domain 1A (*ARID1A*) (12.4%), *ATM* (4%), BRCA1 DNA repair associated (*BRCA1*) (3%), and BRCA2 DNA repair associated (*BRCA2*) (4.5%) [18]. More recently, 13% of patients with BC were found to harbor germline variants, 75% of which were located in DDR genes, mainly in *BRCA2*, mutS homolog 2 (*MSH2*), *BRCA1*, checkpoint kinase 2 (*CHEK2*), ERCC excision repair 3 (*ERCC3*), nibrin (*NBN*), and RAD50 double strand break repair protein (*RAD50*) [19]. In this line, a study by our group in 57 MIBC patients treated with NAC, increased *BRCA1* mRNA expression negatively correlated with pathological response and survival [20].

DDR is a complex process involving several different DNA repair pathways, making it necessary to analyze extensive panels of genes if we are to determine the predictive and prognostic value of the genes involved in each pathway. An MSKCC study analyzed a panel of 34 DDR genes in 100 patients with advanced BC treated with platinum-based chemotherapy and detected at least one alteration in one of the genes in 47 patients. Median overall survival was significantly higher in these patients than in those with no alterations (23.7 vs. 13.0 months, $p = 0.006$). Interestingly, the survival benefit was observed in both cisplatin- and carboplatin-treated patients [21]. A recent phase II trial in 49 patients treated with neoadjuvant dose-dense cisplatin plus gemcitabine analyzed a panel of 29 DDR genes and found that the presence of deleterious mutations, including *ERCC2* mutations, was associated with response to chemotherapy, with a positive predictive value of 89% and a two-year relapse-free survival of 100% [22].

In summary, current evidence indicates that the analysis of alterations in DNA repair pathways can provide prognostic and predictive information in BC patients. However, prospective studies including a larger number of patients are required to confirm these findings. In addition, given that cisplatin is contraindicated in approximately 50% of patients, it is important to analyze these biomarkers in patients treated with carboplatin as well. Finally, the study of these alterations will pave the way for the discovery of new prognostic and predictive biomarkers as well as the incorporation of new biological therapies, such as PARP inhibitors, which have been shown to be effective in ovarian and breast cancer patients harboring mutations in HR genes [23].

3. Therapeutic Implications of BC Molecular Subtypes

Several research groups have proposed various classifications of BC molecular subtypes based on the two reference subtypes, luminal and basal (Table 1). A group from Lund University analyzed a large number of non-MIBC and MIBC tumors and proposed five subtypes: urobasal A, urobasal B, genomically unstable, infiltrated, and squamous-like [24]. Urobasal A and B are characterized by the expression of biomarkers usually expressed in the normal urothelium, while the squamous-like subtype expresses keratin 5 (KRT5), keratin 6 (KRT6), and keratin 14 (KRT14), which are specific to squamous differentiation. The infiltrated subtype is characterized by stromal and immune cell infiltration. A group from the University of North Carolina (UNC) proposed another classification in which the basal subtype presents sarcomatoid characteristics and expresses high levels of both epidermal growth factor receptor (EGFR) and its ligands, while the luminal subtype expresses epithelial markers (E-cadherin (CDH1) and miR-200) and alterations in fibroblast growth factor receptor 3 (FGFR3) [25]. An MD Anderson (MDA) group added a third subtype, called p53-like, which is characterized by the presence of stromal markers and the activation of tumor protein p53 (TP53) [26]. The Cancer Genome Atlas (TCGA) proposed a classification based on four molecular subtypes called clusters (I–IV) [7]. Cluster I corresponds to the luminal phenotype and presents characteristics of papillary tumors, cluster II has the luminal phenotype but with a predominance of p53-like characteristics, and clusters III and IV correspond mainly to the basal subtype defined in the UNC and MD Anderson classifications [25,26]. A recent update of the TCGA study [27] defined five molecular subtypes: luminal papillary (35%), luminal infiltrated (19%), luminal (6%), basal-squamous (35%), and neuronal (5%). The TCGA luminal subtypes are characterized by a high expression of urothelial differentiation markers, such as forkhead box A1 (*FOXA1*), GATA binding protein 3 (*GATA3*), and peroxisome proliferator activated receptor gamma (*PPARG*). The luminal-papillary subtype has *FGFR3* mutations, amplifications, overexpression, and FGFR3-TACC3 fusions. The luminal-infiltrated subtype, which corresponds to cluster II in the original TCGA classification [7], is characterized by elevated expression of epithelial-mesenchymal transition (EMT) markers, such as twist family bHLH transcription factor 1 (*TWIST1*) and zinc finger E-box-binding homeobox 1 (*ZEB1*), and moderate expression of the immune markers Programmed death ligand 1 (*PDL1*), and cytotoxic T-lymphocyte associated protein 4 (*CTLA4*). The luminal subtype presents high expression of the keratin 20 (*KRT 20*). The basal-squamous subtype is defined by the expression of CD44 antigen (*CD44*), *KRT5*, *KRT6*, *KRT14*, is enriched in *TP53* mutations, and has the highest expression of the immune markers *PD-L1*, Programmed cell death 1 (*PD-1*) and *CTLA4*. Finally, the neuronal subtype has high expression of neuroendocrine and neuronal markers [27]. A Canadian study proposed four subtypes: basal, luminal, luminal-infiltrated, and claudin-low [28]. The claudin-low subtype corresponds to TCGA cluster IV [7] and has characteristics of the basal subtype, with the expression of EMT markers and immune infiltration. Recently, the Bladder Cancer Molecular Taxonomy Group (BCMTG) has proposed a consensus classification based on the analysis of 1750 transcriptomic profiles of the classifications published to date [29]: papillary luminal (24%), unspecified luminal (8%), unstable luminal (15%), stromal rich (15%), basal-SCC (35%), and neuroendocrine-like (3%). A web application of this model allows individual and anonymous classification of tumor samples according to this consensus (http://cit.ligue-cancer.net:3838/apps/consensusMIBC_web/).

Table 1. Summary of the main characteristics of molecular subtypes of bladder cancer according to different molecular classifications.

Molecular Classification	Patients (*n*)	Subtypes	Histological and Molecular Characteristics	Ref.
Lund University	308 BC	Urobasal A	High expression of *FGFR3*, *CCND1*, *TP63*, and *KRT5*	[24]
		Urobasal B		
		Genomically unstable (GU)	Frequent *TP53* mutations. *CCNE* and *ERBB2* expression and low cytokeratin expression	
		Squamous cell carcinoma-like (SCC)	High expression of basal keratins normally not expressed in the urothelium	
		Infiltrated	Stromal and immune cell infiltration	
UNC	262 High grade MIBC	Luminal	Expression of epithelial markers (E-cadherin/CDH1 and miR-200) and alterations in *FGFR3*	[25]
		Basal	Sarcomatoid features. High expression of EGFR and its ligands	
MDA	73 MIBC	Luminal	Features of active PPARγ and estrogen receptor transcription. *FGFR3* mutations	[26]
		Basal	p63 activation and squamous differentiation	
		p53-like	Presence of stromal markers and activation of p53 signature	
TCGA (2014)	131 High grade MIBC	Cluster I	Luminal phenotype; presence of papillary tumors features	[7]
		Cluster II	Tumors with luminal phenotype but with a predominance of p53-like subtype features	
		Cluster III	Correspond to basal subtype defined in the UNC and MD Anderson classifications	
		Cluster IV		
TCGA (2017)	412 T2-4, N0-3, M0-1 MIBC	Luminal papillary (35%)	*FOXA1*, *GATA3*, and *PPARG* expression. FGFR3 alterations	[27]
		Luminal infiltrate (19%)	*FOXA1*, *GATA3*, and *PPARG* expression. Expression of EMT (high) and immune (moderate) markers	
		Luminal (6%)	*FOXA1*, *GATA3*, and *PPARG* expression. High expression of *KRT 20*	
		Basal-SCC (35%)	High expression of immune response markers. *CD44*, *KRT5*, *KRT6* and *KRT14* expression. *TP53* mutations	
		Neuronal (5%)	High expression of neuroendocrine and neuronal markers	
BCMTG	1750 MIBC transcriptomic profiles	Luminal papillary (24%)	Papillary morphology. Expression of *FGFR3* and *PPARG*. Mutations in *FGFR3* and *KDM6A*	[29]
		Luminal non-specified (8%)	Micropapillary morphology. *PPARG* expression. Mutations in *ELF3*	
		Luminal unstable (15%)	Expression of *PPARG*, *E2F3*, and *ERBB2*. Genomic instability. Mutation in *TP53* and *ERCC2*	
		Stroma-rich (15%)	Stromal and immune cell (B cells) infiltration	
		Basal/squamous (35%)	*EGFR* expression. Mutations in *TP53* and *RB1*. Stromal and immune cell (CD8 T and NK cells) infiltration	
		Neuroendocrine-like (3%)	Neuroendocrine differentiation. Loss of TP53 and RB1. Mutations in *TP53* and *RB1*	

The molecular subtypes have been associated with specific clinical-pathological characteristics and differential sensitivity to treatments. Basal-SCC tumors, identified in the TCGA, UNC, and MD Anderson classifications [7,25,26], predominate in women and are associated with more aggressive tumors, more advanced disease stages, worse prognosis, and squamous cell features. In contrast, luminal tumors seem to be less aggressive but more resistant to NAC [27,28]. Recently, Lotan et al. showed that in early-stage MIBC treated with cystectomy, upstaging (≥pT3) is less likely in luminal than non-luminal tumors [30], suggesting that luminal tumors could be managed more conservatively with upfront cystectomy.

These molecular classifications can complement or help reconsider the standard histological classifications, since squamous differentiation might well be underreported. For example, only 42% of BCMTG [29] basal-SCC tumors had squamous cell features in the histological analysis. The histological, genomic, and transcriptional heterogeneity of BC has important clinical implications. Warrick et al. analyzed the intratumoral heterogeneity of different regions of primary MIBC tumors in relation to the Lund molecular subtypes [24] and histological variants. Nearly 40% of the tumors demonstrated molecular heterogeneity among the different histologies, especially the basal-squamous tumors, 78% of which co-occurred with either urothelial-like or genomically unstable tumors [31]. These results emphasize the need for an adequate tissue sampling that selects different areas of the tumor when establishing the molecular subtype.

Several studies have indicated that it is possible to classify BC into molecular subtypes using immunohistochemistry (IHC), which is less complex than transcriptomic analysis and could facilitate the use of molecular subtypes in clinical practice. Markers related to basal subtypes, such as KRT5/6, KRT14 and p63, and those associated with luminal phenotypes, such as GATA3, FOXA1, uroplakin and erb-b2 receptor tyrosine kinase 2 (HER2), have been proposed for an IHC-based classification. A meta-analysis found that by analyzing only GATA3 and KRT5/6 with IHC, it was possible to identify the basal and luminal subtypes with 91% reliability [32]. Recently, Makboul et al. stratified BC patients according to the Lund classification [24] using a simple IHC panel of five biomarkers (FGFR3, CK5, cyclin-B1, HER2, p53). More than 90% of tumors were classified without overlap and the different tumor subtypes significantly correlated with prognosis [33]. The different subtypes have also been correlated with response to chemotherapy. Basal tumors are associated with a better response to cisplatin-based chemotherapy, while tumors classified as p53-like or those in cluster II [7] have been associated with chemoresistance [26]. An MD Anderson study of 60 MIBC patients treated with neoadjuvant dose-dense methotrexate + vinblastine + doxorubicin + cisplatin (M-VAC) plus bevacizumab found that patients with basal tumors had more pathological complete responses (pCR) and longer survival than those with luminal or p53-like tumors. Five-year survival rates for patients with basal, luminal, and p53-like tumors were 91%, 73%, and 36%, respectively, probably due to the greater sensitivity to NAC in basal tumors, since achieving downstaging is a predictive factor for longer survival. Additionally, only patients with p53-like tumors presented bone metastases at disease progression. Interestingly, this study also found a greater frequency of the p53-like subtype in cystectomy samples than in transurethral resection (TUR) samples, especially in luminal tumors, suggesting that NAC can induce switching of tumor subtypes [34]. The Canadian study [28] analyzed the association between their four tumor subtypes (basal, luminal-infiltrated, luminal, claudin-low) and response to NAC. Patients with luminal tumors had the longest overall survival, while those with claudin-low tumors had the shortest, regardless of whether they received NAC or only cystectomy. In contrast, patients with basal tumors had longer survival but did not fare differently from luminal tumors if they were treated with NAC rather than only cystectomy. Recently, the same group has defined four subtypes by transcriptional analysis in residual tumor at cystectomy after NAC: CC1-basal, CC2-luminal, CC3-immune, and CC4-scar-like. The basal and luminal phenotypes observed in the residual disease were similar to the pretreatment subtypes. The CC3-immune tumors had the worst outcome and showed a high immune infiltration, suggesting a potential positive impact for immune checkpoint inhibitors (ICIs) as second-line treatment, whereas the CC4-scar-like tumors showed a low proliferation rate, expressed fibrosis, and had a good prognosis regardless of response to NAC [35]. These findings suggest that establishing molecular subtypes after NAC in residual tumor disease can be useful in selecting adjuvant treatment.

A recent study by our group, using IHC-based hierarchical clustering, classified MIBC patients treated with NAC in three clusters: BASQ-like (FOXA1/GATA3 low; KRT5/6/14 high), luminal-like (FOXA1/GATA3 high; KRT5/6/14 low), and mixed-cluster (FOXA1/GATA3 high; KRT5/6 high; KRT14 low). Patients with BASQ-like tumors were more likely to achieve a pathological response to NAC (OR 3.96; $p = 0.017$) [36].

Taken together, these findings indicate that the molecular classification of BC according to gene expression profiles can play an important role in selecting the most effective treatment for each patient. Thus, basal tumors would benefit most from chemotherapy, while luminal tumors would be associated with better prognosis but poor response to cisplatin-based chemotherapy, indicating that the best treatment option for these patients could be cystectomy. Molecular classification can thus provide additional information to the standard histological classification and better characterize BC for personalized treatment approaches.

In recent years, with the emergence of immunotherapy as a treatment option for BC, several studies have attempted to establish a correlation between tumor subtypes and immunotherapy efficacy. The revised TCGA classification [27] suggested that patients with luminal-infiltrated tumors and especially those with basal tumors can derive the greatest benefit from immunotherapy. Importantly, however, the TCGA patients had localized tumors and had not received any previous treatment, thus, these treatment strategies require validation in future studies. The IMvigor 210 study [37] demonstrated a greater benefit of treatment with atezolizumab, a PD-L1-blocking antibody, in advanced BC classified as TCGA cluster II [7], and in the CheckMate 275 study, basal tumors responded better to nivolumab, a PD-1-blocking antibody [38]. Surprisingly, tumors with high immune infiltration, classified as claudin-low, showed a poor response to immunotherapy [37,38]. This apparent paradox could be explained by the fact that there is a more effective suppression of T cells in cluster IV than in cluster II tumors [39]. Intriguingly, immunotherapy and chemotherapy seem to be effective in complementary patient populations. Patients with luminal-infiltrated tumors (cluster II) would benefit from immunotherapy, while in those with basal tumors (cluster IV), chemotherapy may be the treatment of choice. Although patients with neuronal-subtype tumors generally have a worse prognosis, a recent analysis of the IMvigor 210 trial showed that TCGA neuronal-subtype tumors [27] responded better to atezolizumab [40]. Moreover, this did not seem to be associated with other parameters related to immunotherapy response; for instance, the tumor mutational burden (TMB) and the load of tumor neo-antigens were lower in these tumors than in the other subtypes and none of the tumors were immunoinflammatory. In contrast, the neuronal subtype had low levels of transforming growth factor beta 1 (TGF-β1), which has been associated with improved response to immunotherapy [41]. In summary, while a molecular classification can help to select the best treatment option for each patient, it will be necessary to take into consideration other factors that may affect response to either chemotherapy or immunotherapy.

4. Predictive Biomarkers of Immunotherapy Response

The emergence of immunotherapy has highlighted the importance of biomarkers when deciding on the optimal treatment for each patient. In addition to molecular subtypes, many potential biomarkers have been correlated with the response to immunotherapy: PD-L1 expression, $CD8^+$ T-cell infiltration, DDR gene alterations, TMB, and immune and stromal gene expression signatures such as the interferon gamma (IFN-γ) signature [42]. To date, unfortunately, none of these markers has shown sufficiently consistent results to warrant incorporation into the routine management of BC.

PD-L1 expression is detected in 20–30% of bladder tumors and is associated with more advanced disease and worse prognosis [43]. Studies of advanced BC have shown conflicting results regarding the role of PD-L1 as a predictive biomarker of response to immunotherapy [44]. Importantly, since PD-L1 is a dynamic biomarker both in space and time, the analysis of a small tumor fragment in a biopsy may not be representative of the PD-L1 expression in the whole tumor. Moreover, prior treatment may influence PD-L1 expression. Therefore, IHC results of PD-L1 expression must be interpreted in the context of broader biomarker panels when selecting patients to receive immunotherapy.

Some biomarkers, such as the neutrophil/lymphocyte ratio, albumin levels, high C-reactive protein, and Interleukin-6 levels, can be easily incorporated into routine clinical practice, while others, such as gene expression signatures, are more complex [45]. In addition to the potential usefulness of the molecular subtypes in predicting response, the study of DDR pathways may be helpful, since defects in DDR have been associated with an increase in the TMB, and thus, with a greater immune response. An MSKCC study analyzed a panel of 34 DDR genes in patients with advanced BC treated with atezolizumab or nivolumab and found a significant benefit for immunotherapy in patients with deleterious mutations in the genes [46]. In addition, ICIs have recently been shown to be highly effective in tumors with defects in the MMR/microsatellite instability pathway [47]. In an effort to encompass these different biomarkers that may be related to immunotherapy response, an immunogram has recently been proposed that incorporates in seven main axes the different parameters related to immunotherapy response, which will help to predict the efficacy of ICIs in individual patients [48].

The possibility of incorporating immunotherapy in earlier stages of BC, where other treatments are currently available, makes it essential to identify biomarkers to select the most effective therapy for each patient. The solid rationale for exploring the efficacy of immunotherapy in early-stage disease has recently been elegantly reviewed [49]. Early stages have a greater integrity of the immune system and can induce greater T-cell expansion than advanced stages, where increased impairment of T-cell function is more evident and where cancer-associated inflammation has been linked to poor response to immunotherapy. Moreover, the neoadjuvant setting is optimal for exploring the role of potential predictive biomarkers to immunotherapy since tumor tissue can be obtained just before treatment initiation and the genomic profile can be compared before and after therapy.

Two recent phase II trials have explored the role of ICIs in the neoadjuvant setting. In the PURE-01 trial [50], 50 patients, most of whom were eligible for cisplatin therapy, were treated with three cycles of pembrolizumab, a PD-1-blocking antibody, followed by cystectomy. In the ABACUS trial [51], 95 patients who were ineligible for cisplatin-based NAC received two cycles of atezolizumab before cystectomy. A pCR was attained by 42% and 31% of patients in the PURE-01 and ABACUS trials, respectively. Both trials included detailed biomarker analyses to define potential predictive biomarkers of response to ICIs. In the PURE-01 study, a significant association between pCR and PD-L1 expression, TMB, and DDR and *RB1* gene alterations was observed. In the ABACUS trial, in contrast, these biomarkers did not correlate with pathological response; however, the quality of immune infiltration measured by CD8 and granzyme B (GZMB), a surrogate marker of activated CD8 cells, as well as an eight-gene cytotoxic T-cell transcriptional signature, significantly correlated with pCR. In addition, the inflamed and desert immune phenotypes, as described by Mariathasan et al. [41], correlated with response and resistance to atezolizumab, respectively. Interestingly, CD8 levels were higher in responding tumors, while high levels of fibroblast activation protein alpha (FAP), a surrogate marker of cancer-associated fibroblasts related to TGF-β, was associated with resistance to immunotherapy. PD-L1, CD8, GZMB, and FAP expression increased post-therapy. These results suggest a potential predictive role of response to ICIs for these markers although the contradictory findings of the two trials indicate a need for validation in a larger number of patients.

Both the PURE-01 and ABACUS trials showed promising results that suggest a level of efficacy for neoadjuvant immunotherapy comparable to that of NAC, making it a feasible treatment option for cisplatin-ineligible patients. This possibility raises the question of how to select cisplatin-eligible patients for NAC or immunotherapy or NAC-plus-immunotherapy, especially considering that many biomarkers, such as TMB and DDR alterations, are associated with the efficacy of both treatments [21,46]. A study exploring the association between the tumor microenvironment and outcome in MIBC patients found that higher T-cell inflamed and IFN-γ signature scores were associated with improved outcome in patients treated with bladder-sparing trimodality therapy (TMT) but with worse outcome in those treated with NAC-plus-RC, while high stromal infiltration was associated with poor prognosis in patients receiving NAC-plus-RC but not in those treated with TMT [52]. Along the same lines, immune signatures predicted response to neoadjuvant immunotherapy in patients included in the PURE-01 trial but not in patients treated with NAC [53]. An ongoing phase III trial (NCT03732677) exploring the combination of NAC and immunotherapy will shed further light on this issue.

A related question is how to integrate and sequence the different therapeutic options in the multimodality management of MIBC. Intriguingly, the cytotoxic effect of NAC can generate an immune effect through the activation of $CD8^+$ effector T cells and decreasing T_{regs} [54]. The concurrent administration of NAC and immunotherapy could thus hinder the T-cell response if T cells are killed by NAC. This phenomenon may partly explain the limited benefit obtained with NAC-plus-immunotherapy compared to NAC alone in advanced BC [55]. In contrast, a sequential administration of NAC followed by immunotherapy could be a more effective approach. In the TONIC trial in breast cancer, an upregulation of immune-related genes was detected after cisplatin-based chemotherapy, suggesting that NAC may induce a tumor microenvironment more conducive to immunotherapy response [56]. Finally, evidence suggests that neoadjuvant is more effective than adjuvant treatment, based on the greater tumor antigen exposition before tumor resection [49]. The recent results of the IMvigor 010 phase III trial showed that adjuvant atezolizumab did not demonstrate a significant benefit in high-risk MIBC patients treated with cystectomy [57].

5. Conclusions

In recent years, we have greatly broadened our understanding of the molecular biology of BC, which has allowed us to identify new prognostic and predictive biomarkers. We also have at our disposal novel therapeutic options, such as immunotherapy, which can improve patient outcome and quality of life. These new effective drugs show promising results but also highlight the question of how to select the optimal treatment for each patient. There is still no biomarker approved for clinical practice and it is crucial to incorporate into clinical practice all the advances in the field of molecular biology as efficiently and rapidly as possible. Only in this way, will we be able to achieve precision medicine and select the most effective treatment for each individual patient.

Author Contributions: Conceptualization, A.F., V.R.d.P., and J.C.P. Writing—Original draft preparation, A.F., V.R.d.P., and J.C.P. Writing—Review and editing, A.F., V.R.d.P., J.C.P., A.P., C.C., O.E. and O.B. All authors have read and agreed to the published version of the manuscript.

Acknowledgments: We want to acknowledge Renée O'Brate for critical reading and language correction.

References

1. Bellmunt, J.; Fougeray, R.; Rosenberg, J.E.; von der Maase, H.; Schutz, F.A.; Salhi, Y.; Culine, S.; Choueiri, T.K. Long-term survival results of a randomized phase III trial of vinflunine plus best supportive care versus best supportive care alone in advanced urothelial carcinoma patients after failure of platinum-based chemotherapy. *Ann. Oncol.* **2013**, *24*, 1466–1472. [CrossRef]
2. Font, A.; Luque, R.; Villa, J.C.; Domenech, M.; Vazquez, S.; Gallardo, E.; Virizuela, J.A.; Beato, C.; Morales-Barrera, R.; Gelabert, A.; et al. The Challenge of Managing Bladder Cancer and Upper Tract Urothelial Carcinoma: A Review with Treatment Recommendations from the Spanish Oncology Genitourinary Group (SOGUG). *Target Oncol.* **2019**, *14*, 15–32. [CrossRef]
3. Alfred Witjes, J.; Lebret, T.; Comperat, E.M.; Cowan, N.C.; De Santis, M.; Bruins, H.M.; Hernandez, V.; Espinos, E.L.; Dunn, J.; Rouanne, M.; et al. Updated 2016 EAU Guidelines on Muscle-invasive and Metastatic Bladder Cancer. *Eur. Urol.* **2017**, *71*, 462–475. [CrossRef]

4. Reardon, Z.D.; Patel, S.G.; Zaid, H.B.; Stimson, C.J.; Resnick, M.J.; Keegan, K.A.; Barocas, D.A.; Chang, S.S.; Cookson, M.S. Trends in the use of perioperative chemotherapy for localized and locally advanced muscle-invasive bladder cancer: A sign of changing tides. *Eur. Urol.* **2015**, *67*, 165–170. [CrossRef] [PubMed]
5. Thompson, R.H.; Boorjian, S.A.; Kim, S.P.; Cheville, J.C.; Thapa, P.; Tarrel, R.; Dronca, R.; Costello, B.; Frank, I. Eligibility for neoadjuvant/adjuvant cisplatin-based chemotherapy among radical cystectomy patients. *BJU Int.* **2014**, *113*, E17–E21. [CrossRef] [PubMed]
6. Bhindi, B.; Frank, I.; Mason, R.J.; Tarrell, R.F.; Thapa, P.; Cheville, J.C.; Costello, B.A.; Pagliaro, L.C.; Karnes, R.J.; Thompson, R.H.; et al. Oncologic Outcomes for Patients with Residual Cancer at Cystectomy Following Neoadjuvant Chemotherapy: A Pathologic Stage matched Analysis. *Eur. Urol.* **2017**, *72*, 660–664. [CrossRef] [PubMed]
7. Cancer Genome Atlas Research, N. Comprehensive molecular characterization of urothelial bladder carcinoma. *Nature* **2014**, *507*, 315–322. [CrossRef]
8. Hyman, D.M.; Taylor, B.S.; Baselga, J. Implementing Genome-Driven Oncology. *Cell* **2017**, *168*, 584–599. [CrossRef]
9. Siddik, Z.H. Cisplatin: Mode of cytotoxic action and molecular basis of resistance. *Oncogene* **2003**, *22*, 7265–7279. [CrossRef]
10. Curtin, N.J. DNA repair dysregulation from cancer driver to therapeutic target. *Nat. Rev. Cancer* **2012**, *12*, 801–817. [CrossRef]
11. Britten, R.A.; Liu, D.; Tessier, A.; Hutchison, M.J.; Murray, D. ERCC1 expression as a molecular marker of cisplatin resistance in human cervical tumor cells. *Int. J. Cancer* **2000**, *89*, 453–457. [CrossRef]
12. Bellmunt, J.; Paz-Ares, L.; Cuello, M.; Cecere, F.L.; Albiol, S.; Guillem, V.; Gallardo, E.; Carles, J.; Mendez, P.; de la Cruz, J.J.; et al. Spanish Oncology Genitourinary, G. Gene expression of ERCC1 as a novel prognostic marker in advanced bladder cancer patients receiving cisplatin-based chemotherapy. *Ann. Oncol.* **2007**, *18*, 522–528. [CrossRef] [PubMed]
13. Pietzak, E.J.; Zabor, E.C.; Bagrodia, A.; Armenia, J.; Hu, W.; Zehir, A.; Funt, S.; Audenet, F.; Barron, D.; Maamouri, N.; et al. Genomic Differences Between "Primary" and "Secondary" Muscle-invasive Bladder Cancer as a Basis for Disparate Outcomes to Cisplatin-based Neoadjuvant Chemotherapy. *Eur. Urol.* **2019**, *75*, 231–239. [CrossRef]
14. Van Allen, E.M.; Mouw, K.W.; Kim, P.; Iyer, G.; Wagle, N.; Al-Ahmadie, H.; Zhu, C.; Ostrovnaya, I.; Kryukov, G.V.; O'Connor, K.W.; et al. Somatic ERCC2 mutations correlate with cisplatin sensitivity in muscle-invasive urothelial carcinoma. *Cancer Discov.* **2014**, *4*, 1140–1153. [CrossRef] [PubMed]
15. Liu, D.; Plimack, E.R.; Hoffman-Censits, J.; Garraway, L.A.; Bellmunt, J.; Van Allen, E.; Rosenberg, J.E. Clinical Validation of Chemotherapy Response Biomarker ERCC2 in Muscle-Invasive Urothelial Bladder Carcinoma. *JAMA Oncol.* **2016**, *2*, 1094–1096. [CrossRef]
16. Plimack, E.R.; Dunbrack, R.L.; Brennan, T.A.; Andrake, M.D.; Zhou, Y.; Serebriiskii, I.G.; Slifker, M.; Alpaugh, K.; Dulaimi, E.; Palma, N.; et al. Defects in DNA Repair Genes Predict Response to Neoadjuvant Cisplatin-based Chemotherapy in Muscle-invasive Bladder Cancer. *Eur. Urol.* **2015**, *68*, 959–967. [CrossRef]
17. Miron, B.; Hoffman-Censits, J.H.; Anari, F.; O'Neill, J.; Geynisman, D.M.; Zibelman, M.R.; Kutikov, A.; Viterbo, R.; Greenberg, R.E.; Chen, D.; et al. Defects in DNA Repair Genes Confer Improved Long-term Survival after Cisplatin-based Neoadjuvant Chemotherapy for Muscle-invasive Bladder Cancer. *Eur. Urol. Oncol.* **2020**. [CrossRef]
18. Heeke, A.L.; Pishvaian, M.J.; Lynce, F.; Xiu, J.; Brody, J.R.; Chen, W.J.; Baker, T.M.; Marshall, J.L.; Isaacs, C. Prevalence of Homologous Recombination-Related Gene Mutations Across Multiple Cancer Types. *JCO Precis. Oncol.* **2018**, *2018*. [CrossRef]
19. Carlo, M.I.; Ravichandran, V.; Srinavasan, P.; Bandlamudi, C.; Kemel, Y.; Ceyhan-Birsoy, O.; Mukherjee, S.; Mandelker, D.; Chaim, J.; Knezevic, A.; et al. Cancer Susceptibility Mutations in Patients with Urothelial Malignancies. *J. Clin. Oncol.* **2020**, *38*, 406–414. [CrossRef]
20. Font, A.; Taron, M.; Gago, J.L.; Costa, C.; Sanchez, J.J.; Carrato, C.; Mora, M.; Celiz, P.; Perez, L.; Rodriguez, D.; et al. BRCA1 mRNA expression and outcome to neoadjuvant cisplatin-based chemotherapy in bladder cancer. *Ann. Oncol.* **2011**, *22*, 139–144. [CrossRef]

21. Teo, M.Y.; Bambury, R.M.; Zabor, E.C.; Jordan, E.; Al-Ahmadie, H.; Boyd, M.E.; Bouvier, N.; Mullane, S.A.; Cha, E.K.; Roper, N.; et al. DNA Damage Response and Repair Gene Alterations Are Associated with Improved Survival in Patients with Platinum-Treated Advanced Urothelial Carcinoma. *Clin. Cancer Res.* **2017**, *23*, 3610–3618. [CrossRef] [PubMed]
22. Iyer, G.; Balar, A.V.; Milowsky, M.I.; Bochner, B.H.; Dalbagni, G.; Donat, S.M.; Herr, H.W.; Huang, W.C.; Taneja, S.S.; Woods, M.; et al. Multicenter Prospective Phase II Trial of Neoadjuvant Dose-Dense Gemcitabine Plus Cisplatin in Patients with Muscle-Invasive Bladder Cancer. *J. Clin. Oncol.* **2018**, *36*, 1949–1956. [CrossRef] [PubMed]
23. Romeo, M.; Pardo, J.C.; Martinez-Cardus, A.; Martinez-Balibrea, E.; Quiroga, V.; Martinez-Roman, S.; Sole, F.; Margeli, M.; Mesia, R. Translational Research Opportunities Regarding Homologous Recombination in Ovarian Cancer. *Int. J. Mol. Sci.* **2018**, *19*, 3249. [CrossRef] [PubMed]
24. Sjodahl, G.; Lauss, M.; Lovgren, K.; Chebil, G.; Gudjonsson, S.; Veerla, S.; Patschan, O.; Aine, M.; Ferno, M.; Ringner, M.; et al. A molecular taxonomy for urothelial carcinoma. *Clin. Cancer Res.* **2012**, *18*, 3377–3386. [CrossRef] [PubMed]
25. Damrauer, J.S.; Hoadley, K.A.; Chism, D.D.; Fan, C.; Tiganelli, C.J.; Wobker, S.E.; Yeh, J.J.; Milowsky, M.I.; Iyer, G.; Parker, J.S.; et al. Intrinsic subtypes of high-grade bladder cancer reflect the hallmarks of breast cancer biology. *Proc. Natl. Acad. Sci. USA* **2014**, *111*, 3110–3115. [CrossRef]
26. Choi, W.; Porten, S.; Kim, S.; Willis, D.; Plimack, E.R.; Hoffman-Censits, J.; Roth, B.; Cheng, T.; Tran, M.; Lee, I.L.; et al. Identification of distinct basal and luminal subtypes of muscle-invasive bladder cancer with different sensitivities to frontline chemotherapy. *Cancer Cell* **2014**, *25*, 152–165. [CrossRef] [PubMed]
27. Robertson, A.G.; Kim, J.; Al-Ahmadie, H.; Bellmunt, J.; Guo, G.; Cherniack, A.D.; Hinoue, T.; Laird, P.W.; Hoadley, K.A.; Akbani, R.; et al. Comprehensive Molecular Characterization of Muscle-Invasive Bladder Cancer. *Cell* **2018**, *174*, 1033. [CrossRef]
28. Seiler, R.; Ashab, H.A.D.; Erho, N.; van Rhijn, B.W.G.; Winters, B.; Douglas, J.; Van Kessel, K.E.; Fransen van de Putte, E.E.; Sommerlad, M.; Wang, N.Q.; et al. Impact of Molecular Subtypes in Muscle-invasive Bladder Cancer on Predicting Response and Survival after Neoadjuvant Chemotherapy. *Eur. Urol.* **2017**, *72*, 544–554. [CrossRef]
29. Kamoun, A.; de Reynies, A.; Allory, Y.; Sjodahl, G.; Robertson, A.G.; Seiler, R.; Hoadley, K.A.; Groeneveld, C.S.; Al-Ahmadie, H.; Choi, W.; et al. Bladder Cancer Molecular Taxonomy, G. A Consensus Molecular Classification of Muscle-invasive Bladder Cancer. *Eur. Urol.* **2020**, *77*, 420–433. [CrossRef]
30. Lotan, Y.; Boorjian, S.A.; Zhang, J.; Bivalacqua, T.J.; Porten, S.P.; Wheeler, T.; Lerner, S.P.; Hutchinson, R.; Francis, F.; Davicioni, E.; et al. Molecular Subtyping of Clinically Localized Urothelial Carcinoma Reveals Lower Rates of Pathological Upstaging at Radical Cystectomy Among Luminal Tumors. *Eur. Urol.* **2019**, *76*, 200–206. [CrossRef]
31. Warrick, J.I.; Sjodahl, G.; Kaag, M.; Raman, J.D.; Merrill, S.; Shuman, L.; Chen, G.; Walter, V.; DeGraff, D.J. Intratumoral Heterogeneity of Bladder Cancer by Molecular Subtypes and Histologic Variants. *Eur. Urol.* **2019**, *75*, 18–22. [CrossRef] [PubMed]
32. Dadhania, V.; Zhang, M.; Zhang, L.; Bondaruk, J.; Majewski, T.; Siefker-Radtke, A.; Guo, C.C.; Dinney, C.; Cogdell, D.E.; Zhang, S.; et al. Meta-Analysis of the Luminal and Basal Subtypes of Bladder Cancer and the Identification of Signature Immunohistochemical Markers for Clinical Use. *EBioMedicine* **2016**, *12*, 105–117. [CrossRef] [PubMed]
33. Makboul, R.; Hassan, H.M.; Refaiy, A.; Abdelkawi, I.F.; Shahat, A.A.; Hameed, D.A.; Morsy, A.; Salah, T.; Ahmed Mohammed, R.A. A Simple Immunohistochemical Panel Could Predict and Correlate to Clinicopathologic and Molecular Subgroups of Urinary Bladder Urothelial Carcinoma. *Clin. Genitourin Cancer* **2019**, *17*, e712–e719. [CrossRef] [PubMed]
34. McConkey, D.J.; Choi, W.; Shen, Y.; Lee, I.L.; Porten, S.; Matin, S.F.; Kamat, A.M.; Corn, P.; Millikan, R.E.; Dinney, C.; et al. A Prognostic Gene Expression Signature in the Molecular Classification of Chemotherapy-naive Urothelial Cancer is Predictive of Clinical Outcomes from Neoadjuvant Chemotherapy: A Phase 2 Trial of Dose-dense Methotrexate, Vinblastine, Doxorubicin, and Cisplatin with Bevacizumab in Urothelial Cancer. *Eur. Urol.* **2016**, *69*, 855–862.
35. Seiler, R.; Gibb, E.A.; Wang, N.Q.; Oo, H.Z.; Lam, H.M.; van Kessel, K.E.; Voskuilen, C.S.; Winters, B.; Erho, N.; Takhar, M.M.; et al. Divergent Biological Response to Neoadjuvant Chemotherapy in Muscle-invasive Bladder Cancer. *Clin. Cancer Res.* **2019**, *25*, 5082–5093. [CrossRef]

36. Font, A.; Domenech, M.; Benitez, R.; Rava, M.; Marques, M.; Ramirez, J.L.; Pineda, S.; Dominguez-Rodriguez, S.; Gago, J.L.; Badal, J.; et al. Immunohistochemistry-Based Taxonomical Classification of Bladder Cancer Predicts Response to Neoadjuvant Chemotherapy. *Cancers* **2020**, *12*, 1784.
37. Rosenberg, J.E.; Hoffman-Censits, J.; Powles, T.; van der Heijden, M.S.; Balar, A.V.; Necchi, A.; Dawson, N.; O'Donnell, P.H.; Balmanoukian, A.; Loriot, Y.; et al. Atezolizumab in patients with locally advanced and metastatic urothelial carcinoma who have progressed following treatment with platinum-based chemotherapy: A single-arm, multicentre, phase 2 trial. *Lancet* **2016**, *387*, 1909–1920. [CrossRef]
38. Sharma, P.; Retz, M.; Siefker-Radtke, A.; Baron, A.; Necchi, A.; Bedke, J.; Plimack, E.R.; Vaena, D.; Grimm, M.O.; Bracarda, S.; et al. Nivolumab in metastatic urothelial carcinoma after platinum therapy (CheckMate 275): A multicentre, single-arm, phase 2 trial. *Lancet Oncol.* **2017**, *18*, 312–322. [CrossRef]
39. Kardos, J.; Chai, S.; Mose, L.E.; Selitsky, S.R.; Krishnan, B.; Saito, R.; Iglesia, M.D.; Milowsky, M.I.; Parker, J.S.; Kim, W.Y.; et al. Claudin-low bladder tumors are immune infiltrated and actively immune suppressed. *JCI Insight* **2016**, *1*, e85902. [CrossRef]
40. Kim, J.; Kwiatkowski, D.; McConkey, D.J.; Meeks, J.J.; Freeman, S.S.; Bellmunt, J.; Getz, G.; Lerner, S.P. The Cancer Genome Atlas Expression Subtypes Stratify Response to Checkpoint Inhibition in Advanced Urothelial Cancer and Identify a Subset of Patients with High Survival Probability. *Eur. Urol.* **2019**, *75*, 961–964. [CrossRef]
41. Mariathasan, S.; Turley, S.J.; Nickles, D.; Castiglioni, A.; Yuen, K.; Wang, Y.; Kadel, E.E., III; Koeppen, H.; Astarita, J.L.; Cubas, R.; et al. TGFbeta attenuates tumour response to PD-L1 blockade by contributing to exclusion of T cells. *Nature* **2018**, *554*, 544–548. [CrossRef] [PubMed]
42. Hussain, S.A.; Birtle, A.; Crabb, S.; Huddart, R.; Small, D.; Summerhayes, M.; Jones, R.; Protheroe, A. From Clinical Trials to Real-life Clinical Practice: The Role of Immunotherapy with PD-1/PD-L1 Inhibitors in Advanced Urothelial Carcinoma. *Eur. Urol. Oncol.* **2018**, *1*, 486–500. [CrossRef] [PubMed]
43. Boorjian, S.A.; Sheinin, Y.; Crispen, P.L.; Farmer, S.A.; Lohse, C.M.; Kuntz, S.M.; Leibovich, B.C.; Kwon, E.D.; Frank, I. T-cell coregulatory molecule expression in urothelial cell carcinoma: Clinicopathologic correlations and association with survival. *Clin. Cancer Res.* **2008**, *14*, 4800–4808. [CrossRef] [PubMed]
44. Aggen, D.H.; Drake, C.G. Biomarkers for immunotherapy in bladder cancer: A moving target. *J. Immunother. Cancer* **2017**, *5*, 94. [CrossRef]
45. Ayers, M.; Lunceford, J.; Nebozhyn, M.; Murphy, E.; Loboda, A.; Kaufman, D.R.; Albright, A.; Cheng, J.D.; Kang, S.P.; Shankaran, V.; et al. IFN-gamma-related mRNA profile predicts clinical response to PD-1 blockade. *J. Clin. Investig.* **2017**, *127*, 2930–2940. [CrossRef]
46. Teo, M.Y.; Seier, K.; Ostrovnaya, I.; Regazzi, A.M.; Kania, B.E.; Moran, M.M.; Cipolla, C.K.; Bluth, M.J.; Chaim, J.; Al-Ahmadie, H.; et al. Alterations in DNA Damage Response and Repair Genes as Potential Marker of Clinical Benefit From PD-1/PD-L1 Blockade in Advanced Urothelial Cancers. *J. Clin. Oncol.* **2018**, *36*, 1685–1694. [CrossRef]
47. Le, D.T.; Uram, J.N.; Wang, H.; Bartlett, B.R.; Kemberling, H.; Eyring, A.D.; Skora, A.D.; Luber, B.S.; Azad, N.S.; Laheru, D.; et al. PD-1 Blockade in Tumors with Mismatch-Repair Deficiency. *N. Engl. J. Med.* **2015**, *372*, 2509–2520. [CrossRef]
48. van Dijk, N.; Funt, S.A.; Blank, C.U.; Powles, T.; Rosenberg, J.E.; van der Heijden, M.S. The Cancer Immunogram as a Framework for Personalized Immunotherapy in Urothelial Cancer. *Eur. Urol.* **2019**, *75*, 435–444. [CrossRef]
49. Versluis, J.M.; Long, G.V.; Blank, C.U. Learning from clinical trials of neoadjuvant checkpoint blockade. *Nat. Med.* **2020**, *26*, 475–484. [CrossRef]
50. Necchi, A.; Anichini, A.; Raggi, D.; Briganti, A.; Massa, S.; Luciano, R.; Colecchia, M.; Giannatempo, P.; Mortarini, R.; Bianchi, M.; et al. Pembrolizumab as Neoadjuvant Therapy Before Radical Cystectomy in Patients With Muscle-Invasive Urothelial Bladder Carcinoma (PURE-01): An Open-Label, Single-Arm, Phase II Study. *J. Clin. Oncol.* **2018**, *36*, 3353–3360. [CrossRef]
51. Powles, T.; Kockx, M.; Rodriguez-Vida, A.; Duran, I.; Crabb, S.J.; Van Der Heijden, M.S.; Szabados, B.; Pous, A.F.; Gravis, G.; Herranz, U.A.; et al. Clinical efficacy and biomarker analysis of neoadjuvant atezolizumab in operable urothelial carcinoma in the ABACUS trial. *Nat. Med.* **2019**, *25*, 1706–1714. [CrossRef] [PubMed]

52. Efstathiou, J.A.; Mouw, K.W.; Gibb, E.A.; Liu, Y.; Wu, C.L.; Drumm, M.R.; da Costa, J.B.; du Plessis, M.; Wang, N.Q.; Davicioni, E.; et al. Impact of Immune and Stromal Infiltration on Outcomes Following Bladder-Sparing Trimodality Therapy for Muscle-Invasive Bladder Cancer. *Eur. Urol.* **2019**, *76*, 59–68. [CrossRef] [PubMed]
53. Necchi, A.; Raggi, D.; Gallina, A.; Ross, J.S.; Fare, E.; Giannatempo, P.; Marandino, L.; Colecchia, M.; Luciano, R.; Bianchi, M.; et al. Impact of Molecular Subtyping and Immune Infiltration on Pathological Response and Outcome Following Neoadjuvant Pembrolizumab in Muscle-invasive Bladder Cancer. *Eur. Urol.* **2020**, *77*, 701–710. [CrossRef]
54. Krantz, D.; Hartana, C.A.; Winerdal, M.E.; Johansson, M.; Alamdari, F.; Jakubczyk, T.; Huge, Y.; Aljabery, F.; Palmqvist, K.; Zirakzadeh, A.A.; et al. Neoadjuvant Chemotherapy Reinforces Antitumour T cell Response in Urothelial Urinary Bladder Cancer. *Eur. Urol.* **2018**, *74*, 688–692. [CrossRef] [PubMed]
55. Galsky, M.D.; Arija, J.A.A.; Bamias, A.; Davis, I.D.; De Santis, M.; Kikuchi, E.; Garcia-Del-Muro, X.; De Giorgi, U.; Mencinger, M.; Izumi, K.; et al. Atezolizumab with or without chemotherapy in metastatic urothelial cancer (IMvigor130): A multicentre, randomised, placebo-controlled phase 3 trial. *Lancet* **2020**, *395*, 1547–1557. [CrossRef]
56. Voorwerk, L.; Slagter, M.; Horlings, H.M.; Sikorska, K.; van de Vijver, K.K.; de Maaker, M.; Nederlof, I.; Kluin, R.J.C.; Warren, S.; Ong, S.; et al. Immune induction strategies in metastatic triple-negative breast cancer to enhance the sensitivity to PD-1 blockade: The TONIC trial. *Nat. Med.* **2019**, *25*, 920–928. [CrossRef]
57. Hussain, M.H.A.; Powles, T.; Albers, P.; Castellano, D.; Daneshmand, S.; Gschwend, J.; Nishiyama, H.; Oudard, S.; Tayama, D.; Davarpanah, N.N.; et al. IMvigor010: Primary analysis from a phase III randomized study of adjuvant atezolizumab (atezo) versus observation (obs) in high-risk muscle-invasive urothelial carcinoma (MIUC). *J. Clin. Oncol.* **2020**, *38*, 5000. [CrossRef]

4

STAT3/5 Inhibitors Suppress Proliferation in Bladder Cancer and Enhance Oncolytic Adenovirus Therapy

Sruthi V. Hindupur [1,†], Sebastian C. Schmid [1,†], Jana Annika Koch [1], Ahmed Youssef [1,2], Eva-Maria Baur [1], Dongbiao Wang [1], Thomas Horn [1], Julia Slotta-Huspenina [3], Juergen E. Gschwend [1], Per Sonne Holm [1] and Roman Nawroth [1,*]

1 Department of Urology, Klinikum rechts der Isar, Technical University of Munich, 81675 Munich, Germany; sruthi.hindupur@tum.de (S.V.H.); sebastian.schmid@tum.de (S.C.S.); jana.koch@tum.de (J.A.K.); ahmed0122@med.bsu.edu.eg (A.Y.); e-m.baur@gmx.de (E.-M.B.); dongbiao.wang@tum.de (D.W.); t.horn@tum.de (T.H.); juergen.gschwend@tum.de (J.E.G.); per.holm@tum.de (P.S.H.)

2 Department of Urology, Beni-suef University, Beni Suef 62511, Egypt

3 Department of Pathology, Klinikum rechts der Isar, Technical University of Munich, 81675 Munich, Germany; julia.slotta-huspenina@tum.de

* Correspondence: roman.nawroth@tum.de

† These authors contributed equally to this work.

Abstract: The JAK-STAT signalling pathway regulates cellular processes like cell division, cell death and immune regulation. Dysregulation has been identified in solid tumours and STAT3 activation is a marker for poor outcome. The aim of this study was to explore potential therapeutic strategies by targeting this pathway in bladder cancer (BC). High STAT3 expression was detected in 51.3% from 149 patient specimens with invasive bladder cancer by immunohistochemistry. Protein expression of JAK, STAT and downstream targets were confirmed in 10 cell lines. Effects of the JAK inhibitors Ruxolitinib and BSK-805, and STAT3/5 inhibitors Stattic, Nifuroxazide and SH-4-54 were analysed by cell viability assays, immunoblotting, apoptosis and cell cycle progression. Treatment with STAT3/5 but not JAK1/2 inhibitors reduced survival, levels of phosphorylated STAT3 and Cyclin-D1 and increased apoptosis. Tumour xenografts, using the chicken chorioallantoic membrane (CAM) model responded to Stattic monotherapy. Combination of Stattic with Cisplatin, Docetaxel, Gemcitabine, Paclitaxel and CDK4/6 inhibitors showed additive effects. The combination of Stattic with the oncolytic adenovirus XVir-N-31 increased viral replication and cell lysis. Our results provide evidence that inhibitors against STAT3/5 are promising as novel mono- and combination therapy in bladder cancer.

Keywords: bladder cancer; JAK-STAT pathway; combination therapy; oncolytic adenovirus; virotherapy; STAT3/5 inhibitor; JAK inhibitor; XVir-N-31

---

1. Introduction

Bladder cancer (BC) is the 10th most common cancer in the world, as of 2018 [1]. Approximately 25% of patients present as muscle invasive bladder cancer (MIBC) at time of diagnosis. Metastasized BC patients face a poor outcome with median survival time of approximately 14 months and the survival rates have remained largely unchanged for the past 30 years until the emergence of immune checkpoint inhibitors (ICB). Checkpoint inhibitors targeting programmed cell death protein 1 (PD-1) or programmed cell death 1 ligand 1 (PD-L1) have demonstrated durable responses in patients with cisplatin-refractory metastasized BC [2]. However, only 13–21% of patients with metastatic BC respond to immune checkpoint inhibition [3–5].

To find new therapeutic approaches, a plethora of compounds are being tested in clinical trials targeting various signalling pathways in MIBC, including inhibitors of EGFR, HER2, VEGF and the

PI3K/AKT/mTOR pathway [6]. Clinical trials so far have demonstrated that only sub-cohorts of patients benefit from those treatment strategies, probably due to required molecular alterations for therapy response [6]. In 2019, the FGFR inhibitor Balversa (Erdafitinib) was approved by the FDA (Food and Drug Administration) for treatment of patients with metastatic bladder cancer harbouring molecular alterations in FGFR2/3, marking it to be the first targeted therapy to be approved in bladder cancer [7]. Most targeted therapies have shown inconsistent results in early phase clinical trials, which could be attributed to suboptimal selection criteria and biomarker selection, and molecular heterogeneity of the disease [6,8]. Thus, it is not only necessary to identify suitable molecular targets but also predictive markers and combination therapies that broaden the spectrum of responders to treatment.

The JAK-STAT pathway is one of the most studied pathways in cellular signal transduction with diverse roles in physiological processes including cell growth and differentiation and immune response via cytokine signalling [9]. Dysregulations in this pathway are implicated in carcinogenesis and are also associated with poor prognosis in various cancers including kidney cancer [10], lung cancer [11], cervical cancer [12] and bladder cancer [13,14]. The JAK (Janus Kinase) protein family consists of JAK1-3 and Tyk2 in mammals. These proteins are non-receptor tyrosine kinases that are associated with transmembrane cytokine receptors. Signalling is initiated upon binding of a wide range of cytokines (interleukins, interferons, growth factors) to their appropriate receptor. This leads to the dimerization of receptors, bringing the JAKs into close proximity and facilitating transphosphorylation. These activated JAK proteins mediate phosphorylation of STAT proteins. The STAT (signal transducer and activator of transcription) protein family comprises of 7 family members (STAT-1, 2, 3, 4, 5a, 5b and 6). The phosphorylated state results in dimerization and eventual translocation to the nucleus where STATs can activate transcription of target genes. STAT3, in particular, plays a role in cell cycle regulation, cytokine signalling and apoptosis. Increased protein level and constitutive activation of STAT3 have also been reported in bladder cancer [13–17]. Elevated and increased nuclear level of STAT3 and p-STAT3 have been reported to be associated with invasiveness of the disease and advanced stages of the cancer [13,17–21]. Using a STAT3 transgenic mouse model, chemical induction of bladder cancer by N-butyl-N-(4-Hydroxybutyl) nitrosamine (BBN) directly resulted in the development of invasive carcinoma from carcinoma in situ, asserting the role of STAT3 in bladder cancer progression [18].

Considering these findings, we explored targeting of the JAK1/2 and STAT3/5 proteins using specific small molecule inhibitors and combined these inhibitors with standard chemotherapy, inhibitors of cell cycle progression and oncolytic adenovirus in preclinical models of bladder cancer. Several inhibitors for JAK and STAT proteins have been developed and JAK inhibitors were approved by the FDA for treatment of auto-immune disorders and myelofibrosis [22,23]. STAT3 inhibitors have shown anti-tumour activity in pre-clinical stages and have been successfully tested in phase-I clinical trials for safety and efficacy in solid tumours [24,25].

Application of targeted therapies as monotherapy has been shown to be largely influenced by a specific genetic background of patients or acquired resistance mechanisms in the clinical setting. These limitations can be improved by the use of combination therapies. STAT3 is implicated in the development of chemotherapy resistance in various cancers. Targeting STAT3 in combination with chemotherapeutics sensitises cells to chemotherapy in oral squamous cell carcinoma [26]. The interference with STAT3 activity has also been linked to cell cycle arrest either in G0/1 or in G2 phase [27,28]. Thus, we addressed the question if the combination of STAT3/5 inhibitors and inhibitors of cell cycle progression might be beneficial for therapy response. Targeted therapies against CDK4/6 pathway in bladder cancer showed promising data in various preclinical studies [29]. CDK4/6 inhibitors were approved by the FDA for the treatment of Hormone Receptor (HR)-positive and Human Epidermal Growth Factor Receptor 2 (HER2)-negative breast cancer. However, most patients inevitably develop resistance for multifactorial reasons [30,31]. Recently, our group demonstrated that the JAK-STAT pathway plays a role in acquired resistance of CDK4/6 inhibitors in bladder cancer [32]. In this study, we extended these data to show the efficiency of CDK4/6 inhibition by combining it with STAT3/5 inhibitors.

In recent years, there has been a surge in oncolytic virotherapy with several oncolytic viruses showing anti-cancer activity in patients [33]. The use of oncolytic viruses is a very promising new strategy in which native or modified viruses selectively target cancer cells and cause tumour elimination not only by viral spread but also by elicitation of an anti-tumour immune response [34]. As one example, Talimogene laherparepvec (T-Vec), a modified type I Herpes simplex virus for the treatment of advanced melanoma, was approved by the FDA [35]. A multitude of viruses from vesicular stomatitis virus, vaccinia virus or adenovirus are at various stages in clinical trials and most of them have a remarkable safety profile. Most side effects are infection-related or nausea and are easily manageable [36]. At preclinical level, it has been shown that oncolytic adenoviruses are successful in treating MIBC [37]. Several other oncolytic viruses have shown efficacy in urothelial carcinomas and some are currently tested in clinical trials [38]. Combination of oncolytic viruses with immune checkpoint inhibitors and targeted therapies has been proven to be a successful strategy to enhance the efficiency of therapy response to oncolytic virus [39,40]. There are studies showing that targeting the JAK-STAT pathway in combination with the oncolytic herpes simplex virus and vesicular stomatitis viruses could enhance their efficiency possibly by modulating IFN signalling [41,42]. Hence, in this study we investigated also the effects upon combining oncolytic adenovirus with STAT3/5 inhibitors in bladder cancer.

2. Results

2.1. *JAK-STAT Pathway is Dysregulated in Bladder Cancer*

Activation of JAK-STAT signalling, mostly by phosphorylation and protein level of STAT3/5 has been described in bladder cancer by several groups [14,15,20,43,44]. We wanted to specifically focus on involvement of JAK-STAT proteins as prognostic marker and also as potential targets for therapy. Thus, we included the 4 JAK family proteins and 7 STAT family proteins and analysed the data in the TCGA cohort consisting of 412 bladder cancer patients to identify molecular alterations in the JAK-STAT signalling pathway related genes (Table S1) [45]. In 54% of the patients, we found alterations in the selected genes (Figure 1A). The alterations in the JAK-STAT pathway did not have a significant effect on overall survival in patients with bladder cancer (Figure 1B). The TCGA cohort analysis showed that alterations in STAT3 were observed in 7%, STAT5A in 8% and STAT5B in 7% of patients. Alterations in JAK1 were observed in 8% and in JAK2 in 15% of patients indicating, that these genes are frequently altered in bladder cancer (Figure 1C). STAT3 and STAT5 are shown to interact majorly with JAK1 and 2. Statistically significant co-occurrence was found in between JAK2-STAT5A, STAT3-STAT5A and STAT3-STAT5B among others (Table S2). As for mutual exclusivity, none of the genes showed any significance.

Subsequently, considering the TCGA analysis results, we also performed immunohistochemistry to determine STAT3 expression. Here, we wanted to confirm that increased expression level of STAT3 protein might serve as a prognostic marker. We used a previously described tissue microarray including tissue specimen from urothelial carcinoma patients with metastatic disease limited to lymph nodes from 149 patients from January 2003 until December 2012. The clinical characteristics of the patients are described in a prior publication [46]. We analysed STAT3 staining in sections from tumour centre. In total, 14/149 showed no staining, 18/149 showed low intensity staining, 34/149 had moderate staining and 74/149 had high intensity staining (Figure 1D). It was established that 9/149 sections were not evaluable due to a technical reason. When correlating the expression with cancer specific survival, we could not observe any significant difference in survival among no/low staining vs. moderate/high staining (Figure 1E). This also correlates with the survival data from the TCGA cohort. However, the high number of patients positively expressing STAT3 qualifies this protein as a potential molecular target.

Inhibitors against JAK1/2 and STAT3/5 are most advanced in clinical use and molecular alterations in STAT3 and STAT5 genes have previously been shown to be altered in various solid cancers [10,12,47,48]. Based on the TCGA results, we decided to analyse expression and activation level of JAK1/2 and STAT3 in a panel of 10 different bladder cancer derived cell lines. Constitutive expression of JAK1/2 protein was detected in all cell lines (Figure 1G). However, phosphorylation of JAK1/2 could not be detected. In all cell lines, expression of STAT3 protein and also its constitutive phosphorylation was detected although at different level in between cell lines.

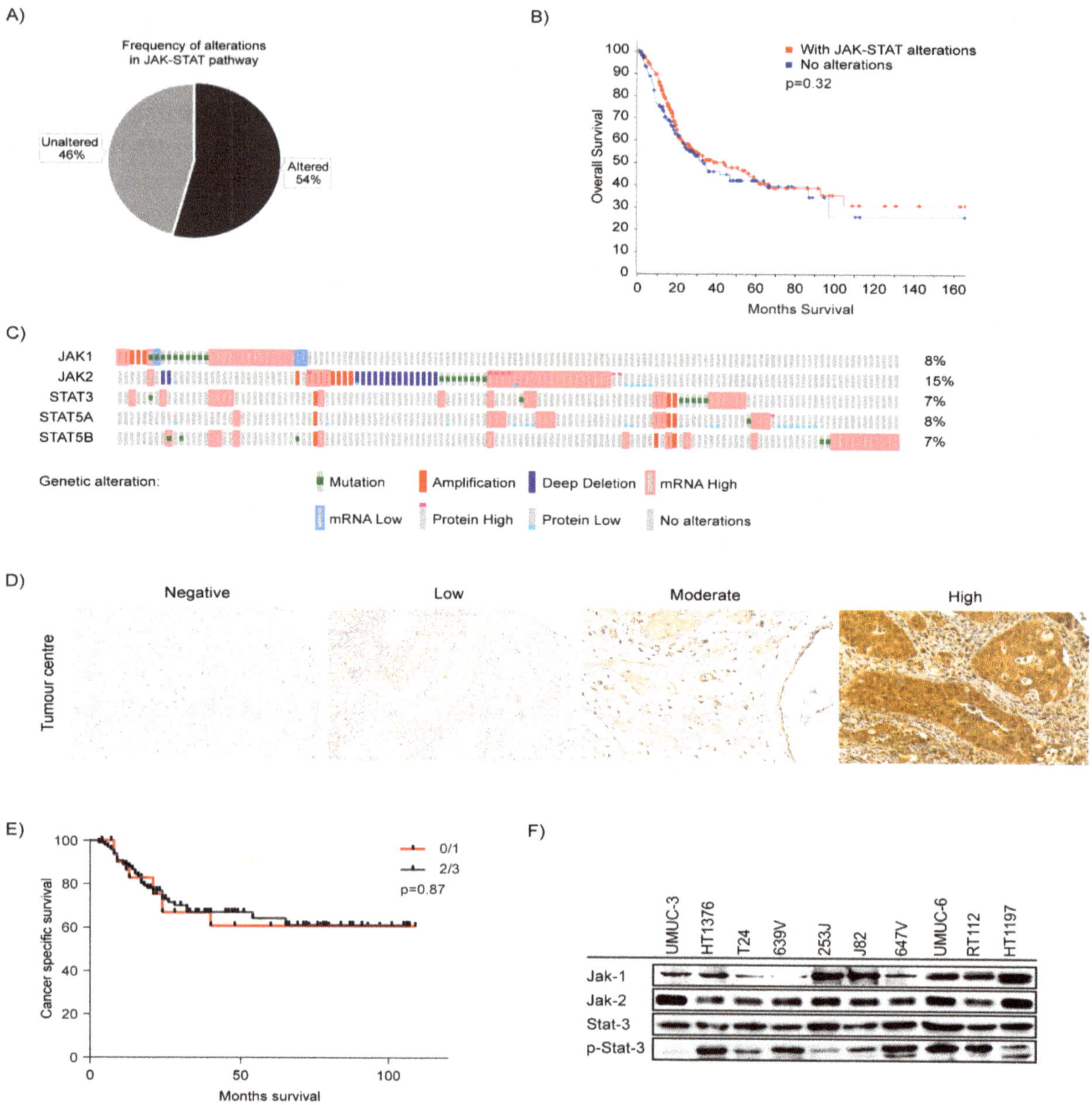

Figure 1. JAK-STAT pathway in bladder cancer: (**A**) TCGA cohort of 412 patients (413 samples) was analysed using cBioPortal. JAK-STAT pathway was altered in 54% of bladder cancer specimens. (**B**) Kalpan-Meier plot depicting overall survival analysis among patients with and without alterations in JAK-STAT pathway in the TCGA cohort. (**C**) Alterations in JAK1, JAK2, STAT3, STAT5A and STAT5B genes—OncoPrint indicates tumours altered with mutations (green bars), amplification (red bars), homozygous deletion (blue bars), high mRNA (red—outlined bars), mRNA low (blue-outlined bars), protein high (bars with red cap), protein low (blue-bottomed bars) and no alterations (grey bars). (**D**) Immunohistochemistry of patient tissues stained for STAT3- images showing staining intensities-Negative (Score-0), Low (Score-1), Moderate (Score-2), High (Score-3). Tissue sections were imaged at 200× magnification. (**E**) Kaplan-Meier plots for cancer specific survival analysis among patients with no or low STAT3 staining vs. moderate/high STAT3 staining. (**F**) Cell lines were analysed for Jak1, Jak2, Stat3 expression and Stat3 phosphorylation by immunoblotting.

2.2. JAK1/2 Inhibitors Have No Effect on Proliferation in Bladder Cancer Cell Lines

We wanted to explore whether upstream inhibition of the JAK-STAT pathway would affect cell viability and used the inhibitors Ruxolitinib targeting JAK1/2 and BSK805 which is a specific JAK2 inhibitor. The effect of these drugs on cell viability was tested in a bladder cancer cell panel of 10 different cell lines. Cells were treated with serial concentrations of Ruxolitinib (0.015–10 μM) and BSK805 (0.0125 to 1 μM). Ruxolitinib did not have any effect on cell viability (Figure 2A and Figure S1). The JAK2 inhibitor, BSK-805 diminished cell growth only on the cell lines T24, J82 and RT112, whereas the other cell lines did not respond (Figure 2B and Figure S2). Overall, the inhibition of JAK1/2 proteins did not substantially interfere with cell growth which might be due to the observation that JAK1/2 protein was also not phosphorylated and thus not activated.

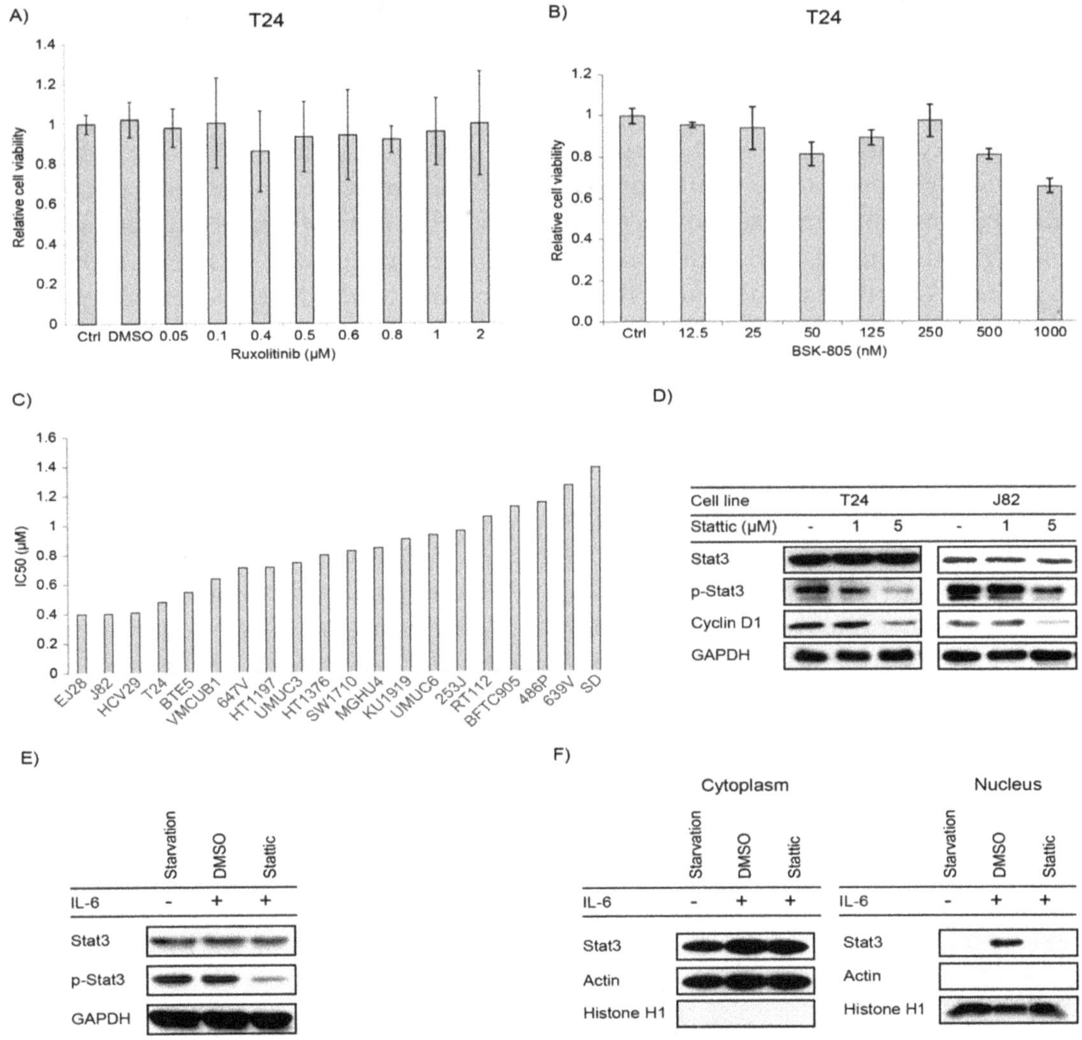

Figure 2. **A**) JAK inhibition by specific inhibitors: T24 cells were treated with increasing concentrations of (**A**) Ruxolitinib and (**B**) BSK-805 and cell viability was assessed by CellTiter-Blue® Cell Viability Assay 72 h after treatment. Error bars S.E. STAT3 inhibition by Stattic: (**C**) Cell viability was assessed by CellTiter-Blue® Cell Viability Assay 72 h after treatment with Stattic and IC50 was determined. Cell lines arranged according to IC50 values. (**D**) T24 and J82 cells were starved for 4 h then activated with 25% FBS and simultaneously treated with serial concentrations of Stattic and DMSO as a control followed by immunoblotting. (**E**) T24 cells were serum starved overnight, treated with 5 μM Stattic (or DMSO) for 3 hours then activated with IL-6 (25 ng/mL) for 30 min before being harvested; protein expression and phosphorylation were analysed by Immunoblotting. (**F**) Cells were treated the same as in (**E**). Compartmental protein extraction was performed, and the lysates were analysed by Immunoblotting.

2.3. STAT3/5 Inhibitors Reduced Proliferation and Downstream Signaling in Bladder Cancer Cell Lines

We also examined effects of STAT3/5 inhibitors on bladder cancer cell growth. Therefore, we applied the specific STAT3/5 inhibitors Stattic and SH-4-54 to 10 different bladder cancer cell lines, and Nifuroxazide in T24 and RT112 cell lines. All inhibitors resulted in dose dependent reduction in cell proliferation in the cell lines tested (Figures S3 and S4). As for Stattic, we extended the number of cell lines to 20 and all cell lines showed a dose-dependent response to Stattic treatment (Figure 2C and Figure S5).

We investigated also the molecular response to Stattic treatment by examining protein levels of total and phosphorylated STAT3. Therefore, we first examined the effect of STAT3 on the constitutive phosphorylation level on T24 and J82 cells which could be suppressed upon treatment in a dose dependent manner (Figure 2D). This effect of Stattic was also confirmed by analysis of the STAT3 downstream effector molecule Cyclin D1, which was downregulated upon treatment.

We also confirmed activity of Stattic on phosphorylation level of STAT3 and its subcellular localization upon an extracellular stimulus, using IL-6. Cells were serum starved, followed by interleukin-6 (IL-6) stimulation. IL-6 stimulation did not result in a further increase in the constitutive STAT3 phosphorylation, but STAT3 phosphorylation could still be suppressed by Stattic (Figure 2E). We then tested the nuclear translocation of STAT3 upon Stattic treatment to evaluate the molecular mechanism of Stattic inhibition. Nuclear and cytoplasmic protein fractions were isolated and the level of total STAT3 and activated STAT3 were analysed. As for control of the purity of the protein compartments, presence of Histone H1 and actin was examined. Interestingly, only after IL-6 treatment we detected a nuclear translocation of STAT3 that was suppressed by Stattic (Figure 2F).

2.4. Stattic Induced G2/M Arrest and Apoptosis in Bladder Cancer Cell Lines

STAT3 and 5 have diverse roles in cells including cell cycle regulation and apoptosis [49]. To investigate whether Stattic influences cell cycle in bladder cancer cells, we treated T24 with Stattic in increasing doses and performed cell cycle analysis measuring BrdU incorporation by flow cytometry, 24 h after treatment. We observed that Stattic induced a G2/M cell cycle arrest in cells (Figure 3A). We also investigated whether Stattic induces apoptosis in a concentration kinetic using T24 cells. Thus, 24 h after treatment, a dose dependent 9-fold increase in Caspase3/7 activity was determined (Figure 3B). From the above results, it is implied that Stattic is acting as a cytostatic and a cytotoxic agent in bladder cancer.

2.5. Stattic Reduced Tumour Growth in 3-Dimensional Xenografts

To further test the effect of Stattic on tumour xenografts, we used the chicken chorioallantoic membrane (CAM) model. As for the purpose of this study, this model reflects characteristics of an immunocompromised mouse model, including the development of a host derived vasculature and extracellular matrix [50]. Hence, we tested the effect of Stattic in vivo by using the CAM model to grow three-dimensional in vivo xenografts of RT112 cells. T24 cells could not be used in the CAM assay as they do not grow well and form very small tumours on the CAM. A significant weight reduction in tumour xenografts, reflecting tumour growth reduction of up to 50% was observed upon treatment with Stattic (Figure 3C). We also performed Ki-67 staining on the CAM tumour tissue sections to estimate the Stattic effect on tumour proliferation in the xenografts. A significant decrease in Ki-67 positive cells was observed in the Stattic treated tumours as compared to untreated tumours (Figure 3D). This correlates with the observed decrease in tumour cell proliferation in vitro.

2.6. Combination of Stattic and Chemotherapeutic Agents Showed Additivity

STAT3 has been shown to be activated in response to chemotherapeutic agents and mediating drug-resistance in several cancers. Hence, we wanted to explore potential options for combination therapy with Stattic and standard chemotherapeutic drugs. We chose 5 bladder cancer cell lines

(HT1376, J82, RT112, SD and T24) with different sensitivities to Stattic monotherapy: J82 as one of the best responder cell lines to Stattic, T24, HT1376 and RT112 as intermediate responder cell lines and SD as lowest responding cell line.

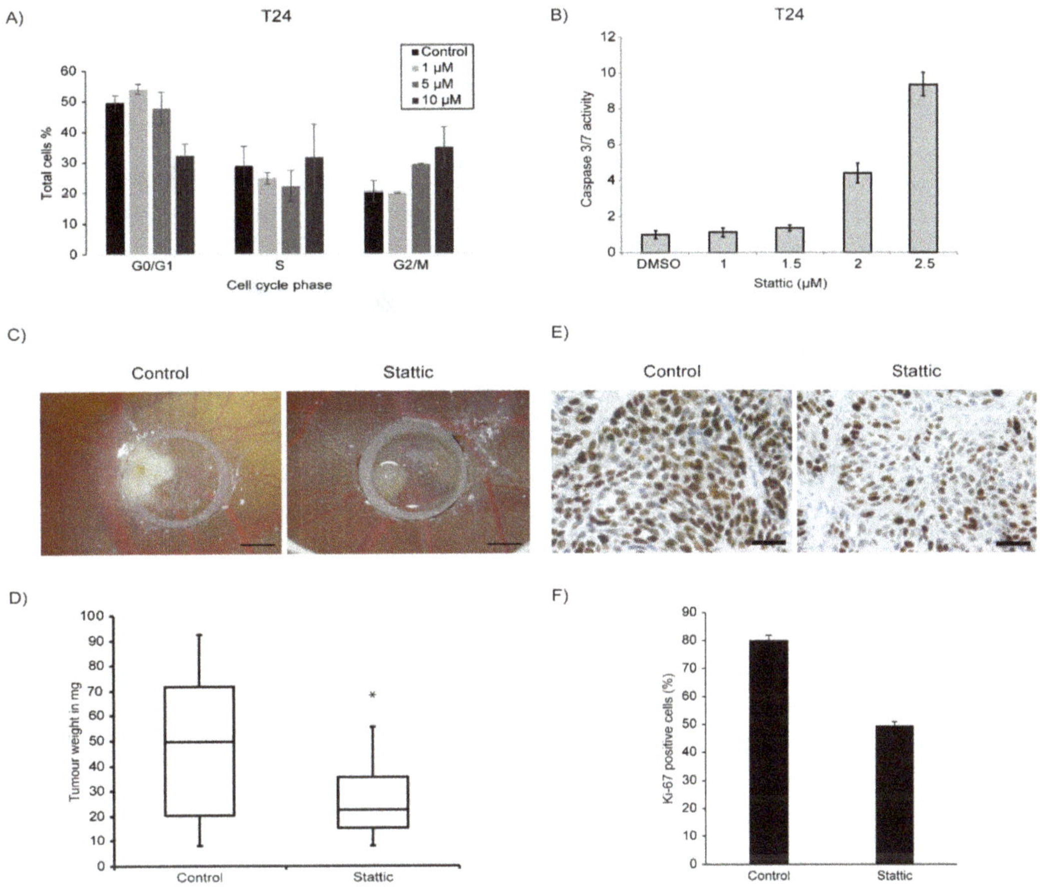

Figure 3. (**A**) Analysis of cell cycle progression in T24 treated with the indicated concentrations of Stattic for 24 h. An increase in G2 population was found with increasing concentration. (**B**) Caspase 3/7 assay for the apoptosis in T24 cells incubated for 24 h with the indicated concentrations of Stattic. The percentage of apoptotic cells was increased in a dose-dependent manner. (**C**) Stattic reduces the bladder cancer cell growth in vivo. Representative images of RT112 cells show tumour formation of Stattic versus control group on the CAM inside a silicone ring, 6 days after seeding of cells. Scale bar equals 2 mm. (**D**) Tumours from indicated cell line were harvested and weighed after Stattic ($n = 21$) or control (DMSO) ($n = 19$) treatment ('*' indicates $p = 0.0069$). (**E**) Tissue sections from the tumours were stained for Ki-67. (**F**) Number of Ki-67 positive cells were counted and compared between Control (DMSO) and Stattic-treated groups. Scale bar equals 4 µm. Error bars S.E.

The cell viability of bladder cancer cell lines in response to the increasing doses of single drugs and combination treatment of Stattic and Cisplatin, Docetaxel, Gemcitabine or Paclitaxel was investigated using the CellTiter-Blue® Cell Viability Assay. Dose response curves for the mono- and combination therapy were generated (Figure S6). Data were analysed using the Chou-Talalay theorem to generate a combination index (CI). According to the theorem, CI values less than 1 indicate a synergistic interaction, while values equal to or greater than 1 indicate additive or antagonistic effects respectively [51]. The combination index was calculated for the combination causing 50% inhibition of cell viability (Fa50). In HT1376 cells, the combination index for all the combinations of Stattic and chemotherapeutic agents were in the range of 1 indicating additivity. In SD cells, the combination index for most of the combinations of Stattic and chemotherapeutic agents were more than 1 indicating antagonism. In T24, J82 and RT112 cells, the combination index varies from additivity to antagonism depending on the combinations (Figure 4).

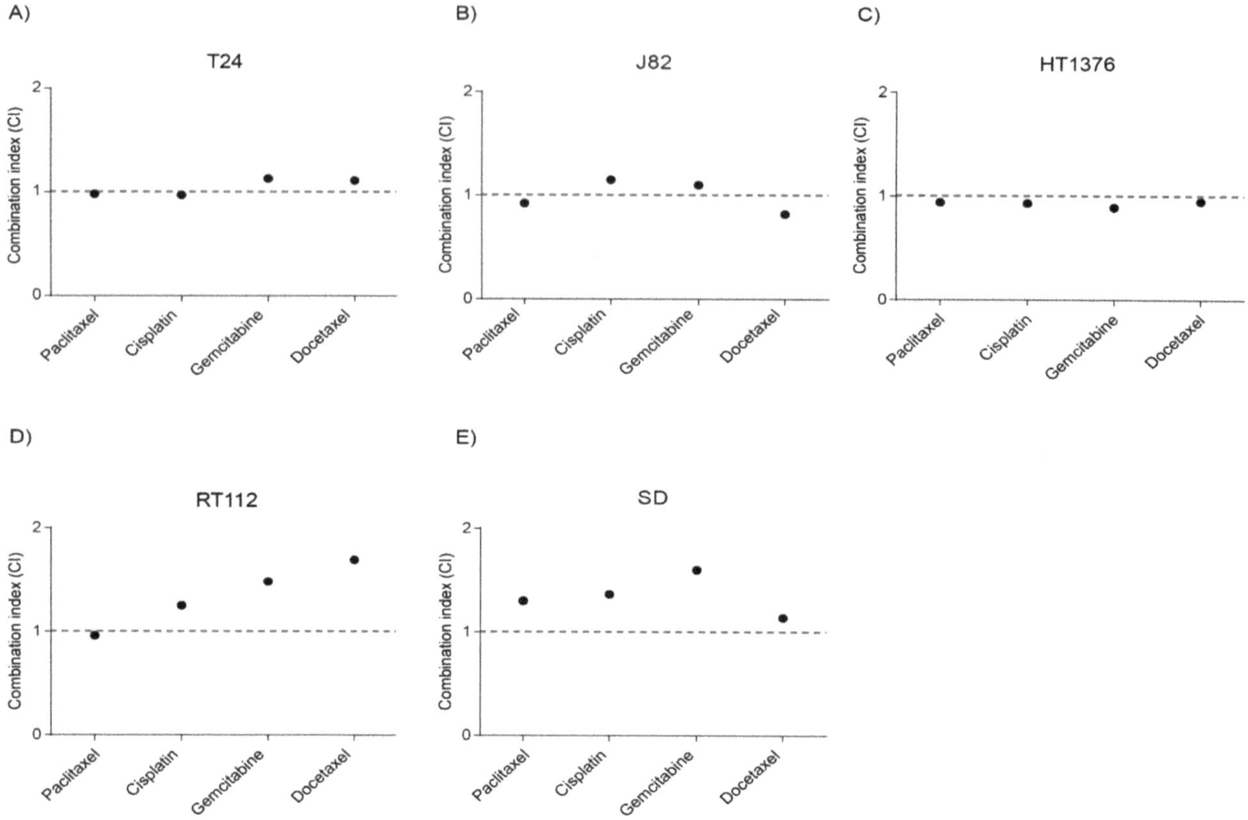

Figure 4. Combination therapy with Stattic and chemotherapeutics. Treatment of the respective cell lines was done for 72 h with Stattic alone and in a fixed ratio combination with Paclitaxel, Cisplatin, Gemcitabine or Docetaxel in (**A**) T24, (**B**) J82, (**C**) HT1376, (**D**) RT112, and (**E**) SD cell lines (See Materials and methods). Combination index (CI) for combining Stattic with Paclitaxel, Cisplatin, Gemcitabine or Docetaxel were plotted. Values were calculated using the Chou-Talalay theorem. CI < 1: synergy, CI = 1; additivity, CI > 1: antagonism.

2.7. Combination of Stattic and CDK4/6 inhibitor Palbociclib Showed Additivity

Our group has previously shown that STAT3 is one of the proteins contributing to therapy resistance to the CDK4/6 inhibitor Palbociclib. Palbociclib induces a G1 arrest in cells. The rational to combine both inhibitors was to induce both G1 and G2 arrest and using Stattic in a supportive role for enhancing Palbociclib activity. We tested this combination before in RT112 and T24 bladder cancer cell lines with slightly controversial results and included here additionally UMUC-3 cells [32]. UMUC-3 cells were treated with increasing doses of Stattic and a fixed concentration of Palbociclib and cell viability was assessed by sulphorhodamine-B assay and the CI was calculated. The combination index was around 1 indicating additive effect of the combination therapy (Figure 5A). In conclusion, the combination of both compounds results in additive activity but requires obviously also specific genetic predisposition as for substantial response limiting it to a subset of patients.

2.8. Stattic Enhanced Oncolytic Virotherapy of the Oncolytic Adenovirus XVir-N-31

Oncolytic virotherapy only recently entered clinical application and received FDA approval with a very favourable response rate and low adverse events [37]. It has been shown that the JAK-STAT pathway is activated upon adenoviral infection. As for viruses, such as vesicular stomatitis virus (VSV), inhibition of JAK by Ruxolitinib has been shown to support viral replication [41]. We combined Stattic with oncolytic adenovirus XVir-N-31 to suppress activation of STAT3/5 and analysed the effect on cell viability [37]. Cells were infected with XVir-N-31 24 h after treatment with Stattic. The combination treatment resulted in enhanced virus-induced cell death in both T24 and UMUC-3 cell lines (Figure 5B). We also observed increased viral replication in combination with Stattic which corresponded with an increase in viral particle formation (Figure 5C,D). Thus, inhibition of STAT3/5 substantially supports replication and viral particle production in cancer cells.

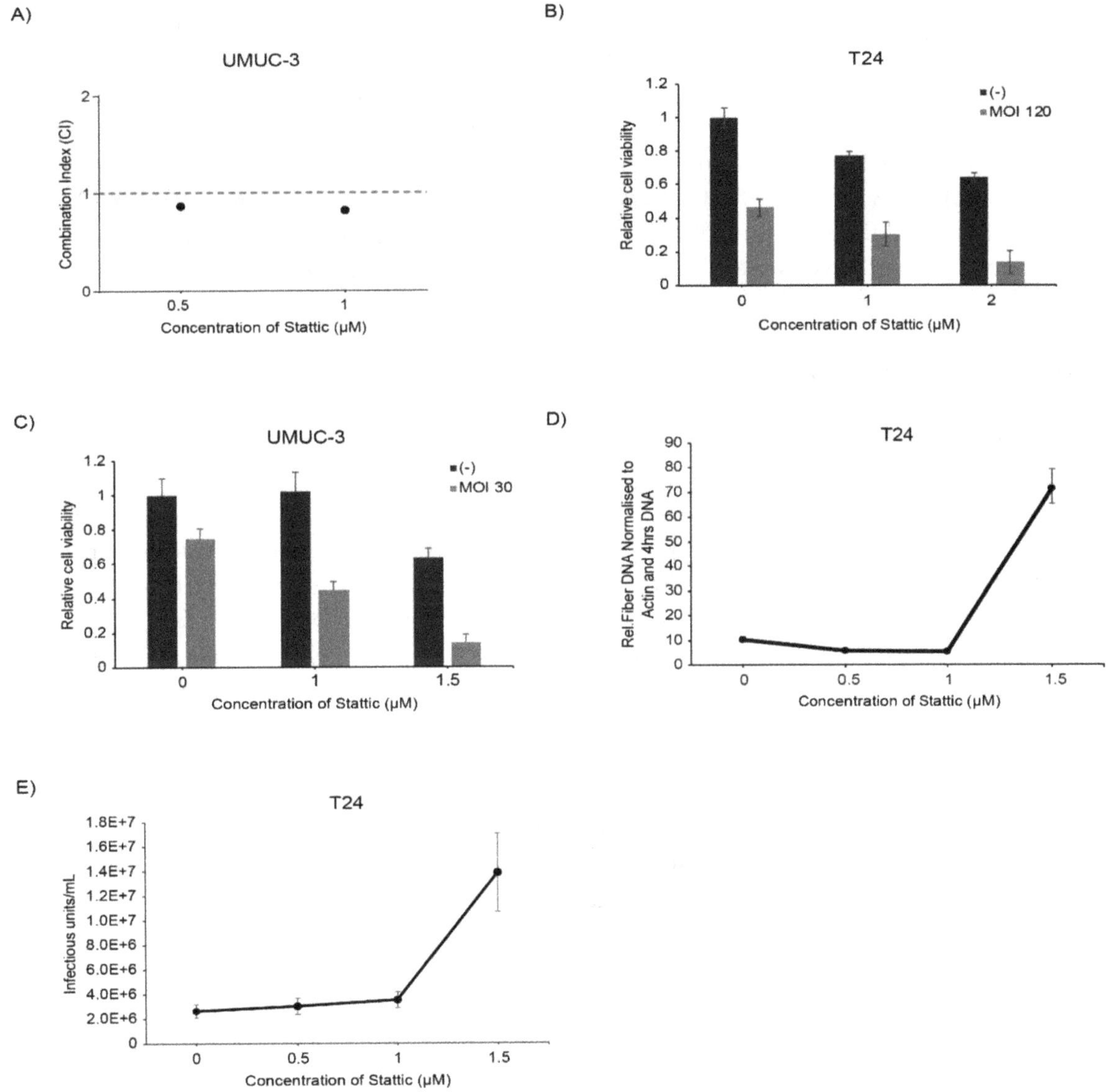

Figure 5. Combination therapy with Stattic and Palbociclib, and oncolytic virotherapy. (**A**) Treatment of the UMUC-3 cells was done for 72 h with Stattic alone at 0.5 μM and 1 μM and in a fixed concentration combination with 0.5 μM Palbociclib. Combination index (CI) for combining Stattic with Palbociclib were plotted. Values were calculated using the Chou-Talalay theorem. (**C**). Cells were treated with Stattic and infected with XVir-N-31 with corresponding multiplicity of infections (MOI) in T24 (**B**) and in UMUC-3 cells (**C**). The MOIs are indicated in the graphs. Cell viability was analysed at 4dpi by sulphorhodamine B assay. Error bars S.E. (**D**,**E**) T24 cells were infected with XVir-N-31 (MOI 50) and treated with increasing concentrations of Stattic (**D**) Viral replication was analysed at 48 h by qPCR of fibre DNA, and (**E**) the increase in viral titre upon Stattic inhibition is measured by hexon titre test and represented as infectious units/mL (IFU/mL).

3. Discussion

In this study, we analysed the potential use of targeting the JAK-STAT pathway for therapy in bladder cancer. It has been observed that expression level of STAT3 correlates with invasion and poor prognosis in bladder cancer [17–19,44]. However, other groups could not confirm the prognostic value of STAT3 expression level [14]. We analysed molecular alterations in JAK/STAT proteins in the TCGA dataset including 412 patient specimens of muscle invasive bladder cancer. This analysis revealed that genetic alterations in the molecular members of the JAK-STAT pathway are frequently found in bladder cancer but they are not suitable markers for prognosis. Analysis of STAT3 protein expression level on a TMA confirmed that most primary tumours of muscle invasive disease express high level of STAT3 but in this cohort STAT3 failed to be a prognostic marker for survival. In conclusion, the data presented here question the prognostic value of STAT3 in bladder cancer.

Previously, the JAK2 tyrosine kinase inhibitor AG490 has been tested in bladder cancer with positive results [52]. We wanted to further analyse if these data could be confirmed using the JAK1/2 inhibitor Ruxolitinib and the specific JAK2 inhibitor BSK-805. Surprisingly, our data are in contradiction to the described observations as we do not observe anti-tumour effects of JAK1/2 inhibition on cell proliferation. An explanation for the observed difference is the specificity of the inhibitors used. AG490 is a tyrosine kinase inhibitor that targets molecules such as EGFR, HER2 or STAT5a/b besides JAK2 whereas Ruxolitinib and BSK-805 are highly selective for JAK proteins [53,54]. Thus, the effects observed upon AG490 treatment could possibly be attributed to the broader spectrum of target molecules of this compound. This observation is very important, since a lower substrate specificity often results in a different response to a drug and is therefore not representative for interfering with a specific molecule which also complicates the identification of predictive biomarker [55]. Also, all bladder cancer cell lines tested by immunoblotting did not show any constitutive phosphorylation of JAK1/2 which might explain the lack of response. In conclusion, our data imply that JAK proteins are not suitable targets for monotherapy in bladder cancer therapy.

Furthermore, we analysed the role of STAT3/5 in bladder cancer cell lines using 3 different STAT3/5 inhibitors Stattic, SH-4-54 and Nifuroxazide. Stattic is a specific STAT3 inhibitor with a lower affinity towards STAT5 [56] and SH-4-54 is a dual inhibitor of STAT3/5 [57]. Nifuroxazide, besides being an inhibitor for STAT3 also inhibits JAK2 and TYK2 [58]. We observed that with these inhibitors proliferation in bladder cancer was greatly reduced which is in line with previous studies on STAT3 inhibition [13,59,60]. Some of the downstream target molecules of STAT3 include anti-apoptotic proteins Bcl-xL. Previously, studies have demonstrated that disrupting STAT3 signalling led to a decrease in anti-apoptotic proteins. Consistent with these findings, we observed a dose-dependent increase in the percentage of apoptotic cells and also a significant increase in cells in G2 phase, which is consistent with prior reports [27].

Combination therapies are a useful approach to overcome limitations of monotherapy options or to enhance the efficiencies. Over the years, there is growing evidence of a connection between STAT3 and chemotherapy resistance [26]. Several studies have shown STAT3 involvement in the development of resistance for chemotherapy in various cancers. It has been demonstrated that STAT3 inhibition sensitized for example squamous cell carcinoma to chemotherapy [61]. In our study, we show that STAT3 inhibition has an additive effect when combined with the most frequently used chemotherapeutic drugs approved for bladder cancer suggesting that this combination might be applicable in patients with STAT3 mediated chemo resistance.

Previously, our group applied a genome wide CRISPR-dCas9 screen to identify acquired resistance mechanisms to the CDK4/6 inhibitor Palbocicib in bladder cancer cell lines [32]. One of the results was an implication of the JAK-STAT signalling pathway in conferring resistance to CDK4/6 inhibitors. The combination therapy with Stattic and Palbociclib showed additive effects in T24 and UMUC-3 but antagonism in RT112 cell lines. Thus, the combination of STAT inhibitors with CDK4/6 inhibitors might not be a general treatment option but should be beneficial for a subset of patients that need to be defined by a detailed analysis of the underlying molecular mechanisms that regulate therapy response in this combination. In conclusion, we show that targeting of STAT3 along with chemotherapy or CDK4/6 inhibitors provide potential combination therapy options in order to improve therapy efficacy in bladder cancer.

In recent years, the development of oncolytic viruses entering clinical trials has dramatically gained momentum [33]. One of the obstacles for inducing an effective therapy response is successful replication of the virus in tumour cells [62]. Thus, a further aim of this study was to combine oncolytic virotherapy with JAK/STAT inhibitors and analyse the effects on virus induced cell death and viral replication. It has been shown that Ruxolitinib enhances replication of VSV but since we could not detect phosphorylation of JAK proteins nor effects on cell viability, we focused on STAT3 inhibitors. Numerous cytokines are released upon virus infection including IFNs and IL-6, which then stimulate the expression of genes that are involved in anti-viral response via direct or indirect mechanisms. It is shown that interferon signalling inhibits adenoviral DNA replication by inhibiting viral early gene expression in normal cells, but not in cancer cells [63,64]. In a STAT2 knockout Syrian hamster model, human adenovirus 5 replicated a 100–1000-fold higher than in the wildtype. The infected cells in the knockout hamsters show interrupted Type I interferon pathway which is implied to be the reason for enhanced replication of virus [65]. Pre-treatment with Ruxolitinib enhanced the viral replication of oncolytic Herpes Simplex Virus (oHSV) in malignant peripheral nerve sheath tumours. Pre-treatment of mice with Ruxolitinib reduced Interferon stimulated genes expression making the tumours susceptible to oHSV infection [42]. Combination of Ruxolitinib and oncolytic vesicular stomatitis virus therapy resulted in enhanced oncolysis and viral replication in non-small cell lung cancer [41].

In this study, combination of STAT3/5 inhibitors with an oncolytic adenovirus resulted in enhancement in virus induced cell death, viral replication and viral particle formation. STAT3/5 inhibition leads to reduction in expression of downstream molecules which also include interleukins and interferons. STAT3/5 inhibition also results in G2 arrest as described. There is evidence for enhanced adenoviral replication upon G2/M arrest [66], which might also be the reason for observed enhancement in viral replication and particle formation upon STAT3/5 inhibition. Further research is required to elucidate the exact mechanisms by which the adenovirus interacts with JAK-STAT pathway and cell cycle. It would also be beneficial to study the viral gene expression analysis to explore the interactions between the viral and cellular genes at various phases of infection.

In conclusion, our study shows that STAT3/5 inhibition reduces cell proliferation both in vitro and in vivo but specific JAK inhibition has no effect on bladder cancer cell lines. We show potential combination therapy options with Stattic and chemotherapeutics, and Stattic and CDK4/6 inhibitor Palbociclib. We also demonstrate enhancement in oncolytic effect of adenoviruses upon combination with STAT3/5 inhibitors. These results indicate that STAT3/5 inhibition, but not JAK1/2 inhibition could be a potentially effective therapeutic strategy in bladder cancer.

4. Materials and Methods

4.1. Patient Material, Tissue Microarray and Immunohistochemistry

Patient characteristics and the details of tissue microarray and immunohistochemistry have been published before [46].

4.2. Cell Lines and Adenovirus

UMUC-3, SW17110, MGHU4, UMUC-6, 639V, SD, J82, VMCUB-1, 647V and BFTC-805 were obtained from Düsseldorf. HCV-29 and KU19-19 were obtained from Leeds, UK. HT1197 was obtained from SIGMA/ECACC, England. BTE-5 were obtained from Uniklinik, Essen. HT-1376, 253J, RT112 and 486P were a kind gift from Homburg. T24, EJ28 and Hek293 cells were from ATCC, VA, USA. Cells were cultured in either RPMI supplemented with 10% foetal bovine serum (FBS), 1% NEAA (Biochrom, Berlin, Germany), penicillin and streptomycin or Dulbecco's modified Eagle's medium supplemented with

10% foetal bovine serum and penicillin-streptomycin, at 5% or 10% CO2, respectively. The oncolytic adenovirus XVir-N-31 was kindly provided by Prof. Holm [37].

4.3. *Small Molecule Inhibitors and Chemotherapeutics*

Stock solutions of Ruxolitinib, BSK-805, Stattic, SH-4- 54 and Nifuroxazide (Selleckchem, Munich, Germany) were prepared in dimethyl sulfoxide (DMSO). Palbociclib (Selleckchem, Munich, Germany) stock solution was prepared in water. Chemotherapeutic drugs Paclitaxel, Docetaxel and Gemcitabine (Sigma Aldrich Chemie GmbH, Munich, Germany) stock solutions were prepared in DMSO. Working concentrations were freshly prepared in medium for immediate use. Cisplatin (Sigma Aldrich Chemie GmbH, Munich, Germany) was prepared fresh in H_2O.

4.4. *Cell Viability, Cell Cycle Analysis and Apoptosis Assays*

Cell viability upon small molecule inhibitors monotherapy, and combination treatment of Stattic and chemotherapy were performed after exposure to inhibitors for indicated time periods by Cell-Titer Blue® assay (Promega, Madison, WI, USA) according to manufacturer's protocol and absolute IC50 was calculated. For combination treatments of Stattic and Palbociclib and with adenovirus XVir-N-31, a Sulphorhodamine B (SRB) assay was performed. In brief, cells were fixed with 10% trichloroacetic acid, stained with 0.05% SRB and rinsed with 1% acetic acid and allowed to dry. Dried SRB was dissolved in 10 mM tris base and absorbance was measured at 590 nm. These assays were conducted in 12-well plates, seeding 1×10^4 cells/well. For Stattic and Palbociclib treatment, cells were incubated for 3 days post treatment.

The effect of virus induced cell killing in combination with small molecule inhibitors was analysed in 12-well plates. In total, $0.25–0.5 \times 10^5$ cells were seeded and infected with increasing concentrations (multiplicity of infection, MOI) of the adenovirus XVir-N-31 one day after treatment with Stattic in 200µl medium without FBS. At 1hpi, complete medium with or without Stattic was added to the cells. Cells were fixed 4 days post infection and cell viability was analysed by SRB assay.

Apoptosis (Caspase-Glo® 3/7 Assay-Promega) and cell cycle analysis (7-AAD, Thermo Fisher Scientific) were performed according to the manufacturer's protocol.

4.5. *Combination Index Analysis and Bladder Cancer Molecular Alteration Analysis*

For combination therapy with Stattic and chemotherapeutics, fixed ratio combinations were used. The fixed ratio combinations are as follows: For T24 cells: S:P (Stattic: Paclitaxel) at 122.2:1, S:C (Stattic and Cisplatin) at 1:2.1, S:G (Stattic and Gemcitabine) at 1:2.1 and S:D (Stattic: Docetaxel) at 1447.4:1; for J82 cells: S:P (Stattic: Paclitaxel) at 33.3:1, S:C (Stattic and Cisplatin) at 1:1, S:G (Stattic and Gemcitabin) at 25:1 and S:D (Stattic: Docetaxel) at 250:1; for HT1376 cells: S:P(Stattic:Paclitaxel) at 176:1, S:C (Stattic and Cisplatin) at 1:5.68, S:G (Stattic and Gemcitabine) at 149.15:1 and S:D (Stattic: Docetaxel) at 352:1; for RT112 cells: S:P(Stattic:Paclitaxel) at 500:1, S:C (Stattic and Cisplatin) at 1:1, S:G (Stattic and Gemcitabine) at 50:1 and S:D (Stattic: Docetaxel) at 2000:1; for SD cells: S:P(Stattic:Paclitaxel) at 444.4:1, S:C (Stattic and Cisplatin) at 1:1, S:G (Stattic and Gemcitabine) at 160:1 and S:D (Stattic: Docetaxel) at 4000:1. The combination index (CI) was assessed with the Chou–Talalay combination index (CI) theorem [51]. CI value of 1 was defined as additivity, CI < 1 as synergistic and CI >1 as antagonistic effects. The analysis was performed with CompuSyn software (Combosyn, NJ, USA). The Cancer Genome Atlas (TCGA) analysis was performed on cBioPortal (https://www.cbioportal.org/).

4.6. *Immunoblot Analysis*

Cells were seeded in 10 cm tissue culture plates and allowed to grow till 50–60% confluency. The medium was then changed with FBS-free medium overnight. Stattic was applied in indicated concentrations for 3 h and cells were stimulated by supplementing with IL-6 (25ng/mL) for 30 min. Then protein extraction (either total or compartmental) was performed. Cells were lysed on ice in protein lysis buffer comprising of 1% sodium dodecyl sulphate, 1 mM sodium orthovanadate and 10 mM tris, pH 7.4. Lysates were sheared using a 27-gauge needle (BD Biosciences®) until no viscosity was observed. The sheared lysates were then centrifuged at 30,000 RCF at 4 °C for total lysates. For compartmentalisation, cells were harvested by trypsin, pelleted then washed twice in phosphate-buffered saline, pelleted again by spinning at 600 RCF in microcentrifuge at 4 °C for 4 min. The pellet was resuspended in lysis buffer. After 5 min on ice, the lysates were spun at 600 RCF in microcentrifuge at 4 °C for 4 min. The supernatants were used as cytoplasmic extracts. The pelleted nuclei were briefly washed in lysis buffer without NP-40. The nuclear pellet was then resuspended in 50–100 μL nuclear extract buffer (20 mM Tris-HCl (pH 8.0), 420 mM NaCl, 1.5 mM $MgCl_2$, 0.2 mM EDTA, 25% glycerol) After a 10-min incubation at 4 °C, the nuclei were briefly vortexed and spun at 18300 RCF in microcentrifuge at 4 °C for 15 min. The supernatant was then removed and used as a nuclear extract. The primary antibodies used included: Stat3 (#9139), p-Stat3 (#9145), Jak1 (#3344), p-Jak1 (#3331), Jak2 (#3230), p-Jak2 (#3771), cyclin-D1(#2922) and GAPDH (#2118) from Cell Signaling Technology, Danvers, MA, USA. Actin (#A2066) from Sigma, Saint Louis, Missouri, USA and histone H1 (#05-457) from Millipore corporation, Temecula, CA, USA.

4.7. *CAM Assay and Immunohistochemistry (IHC)*

The CAM assay was performed as described previously [50]. In brief, 2 million cells were seeded on embryonic day 8 on the CAM. Topical treatment using 2 μM Stattic was performed daily from day 10 after the formation of visible xenografts. The control tumours were treated with PBS. On day 15, the tumours were harvested: embryos were transferred to a Styrofoam box containing dry ice and suffocated. Tumours were then removed from the CAM, immersed in a petri dish filled with ice-cold PBS and trimmed under a stereo microscope (Leica) with micro scissors to remove as much of the attached CAM as possible. The tumours were immersed in pre-weighed 1.5 mL reaction tubes containing PBS and weighed on a fine balance. IHC was done with Ki-67 (No. M7240, Dako Deutschland, Hamburg, Germany) using heat induced epitope retrieval with 0.01 M citrate buffer at pH 6.0.

4.8. *Viral Replication and Particle Formation*

Thus, 5×10^4 cells were seeded in 6-well plates and treated with specified concentrations of Stattic. Viral infection was performed a day after the inhibitor treatment in the same manner as described for cell viability assay. DNA lysates were made 4–48 h after infection for viral replication analysis and lysates and supernatant were collected at 72 h for viral particle formation analysis. Viral replication was analysed by real time PCR for fibre DNA using the ΔΔCT-method. Actin was used as the housekeeping gene. Viral titres in the lysates were measured in Hek293 cells seeded in 24-well plates by hexon staining. The protocols for viral replication analysis and hexon titre test were performed as described [37].

4.9. *Statistical Analysis*

All the cell error bars in cell viability assays, apoptosis assays are presented as mean ± standard error. Statistical analysis for patient's survival analysis and CAM assay was performed using SPSS software. $p < 0.05$ was considered as significant.

Author Contributions: Conceptualization: S.C.S. and R.N., Methodology: S.H., J.A.K., S.C.S., validation: J.S.-H., P.S.H., T.H. and R.N., formal analysis: S.C.S., A.Y., E.-M.B., D.W. and S.V.H., investigation: S.C.S., A.Y., E.-M.B., D.W. and S.V.H., resources: J.E.G., data curation: R.N., writing-original draft preparation: S.V.H. and R.N., writing review and editing: R.N., P.S.H., T.H. and J.E.G., supervision: R.N., funding acquisition: S.C.S, R.N. All authors have read and agreed to the published version of the manuscript.

Acknowledgments: Not applicable.

Abbreviations

CAM	Chorioallantoic Membrane
FGFR	Fibroblast Growth Factor Receptor
JAK	Janus Kinase
STAT	Signal Transducer and Activator of Transcription
TCGA	The Cancer Genome Atlas

References

1. Bray, F.; Ferlay, J.; Soerjomataram, I.; Siegel, R.L.; Torre, L.A.; Jemal, A. Global cancer statistics 2018: GLOBOCAN estimates of incidence and mortality worldwide for 36 cancers in 185 countries. *CA Cancer J. Clin.* **2018**, *68*, 394–424. [CrossRef] [PubMed]
2. Apolo, A.B. Determining superior first-line therapy in metastatic bladder cancer. *Nat. Rev. Urol.* **2019**, *16*, 698–699. [CrossRef] [PubMed]
3. Boegemann, M.; Aydin, A.M.; Bagrodia, A.; Krabbe, L.M. Prospects and progress of immunotherapy for bladder cancer. *Expert Opin. Biol. Ther.* **2017**, *17*, 1417–1431. [CrossRef] [PubMed]
4. Koshkin, V.S.; Grivas, P. Emerging Role of Immunotherapy in Advanced Urothelial Carcinoma. *Curr. Oncol. Rep.* **2018**, *20*, 48. [CrossRef]
5. Duplisea, J.J.; Dinney, C.P.N. Should chemotherapy still be used to treat all muscle invasive bladder cancer in the "era of immunotherapy"? *Expert Rev. Anticancer Ther.* **2019**, *19*, 543–545. [CrossRef]
6. Grivas, P.; Yu, E.Y. Role of Targeted Therapies in Management of Metastatic Urothelial Cancer in the Era of Immunotherapy. *Curr. Treat Options Oncol.* **2019**, *20*, 67. [CrossRef]
7. Loriot, Y.; Necchi, A.; Park, S.H.; Garcia-Donas, J.; Huddart, R.; Burgess, E.; Fleming, M.; Rezazadeh, A.; Mellado, B.; Varlamov, S.; et al. Erdafitinib in Locally Advanced or Metastatic Urothelial Carcinoma. *N. Engl. J. Med.* **2019**, *381*, 338–348. [CrossRef]
8. Da Costa, J.B.; Gibb, E.A.; Nykopp, T.K.; Mannas, M.; Wyatt, A.W.; Black, P.C. Molecular tumor heterogeneity in muscle invasive bladder cancer: Biomarkers, subtypes, and implications for therapy. *Urol. Oncol.* **2018**, 1–8. [CrossRef]
9. Hammaren, H.M.; Virtanen, A.T.; Raivola, J.; Silvennoinen, O. The regulation of JAKs in cytokine signaling and its breakdown in disease. *Cytokine* **2019**, *118*, 48–63. [CrossRef]
10. Guo, C.; Yang, G.; Khun, K.; Kong, X.; Levy, D.; Lee, P.; Melamed, J. Activation of Stat3 in renal tumors. *Am. J. Transl. Res.* **2009**, *1*, 283.
11. Tong, M.; Wang, J.; Jiang, N.; Pan, H.; Li, D. Correlation between p-STAT3 overexpression and prognosis in lung cancer: A systematic review and meta-analysis. *PLoS ONE* **2017**, *12*, e0182282. [CrossRef] [PubMed]
12. Takemoto, S.; Ushijima, K.; Kawano, K.; Yamaguchi, T.; Terada, A.; Fujiyoshi, N.; Nishio, S.; Tsuda, N.; Ijichi, M.; Kakuma, T.; et al. Expression of activated signal transducer and activator of transcription-3 predicts poor prognosis in cervical squamous-cell carcinoma. *Br. J. Cancer* **2009**, *101*, 967–972. [CrossRef] [PubMed]
13. Chen, C.L.; Cen, L.; Kohout, J.; Hutzen, B.; Chan, C.; Hsieh, F.C.; Loy, A.; Huang, V.; Cheng, G.; Lin, J. Signal transducer and activator of transcription 3 activation is associated with bladder cancer cell growth and survival. *Mol. Cancer* **2008**, *7*, 78. [CrossRef] [PubMed]
14. Degoricija, M.; Situm, M.; Korac, J.; Miljkovic, A.; Matic, K.; Paradzik, M.; Marinovic Terzic, I.; Jeroncic, A.; Tomic, S.; Terzic, J. High NF-kappaB and STAT3 activity in human urothelial carcinoma: a pilot study. *World J. Urol.* **2014**, *32*, 1469–1475. [CrossRef] [PubMed]
15. Shen, H.B.; Gu, Z.Q.; Jian, K.; Qi, J. CXCR4-mediated Stat3 activation is essential for CXCL12-induced cell invasion in bladder cancer. *Tumor Biol.* **2013**, *34*, 1839–1845. [CrossRef] [PubMed]

16. Yang, X.; Ou, L.; Tang, M.; Wang, Y.; Wang, X.; Chen, E.; Diao, J.; Wu, X.; Luo, C. Knockdown of PLCepsilon inhibits inflammatory cytokine release via STAT3 phosphorylation in human bladder cancer cells. *Tumor Biol.* **2015**, *36*, 9723–9732. [CrossRef]
17. Gatta, L.B.; Melocchi, L.; Bugatti, M.; Missale, F.; Lonardi, S.; Zanetti, B.; Cristinelli, L.; Belotti, S.; Simeone, C.; Ronca, R.; et al. Hyper-Activation of STAT3 Sustains Progression of Non-Papillary Basal-Type Bladder Cancer via FOSL1 Regulome. *Cancers* **2019**, *11*, 1219. [CrossRef]
18. Ho, P.L.; Lay, E.J.; Jian, W.; Parra, D.; Chan, K.S. Stat3 activation in urothelial stem cells leads to direct progression to invasive bladder cancer. *Cancer Res.* **2012**, *72*, 3135–3142. [CrossRef]
19. Mitra, A.P.; Pagliarulo, V.; Yang, D.; Waldman, F.M.; Datar, R.H.; Skinner, D.G.; Groshen, S.; Cote, R.J. Generation of a concise gene panel for outcome prediction in urinary bladder cancer. *J. Clin. Oncol.* **2009**, *27*, 3929–3937. [CrossRef]
20. Sun, Y.; Cheng, M.K.; RL Griffiths, T.; Kilian Mellon, J.; Kai, B.; Kriajevska, M.; M Manson, M. Inhibition of STAT Signalling in Bladder Cancer by Diindolylmethane-Relevance to Cell Adhesion, Migration and Proliferation. *Curr. Cancer Drug Targets* **2013**, *13*, 57–68. [CrossRef]
21. Vlahou, A.; Gromova, I.; Svensson, S.; Gromov, P.; Moreira, J.M. Identification of BLCAP as a novel STAT3 interaction partner in bladder cancer. *PLoS ONE* **2017**, *12*. [CrossRef]
22. Groner, B.; von Manstein, V. Jak Stat signaling and cancer: Opportunities, benefits and side effects of targeted inhibition. *Mol. Cell. Endocrinol.* **2017**, *451*, 1–14. [CrossRef] [PubMed]
23. Kontzias, A.; Kotlyar, A.; Laurence, A.; Changelian, P.; O'Shea, J.J. Jakinibs: A new class of kinase inhibitors in cancer and autoimmune disease. *Curr. Opin. Pharmacol.* **2012**, *12*, 464–470. [CrossRef] [PubMed]
24. Wong, A.L.A.; Hirpara, J.L.; Pervaiz, S.; Eu, J.Q.; Sethi, G.; Goh, B.C. Do STAT3 inhibitors have potential in the future for cancer therapy? *Expert Opin. Investig. Drugs* **2017**, *26*, 883–887. [CrossRef] [PubMed]
25. Yang, L.; Lin, S.; Xu, L.; Lin, J.; Zhao, C.; Huang, X. Novel activators and small-molecule inhibitors of STAT3 in cancer. *Cytokine Growth Factor Rev.* **2019**, *49*, 10–22. [CrossRef]
26. Zhao, C.; Li, H.; Lin, H.J.; Yang, S.; Lin, J.; Liang, G. Feedback Activation of STAT3 as a Cancer Drug-Resistance Mechanism. *Trends Pharmacol. Sci.* **2016**, *37*, 47–61. [CrossRef]
27. Shao, D.; Ma, J.; Zhou, C.; Zhao, J.N.; Li, L.L.; Zhao, T.J.; Ai, X.L.; Jiao, P. STAT3 down-regulation induces mitochondria-dependent G2/M cell cycle arrest and apoptosis in oesophageal carcinoma cells. *Clin. Exp. Pharmacol. Physiol.* **2017**, *44*, 413–420. [CrossRef]
28. Zhou, C.; Ma, J.; Su, M.; Shao, D.; Zhao, J.; Zhao, T.; Song, Z.; Meng, Y.; Jiao, P. Down-regulation of STAT3 induces the apoptosis and G1 cell cycle arrest in esophageal carcinoma ECA109 cells. *Cancer Cell Int.* **2018**, *18*, 53. [CrossRef]
29. Sathe, A.; Koshy, N.; Schmid, S.C.; Thalgott, M.; Schwarzenbock, S.M.; Krause, B.J.; Holm, P.S.; Gschwend, J.E.; Retz, M.; Nawroth, R. CDK4/6 Inhibition Controls Proliferation of Bladder Cancer and Transcription of RB1. *J. Urol.* **2016**, *195*, 771–779. [CrossRef]
30. Sobhani, N.; D'Angelo, A.; Pittacolo, M.; Roviello, G.; Miccoli, A.; Corona, S.P.; Bernocchi, O.; Generali, D.; Otto, T. Updates on the CDK4/6 Inhibitory Strategy and Combinations in Breast Cancer. *Cells* **2019**, *8*, 321. [CrossRef]
31. McCartney, A.; Migliaccio, I.; Bonechi, M.; Biagioni, C.; Romagnoli, D.; De Luca, F.; Galardi, F.; Risi, E.; De Santo, I.; Benelli, M.; et al. Mechanisms of Resistance to CDK4/6 Inhibitors: Potential Implications and Biomarkers for Clinical Practice. *Front. Oncol.* **2019**, *9*, 666. [CrossRef] [PubMed]
32. Tong, Z.; Sathe, A.; Ebner, B.; Qi, P.; Veltkamp, C.; Gschwend, J.E.; Holm, P.S.; Nawroth, R. Functional genomics identifies predictive markers and clinically actionable resistance mechanisms to CDK4/6 inhibition in bladder cancer. *J. Exp. Clin. Cancer Res.* **2019**, *38*, 322. [CrossRef]
33. Harrington, K.; Freeman, D.J.; Kelly, B.; Harper, J.; Soria, J.C. Optimizing oncolytic virotherapy in cancer treatment. *Nat. Rev. Drug Discov.* **2019**, *18*, 689–706. [CrossRef] [PubMed]
34. Fukuhara, H.; Ino, Y.; Todo, T. Oncolytic virus therapy: A new era of cancer treatment at dawn. *Cancer Sci.* **2016**, *107*, 1373–1379. [CrossRef] [PubMed]
35. Conry, R.M.; Westbrook, B.; McKee, S.; Norwood, T.G. Talimogene laherparepvec: First in class oncolytic virotherapy. *Hum. Vaccines Immunother.* **2018**, *14*, 839–846. [CrossRef] [PubMed]

36. Matsuda, T.; Karube, H.; Aruga, A. A Comparative Safety Profile Assessment of Oncolytic Virus Therapy Based on Clinical Trials. *Ther. Innov. Regul. Sci.* **2018**, *52*, 430–437. [CrossRef] [PubMed]
37. Lichtenegger, E.; Koll, F.; Haas, H.; Mantwill, K.; Janssen, K.P.; Laschinger, M.; Gschwend, J.; Steiger, K.; Black, P.C.; Moskalev, I.; et al. The Oncolytic Adenovirus XVir-N-31 as a Novel Therapy in Muscle-Invasive Bladder Cancer. *Hum. Gene Ther.* **2019**, *30*, 44–56. [CrossRef]
38. Taguchi, S.; Fukuhara, H.; Homma, Y.; Todo, T. Current status of clinical trials assessing oncolytic virus therapy for urological cancers. *Int. J. Urol.* **2017**, *24*, 342–351. [CrossRef]
39. LaRocca, C.J.; Warner, S.G. Oncolytic viruses and checkpoint inhibitors: combination therapy in clinical trials. *Clin. Transl. Med.* **2018**, *7*, 35. [CrossRef]
40. Jiang, H.; Gomez-Manzano, C.; Rivera-Molina, Y.; Lang, F.F.; Conrad, C.A.; Fueyo, J. Oncolytic adenovirus research evolution: from cell-cycle checkpoints to immune checkpoints. *Curr. Opin. Virol.* **2015**, *13*, 33–39. [CrossRef]
41. Patel, M.R.; Dash, A.; Jacobson, B.A.; Ji, Y.; Baumann, D.; Ismail, K.; Kratzke, R.A. JAK/STAT inhibition with ruxolitinib enhances oncolytic virotherapy in non-small cell lung cancer models. *Cancer Gene Ther.* **2019**, *26*, 411–418. [CrossRef] [PubMed]
42. Ghonime, M.G.; Cassady, K.A. Combination Therapy Using Ruxolitinib and Oncolytic HSV Renders Resistant MPNSTs Susceptible to Virotherapy. *Cancer Immunol. Res.* **2018**, *6*, 1499–1510. [CrossRef] [PubMed]
43. Huang, W.T.; Yang, S.F.; Wu, C.C.; Chen, W.T.; Huang, Y.C.; Su, Y.C.; Chai, C.Y. Expression of signal transducer and activator of transcription 3 and suppressor of cytokine signaling in urothelial carcinoma. *Kaohsiung J. Med. Sci.* **2009**, *25*, 640–646. [CrossRef]
44. Chan, K.S.; Espinosa, I.; Chao, M.; Wong, D.; Ailles, L.; Diehn, M.; Gill, H.; Presti, J., Jr.; Chang, H.Y.; van de Rijn, M.; et al. Identification, molecular characterization, clinical prognosis, and therapeutic targeting of human bladder tumor-initiating cells. *Proc. Natl. Acad. Sci. USA* **2009**, *106*, 14016–14021. [CrossRef]
45. Robertson, A.G.; Kim, J.; Al-Ahmadie, H.; Bellmunt, J.; Guo, G.; Cherniack, A.D.; Hinoue, T.; Laird, P.W.; Hoadley, K.A.; Akbani, R.; et al. Comprehensive Molecular Characterization of Muscle-Invasive Bladder Cancer. *Cell* **2017**, *171*, 540–556. [CrossRef]
46. Horn, T.; Laus, J.; Seitz, A.K.; Maurer, T.; Schmid, S.C.; Wolf, P.; Haller, B.; Winkler, M.; Retz, M.; Nawroth, R.; et al. The prognostic effect of tumour-infiltrating lymphocytic subpopulations in bladder cancer. *World J. Urol.* **2016**, *34*, 181–187. [CrossRef]
47. Horiguchi, A.; Oya, M.; Shimada, T.; Uchida, A.; Marumo, K.; Murai, M. Activation of signal transducer and activator of transcription 3 in renal cell carcinoma—A study of incidence and its association with pathological features and clinical outcome. *J. Urol.* **2002**, *168*, 762–765. [CrossRef]
48. Igelmann, S.; Neubauer, H.A.; Ferbeyre, G. STAT3 and STAT5 Activation in Solid Cancers. *Cancers* **2019**, *11*, 1428. [CrossRef]
49. Fukada, T.; Ohtani, T.; Yoshida, Y.; Shirogane, T.; Nishida, K.; Nakajima, K.; Hibi, M.; Hirano, T. STAT3 orchestrates contradictory signals in cytokine-induced G1 to S cell-cycle transition. *EMBO J.* **1998**, *17*, 6670–6677. [CrossRef]
50. Skowron, M.A.; Sathe, A.; Romano, A.; Hoffmann, M.J.; Schulz, W.A.; van Koeveringe, G.A.; Albers, P.; Nawroth, R.; Niegisch, G. Applying the chicken embryo chorioallantoic membrane assay to study treatment approaches in urothelial carcinoma. *Urol. Oncol.* **2017**, *35*, 544.e11–544.e23. [CrossRef]
51. Chou, T.C. Drug combination studies and their synergy quantification using the Chou-Talalay method. *Cancer Res.* **2010**, *70*, 440–446. [CrossRef] [PubMed]
52. Joung, Y.H.; Na, Y.M.; Yoo, Y.B.; Darvin, P.; Sp, N.; Kang, D.Y.; Kim, S.Y.; Kim, H.S.; Choi, Y.H.; Lee, H.K.; et al. Combination of AG490, a Jak2 inhibitor, and methylsulfonylmethane synergistically suppresses bladder tumor growth via the Jak2/STAT3 pathway. *Int. J. Oncol.* **2014**, *44*, 883–895. [CrossRef] [PubMed]
53. Quintás-Cardama, A.; Vaddi, K.; Liu, P.; Manshouri, T.; Li, J.; Scherle, P.A.; Caulder, E.; Wen, X.; Li, Y.; Waeltz, P.; et al. Preclinical characterization of the selective JAK1/2 inhibitor INCB018424: therapeutic implications for the treatment of myeloproliferative neoplasms. *Blood* **2010**, *115*, 3109–3117. [CrossRef] [PubMed]
54. Baffert, F.; Régnier, C.H.; De Pover, A.; Pissot-Soldermann, C.; Tavares, G.A.; Blasco, F.; Brueggen, J.; Chène, P.; Drueckes, P.; Erdmann, D.; et al. Potent and Selective Inhibition of Polycythemia by the Quinoxaline JAK2 Inhibitor NVP-BSK805. *Mol. Cancer Ther.* **2010**, *9*, 1945–1955. [CrossRef]

55. Knudsen, E.S.; Witkiewicz, A.K. The Strange Case of CDK4/6 Inhibitors: Mechanisms, Resistance, and Combination Strategies. *Trends Cancer* **2017**, *3*, 39–55. [CrossRef] [PubMed]
56. Schust, J.; Sperl, B.; Hollis, A.; Mayer, T.U.; Berg, T. Stattic: A small-molecule inhibitor of STAT3 activation and dimerization. *Chem. Biol.* **2006**, *13*, 1235–1242. [CrossRef] [PubMed]
57. Haftchenary, S.; Luchman, H.A.; Jouk, A.O.; Veloso, A.J.; Page, B.D.; Cheng, X.R.; Dawson, S.S.; Grinshtein, N.; Shahani, V.M.; Kerman, K.; et al. Potent Targeting of the STAT3 Protein in Brain Cancer Stem Cells: A Promising Route for Treating Glioblastoma. *ACS Med. Chem. Lett.* **2013**, *4*, 1102–1107. [CrossRef]
58. Nelson, E.A.; Walker, S.R.; Kepich, A.; Gashin, L.B.; Hideshima, T.; Ikeda, H.; Chauhan, D.; Anderson, K.C.; Frank, D.A. Nifuroxazide inhibits survival of multiple myeloma cells by directly inhibiting STAT3. *Blood* **2008**, *112*, 5095–5102. [CrossRef]
59. Zhang, H.; Ye, Y.L.; Li, M.X.; Ye, S.B.; Huang, W.R.; Cai, T.T.; He, J.; Peng, J.Y.; Duan, T.H.; Cui, J.; et al. CXCL2/MIF-CXCR2 signaling promotes the recruitment of myeloid-derived suppressor cells and is correlated with prognosis in bladder cancer. *Oncogene* **2016**, *36*, 2095–2104. [CrossRef]
60. Tsujita, Y.; Horiguchi, A.; Tasaki, S.; Isono, M.; Asano, T.; Ito, K.; Asano, T.; Mayumi, Y.; Kushibiki, T. STAT3 inhibition by WP1066 suppresses the growth and invasiveness of bladder cancer cells. *Oncol. Rep.* **2017**, *38*, 2197–2204. [CrossRef]
61. Zhou, X.; Ren, Y.; Liu, A.; Jin, R.; Jiang, Q.; Huang, Y.; Kong, L.; Wang, X.; Zhang, L. WP1066 sensitizes oral squamous cell carcinoma cells to cisplatin by targeting STAT3/miR-21 axis. *Sci. Rep.* **2014**, *4*, 7461. [CrossRef]
62. Chiocca, E.A.; Rabkin, S.D. Oncolytic viruses and their application to cancer immunotherapy. *Cancer Immunol. Res.* **2014**, *2*, 295–300. [CrossRef] [PubMed]
63. Chahal, J.S.; Qi, J.; Flint, S.J. The human adenovirus type 5 E1B 55 kDa protein obstructs inhibition of viral replication by type I interferon in normal human cells. *PLoS Pathog.* **2012**, *8*, e1002853. [CrossRef] [PubMed]
64. Zheng, Y.; Stamminger, T.; Hearing, P. E2F/Rb Family Proteins Mediate Interferon Induced Repression of Adenovirus Immediate Early Transcription to Promote Persistent Viral Infection. *PLoS Pathog.* **2016**, *12*, e1005415. [CrossRef] [PubMed]
65. Toth, K.; Lee, S.R.; Ying, B.; Spencer, J.F.; Tollefson, A.E.; Sagartz, J.E.; Kong, I.K.; Wang, Z.; Wold, W.S. STAT2 Knockout Syrian Hamsters Support Enhanced Replication and Pathogenicity of Human Adenovirus, Revealing an Important Role of Type I Interferon Response in Viral Control. *PLoS Pathog.* **2015**, *11*, e1005084. [CrossRef]
66. Steinwaerder, D.S.; Carlson, C.A.; Lieber, A. DNA Replication of First-Generation Adenovirus Vectors in Tumor Cells. *Hum. Gene Ther.* **2000**, *11*, 1933–1948. [CrossRef]

5

Biomarkers for Predicting Clinical Outcomes of Chemoradiation-Based Bladder Preservation Therapy for Muscle-Invasive Bladder Cancer

Fumitaka Koga *, Kosuke Takemura and Hiroshi Fukushima

Department of Urology, Tokyo Metropolitan Cancer and Infectious diseases Center Komagome Hospital, 3-18-22 Honkomagome, Bunkyo-ku, Tokyo 113-8677, Japan; takemura-uro@cick.jp (K.T.); fukuuro@tmd.ac.jp (H.F.)

* Correspondence: f-koga@cick.jp

Abstract: Chemoradiation-based bladder preservation therapy (BPT) is currently a curative option for non-metastatic muscle-invasive bladder cancer (MIBC) patients at favorable risk or an alternative to radical cystectomy (RC) for those who are unfit for RC. In BPT, only patients who achieve complete response (CR) after chemoradiation have a favorable prognosis and quality of life with a preserved functional bladder. Thus, predicting CR and favorable prognosis is important for optimal patient selection for BPT. We reviewed biomarkers for predicting the clinical outcomes of chemoradiation-based BPT. The biomarkers studied were categorized into those related to apoptosis, cell proliferation, receptor tyrosine kinases, DNA damage response genes, hypoxia, molecular subtype, and others. Among these biomarkers, the Ki-67 labeling index (Ki-67 LI) and meiotic recombination 11 may be used for selecting BPT or RC. Ki-67 LI and erythroblastic leukemia viral oncogene homolog 2 (erbB2) may be used for predicting both the chemoradiation response and the prognosis of patients on BPT. Concurrent use of trastuzumab and a combination of carbogen and nicotinamide can overcome chemoradiation resistance conferred by erbB2 overexpression and tumor hypoxia. Further studies are needed to confirm the practical utility of these biomarkers for progress on biomarker-directed personalized management of MIBC patients.

Keywords: biomarker; chemoradiation; prognosis; bladder preservation; bladder neoplasm; urothelial carcinoma

---

1. Introduction

Bladder cancer is the second most common malignancy of the genitourinary tract after prostate cancer in the United States, with approximately 81,000 new cases and 17,000 deaths each year as of 2018 [1]. Approximately 75% of bladder cancer patients present with non-muscle-invasive bladder cancer confined to the mucosa and submucosa (Tis, Ta, and T1), while the rest present with muscle-invasive bladder cancer (MIBC) [2]. The reference standard of care for MIBC patients has long been radical cystectomy (RC) with urinary diversion and lymph node dissection. However, this surgical procedure is complex and invasive and could have long-term adverse effects on urinary, gastrointestinal, and sexual functions. A recent systematic review on the surgical outcomes of robot-assisted laparoscopic RC demonstrated a 90-day overall complication rate of 59%, a 90-day major complication rate of 15%, and a 90-day mortality rate of 3% [3]. The long-term adverse effects on urinary, gastrointestinal, and sexual functions significantly compromised quality of life (QOL) in patients undergoing RC and urinary diversion when compared with those retaining their native bladders [4].

Bladder preservation therapy (BPT), consisting of transurethral resection, chemotherapy, and radiation, has yielded oncological outcomes and QOL comparable to or more favorable than RC when select MIBC patients undergo BPT [5]. Because of the lack of randomized control trials, BPT used to be an alternative to RC for MIBC patients medically unfit for RC. However, accumulated clinical evidence reported from centers of excellence has demonstrated favorable oncological and QOL outcomes [6–8]. Consequently, guidelines of the American Urological Association, American Society of Clinical Oncology, American Society for Radiation Oncology, and Society of Urologic Oncology mention that chemoradiation-based BPT should be offered as an option of standard therapies for non-metastatic MIBC patients who desire to retain their bladders and for whom RC is not a treatment option [2].

MIBC patients with favorable oncological and QOL outcomes after BPT are those achieving complete response (CR) to chemoradiation; such patients account for 50–90% of MIBC patients treated with chemoradiation-based BPT [5]. Although those who do not achieve CR are advised to undergo salvage RC, MIBC patients who do not achieve CR to chemoradiation show unfavorable cancer-specific survival (CSS) regardless of salvage RC with curative intent due to metastatic recurrences [5,9]; such patients may benefit from neoadjuvant chemotherapy plus RC in terms of CSS. Thus, prediction of chemoradiation response enables selection of optimal candidates for BPT and may ultimately improve prognosis and QOL of MIBC patients.

In this study, we conducted a non-systematic review to identify studies investigating biomarkers associated with chemoradiation response and prognosis on chemoradiation-based BPT among MIBC patients. Some biomarkers can be used as targets for therapeutic intervention to improve clinical outcomes by modifying the functions of biomarkers (e.g., concurrent use of trastuzumab for erythroblastic leukemia viral oncogene homolog 2 (erbB2)-overexpressing tumors to improve chemoradiation response).

2. Current Practice on Bladder Preservation Therapy in Muscle-Invasive Bladder Cancer Patients

BPT in the form most widely utilized and recommended by guidelines comprises transurethral resection and chemoradiation. Randomized controlled phase III trials demonstrated oncological advantages of concurrent administration of chemotherapeutic agents over radiotherapy alone in non-metastatic MIBC patients. In a Canadian trial reported in 1996, adding cisplatin as a radiosensitizer significantly improved local control [10]. However, this study did not have adequate power to show the survival advantages of chemoradiation over radiotherapy alone. A randomized trial in the United Kingdom investigated fluorouracil and mitomycin-C as radiosensitizers in MIBC patients [11]. The concurrent use of these agents significantly improved the 2-year locoregional disease-free survival from 54% to 67%. In this trial, the 5-year overall survival (OS) improved from 35% to 48% but there was no statistical significance. Case series and phase I/II studies demonstrated possible activity of gemcitabine [12] and paclitaxel [13] as radiosensitizers for MIBC.

2.1. Indications

Indications of BPT in MIBC patients are quite different according to whether they are fit for RC or not. BPT for those who are fit for RC and who desire their native bladders is regarded as selective BPT. On the other hand, those who are unfit for RC due to severe comorbidity or poor performance status receive BPT as an alternative to RC.

Selective BPT is generally given to patients with low-risk MIBC in whom favorable oncological outcomes are expected to be comparable to those of RC. Favorable clinical features of MIBC include small, solitary and non-metastatic low stage (clinical T2N0) diseases, the absence of hydronephrosis, and the absence of extensive carcinoma in situ [5]. Such tumors are amenable to complete transurethral resection prior to chemoradiation; indeed, the visibly complete transurethral resection of primary tumors is associated with favorable prognosis in patients treated with BPT [5,8].

In contrast to the RC-fit patients, those unfit for RC would receive BPT with chemoradiation as a curative option alternative to RC. These patients would have diseases of higher risks than those who are subjected to selective BPT. Therefore, RC-unfit patients treated with BPT generally have a worse prognosis than those treated with selective BPT.

2.2. Therapeutic Protocols

Two typical templates for chemoradiation were reported: Split- or single-course protocol [5]. A split-course protocol consists of induction chemoradiation of 40–45 Gy, followed by evaluation of any residual tumor with imaging studies and transurethral biopsy, and then consolidative chemoradiation of 20–25 Gy if CR is achieved. Patients who do not achieve CR undergo salvage RC. In contrast, a single-course protocol includes full-dose chemoradiation of 55–65 Gy followed by response evaluation and surveillance if CR is achieved. Although salvage RC is planned for patients who do not achieve CR, high-dose (>60 Gy) pelvic irradiation increases both the morbidity and mortality of RC; in patients undergoing salvage RC after high-dose radiotherapy, mortality rates range from 6% to 33%, higher than the rates reported in published contemporary RC series for non-irradiated subjects, which range up to 4% [5]. The split-course protocol places priority on cancer control by carrying out salvage RC with minimal delay for non-CR patients in selective BPT. A lower dose of preoperative irradiation also reduces the risk of RC-associated complications for non-CR patients after induction chemoradiation [14]. However, splitting of radiotherapy could reduce antitumor effects of the split-course protocol compared with those of the single-course protocol. In this respect, the single-course protocol is more suitable than the split-course protocol for BPT in patients unfit for RC.

Other protocols involve consolidative partial cystectomy with pelvic lymph node dissection following induction chemoradiation [15,16] and intraarterial chemotherapy [17] to increase therapeutic intensity.

2.3. Prognosis

A published series of chemoradiation-based BPT reported OS comparable to that of RC (50–70% at 5 years) while preserving the native bladder in 40–60% of MIBC patients [5]. There is no randomized controlled trial comparing outcomes between BPT and RC in MIBC patients. Recently, 3 studies retrospectively compared prognosis of MIBC patients between BPT and RC using a propensity score matching analysis: 2 studies derived from the National Cancer Database (NCD) [18,19] and one study from a Canadian multidisciplinary bladder cancer clinic [20]. The 2 NCD studies demonstrated more favorable OS for RC than that for BPT. Because of the lack of adjustment for performance status, an established prognostic factor in MIBC patients, in these NCD studies, the results would be biased by patients who were unfit for RC due to poor performance status and thus received BPT [18,19]. In the Canadian study, subjects were matched for more prognostic factors including performance status than those of the NCD studies, and BPT yielded OS and CSS similar to RC after propensity score matching [20].

2.4. Clinicopathologic Factors Associated with Outcomes of Bladder Preservation Therapy

Clinicopathologic parameters associated with outcomes of chemoradiation-based BPT are classified into tumor and therapeutic factors. The clinical tumor parameters associated with favorable chemoradiation response include small tumor size (<5 cm), clinical T2 stage, unifocal disease, and the absence of hydronephrosis [8,16]. The most important therapeutic parameter is completeness of transurethral resection [8]. Thus, it is mandatory to attempt transurethral resection of tumors as thoroughly as is safely possible for candidates of BPT. Prognostic factors after BPT include completeness of transurethral resection, clinical T stage, and lymphovascular invasion [8].

Coen et al. developed comprehensive nomograms predicting outcomes of BPT including therapeutic response to chemoradiation, CSS, and bladder-intact disease-free survival in a cohort of 325 MIBC patients who were treated with selective BPT of split-course chemoradiation [21]. The most important clinical parameters for CR after chemoradiation are the absence of hydronephrosis and complete transurethral resection followed by younger age (<65 years) and female gender. For

CSS, the most favorable parameters include clinical T2 disease (versus T3–4) and the absence of hydronephrosis followed by histological grade 2 disease (versus grade 3). For favorable bladder-intact disease-free survival, the most relevant parameter is the absence of hydronephrosis followed by complete transurethral resection, clinical T2 disease, and younger age (<65 years). Such nomograms may assist patients and clinicians making treatment decisions.

3. Biomarkers Associated with Chemoradiation Response and Prognosis

Summaries of studies that reported emerging biomarkers associated with chemoradiation response and prognosis on BPT for MIBC are listed in Tables 1 and 2, respectively. These biomarkers are categorized as follows: (1) apoptosis-related biomarkers, (2) cell proliferation-related biomarkers, (3) receptor tyrosine kinases (RTK), (4) DNA damage response (DDR)-related biomarkers, (5) hypoxia-related biomarkers, (6) molecular subtypes, and (7) others.

Table 1. Biomarkers associated with chemoradiation response.

Biomarkers	Samples Used (No. Patients)	Chemoradiation Regimen	Associations with Response	Study Type	Reference
Apoptosis-related					
Apoptotic index	Tumor tissues ($n = 70$)	RT 59.4 Gy + cisplatin	Higher apoptotic index was associated with a higher CR rate (86% vs. 57%, $p = 0.02$)	Retrospective	[22]
bax/bcl-2 ratio	Tumor tissues ($n = 62$)	RT 40.5 Gy (median) + cisplatin	Higher Bax/Bcl-2 ratio was associated with a higher CR rate ($p = 0.029$)	Retrospective	[23]
Cell proliferation-related					
Ki-67 LI	Tumor tissues ($n = 70$)	RT 59.4 Gy + cisplatin	Higher Ki-67 LI was associated with a higher CR rate (86% vs. 57%, $p = 0.02$)	Retrospective	[22]
Ki-67 LI	Tumor tissues ($n = 94$)	RT 40 Gy + cisplatin, 69 (73%) underwent partial or salvage radical cystectomy	Higher Ki-67 LI (continuous variable) was associated with a higher CR rate ($p = 0.0004$)	Retrospective	[24]
ADC value	MRI ($n = 23$)	RT 40 Gy + cisplatin	Sensitivity/specificity/accuracy = 92/90/91% when ADC < 0.74×10^{-3} mm^2/s	Retrospective	[25]
RTKs					
erbB2	Tumor tissues ($n = 55$)	RT 40 Gy + cisplatin + other agents	CR rates, 50% vs. 81% for positive vs. negative ($p = 0.026$)	Retrospective	[26]
erbB2	Tumor tissues ($n = 119$)	RT 40 Gy + cisplatin	CR rates, 29% vs. 53% for positive vs. negative ($p = 0.01$)	Retrospective	[27]
erbB2	Tumor tissues ($n = 66$)	RT 64.8 Gy + paclitaxel with (group 1: erbB2+) or without trastuzumab (group 2: erbB2-)	CR rates, 72% for group 1 and 68% for group 2	Prospective	[28]
DDR-related					
ERCC1	Tumor tissues ($n = 22$)	RT 40-66 Gy + cisplatin or nedaplatin	CR rates, 25% vs. 86% for positive vs. negative ($p = 0.008$)	Retrospective	[29]
Molecular subtype					
Molecular subtype	Tumor tissues ($n = 118$)	RT 40 Gy + cisplatin	CR rates, 52%/45%/15% for GU/SCC-like/Uro ($p < 0.001$)	Retrospective	[30]
Others					
Hsp60	Tumor tissues ($n = 54$)	RT 40 Gy + cisplatin	Positive Hsp60 was associated with better response ($p = 0.05$)	Retrospective	[31]

RT, radiotherapy; CR, complete response; LI, labeling index; ADC, apparent diffusion coefficient; MRI, magnetic resonance imaging; RTK, receptor tyrosine kinases; erbB2, erythroblastic leukemia viral oncogene homolog 2; DDR, DNA damage response; ERCC1, excision repair cross-complementing group 1; GU, genomically unstable subtype; SCC-like, squamous cell cancer-like subtype; Uro, urobasal subtype; Hsp60, heat shock protein 60.

Table 2. Biomarkers associated with prognosis of muscle invasive bladder cancer patients on chemoradiation-based bladder preservation therapy.

Biomarkers	Samples Used (No. Patients)	Chemoradiation Regimen	Associations with Prognosis	Study Type	Reference
Cell proliferation-related					
Ki-67LI	Tumor tissues ($n = 70$)	RT 59.4 Gy + cisplatin	Better CSS with preserved bladder for higher Ki-67 LI (50% vs. 36% at 5-year, $p = 0.04$)	Retrospective	[22]
Ki-67 LI	Tumor tissues ($n = 62$)	RT 40.5 Gy (median) + cisplatin	Worse CSS for high Ki-67 LI of > 20% ($p = 0.014$)	Retrospective	[23]
Ki-67 LI	Tumor tissues ($n = 94$)	RT 40 Gy + cisplatin, 69 (73%) underwent partial or salvage radical cystectomy	Better CSS for high Ki-67 LI of > 20% (HR 0.3, $p = 0.01$)	Retrospective	[24]
RTKs					
EGFR	Tumor tissues ($n = 73$)	RT 40 Gy + cisplatin + other agents	Better CSS for positive EGFR ($p = 0.042$)	Retrospective	[26]
erbB2	Tumor tissues ($n = 119$)	RT 40 Gy + cisplatin	Worse CSS for erbB2 overexpression (56% vs. 87%, $p = 0.001$)	Retrospective	[27]
VEGF-B/C and VEGFR2	Tumor tissues ($n = 43$)	RT 64.8 Gy + cisplatin + other agents	Worse OS for high VEGF-B/C/R2 expression ($p = 0.01$-0.02), higher distant failure rate for high VEGF-R2 expression ($p = 0.01$)	Retrospective	[32]
VEGF-C/NRP2	Tumor tissues ($n = 247$)	RT 56.3 Gy + cisplatin	Worse OS for high NRP2 or VEGFC expression (HR 4.25, $p = 0.023$)	Retrospective	[33]
DDR-related					
MRE11	Tumor tissues ($n = 179$)	RT 55 Gy	Better CSS for high MRE11 expression (HR 0.36, $p = 0.01$)	Retrospective	[34]
ERCC1/XRCC1	Tumor tissues ($n = 157$)	RT 48.6 Gy (median) + cisplatin	Better CSS for positive ERCC1 or XRCC1 (HR 0.64, $p = 0.024$)	Retrospective	[35]
DDR alterations	Tumor tissues ($n = 48$)	RT or chemoradiation (details unavailable)	Trend for better RFS for the presence of DDR alterations (HR 0.37, $p = 0.07$)	Retrospective	[36]
Hypoxia-related					
Necrosis	Tumor tissues ($n = 220$)	RT vs. RT + CON	The presence of necrosis predicted better OS for RT + CON than RT alone (HR 0.43, $p = 0.004$)	Retrospective	[37]
HIF-1α	Tumor tissues ($n = 137$)	RT vs. RT + CON	Positive HIF-1α predicted better DFS for RT + CON than RT alone (HR 0.48, $p = 0.02$)	Retrospective	[38]
Others					
CRP	Serum ($n = 88$)	RT 40 Gy + cisplatin	Worse CSS for high CRP of > 0.5 mg/dL (HR 1.8, $p = 0.046$)	Retrospective	[39]
Lymphocytopenia	Blood ($n = 74$)	RT 52.5 Gy + gemcitabine	Worse RFS for lymphocytopenia of $< 1.5 \times 10^9$/L (HR 3.9, $p = 0.003$)	Retrospective	[40]

LI, labeling index; RT, radiotherapy; CSS, cancer-specific survival; HR, hazard ratio; RTK, receptor tyrosine kinases; EGFR, epidermal growth factor receptor; erbB2, erythroblastic leukemia viral oncogene homolog 2; VEGF(R), vascular endothelial growth factor (receptor); OS, overall survival; NRP2, neutropilin 2; DDR, DNA damage response; MRE11, meiotic recombination 11; ERCC1, excision repair cross-complementing group 1; XRCC1, X-ray repair cross-complementing group 1; RFS, recurrence-free survival; CON, carbogen and nicotinamide; HIF-1α, hypoxia-inducible factor-1α; DFS, disease-free survival; CRP, C-reactive protein.

3.1. Apoptosis-Related Biomarkers

Apoptosis is a key mechanism by which DNA-damaging stimuli, including chemotherapeutic agents and ionizing radiation, exhibit therapeutic effects. Apoptosis-related biomarkers, including apoptotic index (AI), p53, bcl-2, and bax, were investigated in relation to chemoradiation response and prognosis following BPT. Bax and bcl-2 regulate apoptosis downstream of p53 in response to DNA damage, and bax and bcl-2 have a pro-apoptotic and anti-apoptotic effect, respectively [41].

Rodel et al. reported that a higher AI was associated with a higher CR rate (86% vs. 57%, $p = 0.02$) among 70 invasive bladder cancer (cT1-4) patients treated with chemoradiation (59.4 Gy + cisplatin) [22]. However, no significant association with chemoradiation response was observed for immunohistochemical expression p53 or bcl-2. Neither AI, nor p53, nor bcl-2 was associated with CSS in this study. Matsumoto et al. investigated associations of p53, bcl-2, bax, and apoptotic index with clinical response among 62 invasive bladder cancer patients (cT1G3-T4N0) receiving chemoradiation (median dose 40.5 Gy + cisplatin) [23]. They found no significant association between immunohistochemical expression of each biomarker and chemoradiation response. However, higher bax/bcl-2 ratios were significantly associated with higher CR rates ($p = 0.029$). No association with prognosis was observed for any of these biomarkers.

Thus, some apoptosis-related biomarkers (AI and bax/bcl-2 ratios) are predictive of chemoradiation response but not of prognosis of patients treated with BPT.

3.2. *Cell Proliferation-Related Biomarkers*

Ki-67 is an established marker of cell proliferation and a biomarker reflecting the biological aggressiveness of malignancies. In fact, a high Ki-67 labeling index (LI) was an independent risk factor for recurrence and cancer death in bladder cancer patients undergoing RC [42]. In contrast, Ki-67 LI could be a biomarker predicting favorable clinical outcomes for MIBC patients when they are treated with chemoradiation.

Rodel et al. [22] and Tanabe et al. [24] reported that a higher Ki-67 LI was significantly associated with a higher CR rate among bladder cancer patients receiving chemoradiation. These two studies also demonstrated significantly better CSS for patients with tumors of higher Ki-67 LI. However, Matsumoto et al. reported conflicting results; Ki-67 LI was not associated with chemoradiation response and higher Ki-67 LI was significantly associated with worse CSS [23]. In the latter study [10], the total radiation dose of chemoradiation (median 40.5 Gy) and CR rate (34%) were lower than those of a study by Rodel et al. (59.4 Gy and 71%, respectively) [9]. In a study by Tanabe et al., patients received chemoradiation at 40 Gy, and 73% eventually underwent partial cystectomy of the original MIBC site or salvage RC to completely eradicate possible residual cancer cells [12]. The above conflicting results may be attributed to the difference in therapeutic intensity and the probability of the presence of residual disease; residual cancer cells of high Ki-67 LI, which survive chemoradiation at a relatively low dose, may progress and be associated with worse prognosis in a study by Matsumoto et al. [10].

Magnetic resonance imaging (MRI) is routinely used for staging of bladder cancer. Diffusion-weighted MRI is constructed by quantifying the diffusion of water molecules and malignant lesions exhibit high signal intensity in this modality as a result of higher cellularity, tissue disorganization, and decreased extracellular space, all of which restrict water diffusion [43]. The extent of the water diffusion is quantitatively expressed as apparent diffusion coefficient (ADC) values. Yoshida et al. demonstrated that ADC values were inversely correlated with Ki-67 LI in MIBC tissues and that tumors with lower ADC values were more sensitive to chemoradiation [25]. However, the prognostic significance of ADC values has not yet been assessed among MIBC patients treated with BPT.

Taken together, cell proliferation-related biomarkers (Ki-67 LI and ADC values) are likely to be predictive of the chemoradiation response and prognosis of MIBC patients treated with BPT. However, validation studies are needed to confirm the prognostic significance of Ki-67 LI.

3.3. *Receptor Tyrosine Kinases*

Signaling via receptor tyrosine kinases (RTKs) promotes cell proliferation, tumor invasion, and therapeutic resistance [44]. Among RTKs, erbB2, epidermal growth factor receptor (EGFR), and vascular endothelial growth factor (VEGF)-family proteins are associated with clinical outcomes of chemoradiation in MIBC patients. Notably, a biomarker-driven clinical trial was conducted to overcome chemoradiation resistance of erbB2-overexpressing bladder cancer [28].

Chakravarti, et al. investigated the associations of erbB2 and EGFR with chemoradiation response and prognosis following BPT. They reported that positive erbB2 was significantly associated with lower CR rates (50% vs. 81% for negative erbB2, $p = 0.026$) and that positive EGFR was significantly associated with better CSS ($p = 0.042$) [26]. However, the reasons for the association between positive EGFR and better CSS remain to be elucidated. Inoue et al. confirmed the association between erbB2 overexpression and lower CR rates, and demonstrated, for the first time, adverse CSS for erbB2 overexpression among 119 MIBC patients receiving chemoradiation [27]. These data suggest that erbB2 inhibitors improve clinical outcomes of chemoradiation in patients with MIBC overexpressing erbB2. A recent study by Michaelson et al. showed possible improvement of chemoradiation response with erbB2 targeted therapy [28]; 66 evaluable bladder cancer patients were treated with radiation (64.8 Gy) and either paclitaxel + anti-erbB2 monoclonal antibody, trastuzumab (group 1, $n = 20$) or paclitaxel alone (group 2, $n = 46$) according to the presence (group 1) or absence of erbB2 overexpression (group 2) in tumor tissues. The CR rate at 1 year for group 1 was equivalent to that for group 2 (72% vs. 68%, respectively) with comparable toxicity profiles between the 2 groups. In this phase I/II clinical trial, mid- to long-term prognostic outcomes were not reported.

VEGFs have important functions in tumor angiogenesis and lymphangiogenesis, promoting cancer progression [45]. Two studies demonstrated prognostic significance of expression of VEGF family proteins among bladder cancer patients treated with chemoradiation. Lautenschlaeger et al. reported that overexpression of VEGF-B and C and their receptor VEGFR2 were significantly associated with worse OS [32]. However, no association was observed between these biomarkers and the chemoradiation response. Keck et al. demonstrated that overexpression of VEGF-C or its receptor neutropilin-2 was independently associated with worse OS [33]. In this study, the associations of VEGF-C/neutropilin-2 expression with chemoradiation response were not assessed.

3.4. DNA Damage Response-Related Biomarkers

Ionizing radiation induces cell death primarily via DNA double-strand breaks. Upon exposure to ionizing radiation, the damage is detected by the meiotic recombination 11 (MRE11)-RAD50-NBS1 complex, resulting in activation of the DDR pathway [46]. DNA cross-links induced by cisplatin are repaired by the nucleotide excision repair pathway, including excision repair cross-complementing group 1 (ERCC1) [47]. Failure to repair such DNA damage results in tumor cell death.

No DDR-related biomarkers except ERCC1 were associated with chemoradiation response. Kawashima et al. demonstrated that loss of ERCC1 expression was significantly associated with better chemoradiation response (CR rate, 86% vs. 25% for positive ERCC1) in a cohort of 22 MIBC patients [29]. These investigators also showed that loss of ERCC1 expression canceled resistance to ionizing radiation in bladder cancer cells in vitro.

Choudhury et al. reported that higher MRE11 expression was significantly associated with better CSS in 179 invasive bladder cancer patients treated with definitive radiotherapy at 55 Gy (hazard ratio (HR) 0.36, $p = 0.01$) [34]. A trend for an inverse prognostic effect of higher MRE11 expression was observed among patients undergoing RC, and CSS was significantly better for those treated with radiotherapy than RC among patients with tumors of higher MRE11 expression (HR 0.60, $p = 0.02$). This study suggests that MRE11 expression status may allow patient selection for radiotherapy or RC. Sakano et al. reported that positive expression of ERCC1 or X-ray repair cross-complementing group 1 (XRCC1) was significantly associated with better CSS (HR 0.64, $p = 0.024$) among 157 invasive bladder cancer patients undergoing cisplatin-based chemoradiation [35]. Given that chemoradiation sensitivity is a critical surrogate for prognosis among MIBC patients treated with BPT [5,9], findings of this study and the abovementioned ERCC1 study [29] appear to be conflicting. Desai et al. investigated the prognostic impact of DDR gene alterations, which were analyzed using a next-generation sequencing assay, in 48 invasive bladder cancer patients undergoing chemoradiation or radiotherapy [36]. The presence of DDR gene alterations, most commonly identified in *ERCC2*, showed a trend for better bladder or metastatic recurrence-free survival (HR 0.47, $p = 0.070$); this finding is in line with studies on neoadjuvant chemotherapy for MIBC [48,49] and systemic chemotherapy for advanced urothelial carcinoma [50], showing significantly better clinical outcomes for tumors with DDR gene alterations.

Thus, the roles of DNA damage response-related genes or proteins as practical biomarkers for predicting outcomes of chemoradiation seem to be largely unknown. The presence of DDR gene alterations may be a biomarker to predict favorable clinical outcomes of MIBC patients undergoing chemoradiation. MRE11 expression status may be used for selecting BPT or RC. However, further validation studies are needed to confirm the practical utility of DDR-related biomarkers in predicting clinical outcomes of BPT for MIBC patients.

3.5. Hypoxia-Related Biomarkers

Tumor hypoxia contributes to tumor progression, invasion, metastasis, and resistance to chemotherapy and radiotherapy [45]. A phase III clinical trial showed that hypoxia modification with carbogen and nicotinamide (CON) significantly improved prognosis of invasive bladder cancer patients treated with radiotherapy [51]. Ad hoc analyses of this clinical trial identified hypoxia-related biomarkers for predicting patients who benefit from concurrent CON [37,38]. Tumor hypoxia induces hypoxia-inducible factor-1α (HIF-1α) expression and necrosis in bladder cancer tissues. The presence of histological necrosis in tumor tissues was predictive of benefit from CON; radiotherapy + CON showed significantly better OS than radiotherapy alone in the presence of necrosis (HR 0.43, $p = 0.02$) but not in the absence of necrosis (HR 1.64, $p = 0.08$) [37]. Similarly, the addition of CON provided survival benefit for patients with higher HIF-1α-expressing tumors (HR 0.48, $p = 0.02$) but not for those with lower HIF-1α-expressing ones (HR 0.81, $p = 0.5$) [38].

3.6. Molecular Subtypes

Molecular subtypes of bladder cancer can characterize their clinical behaviors and can help predict therapeutic responses to neoadjuvant chemotherapy prior to RC [52,53]. Tanaka et al. demonstrated that molecular subtypes may be used to predict chemoradiation response in 118 MIBC patients [30]. The subtyping model used was the Lund University model, which characterizes three subtypes based on immunohistochemical expression patterns of cyclin B1 and keratin 5: Urobasal (Uro), genomically unstable (GU), and squamous cell cancer-like (SCC-like) [54]. CR rates after chemoradiation (40 Gy + cisplatin) were 52%, 45%, and 15% for GU, SCC-like, and Uro, respectively ($p < 0.001$). Molecular subtypes were not associated with CSS probably because most non-CR patients underwent salvage cystectomy [30].

3.7. Others

Urushibara et al. investigated the associations of heat shock proteins (Hsp), which play key roles in cellular stress responses and can be involved in therapeutic resistance and tumor aggressiveness, with clinical outcomes of 54 invasive bladder cancer patients treated with chemoradiation (40 Gy + cisplatin) [31]. Among Hsp27, Hsp60, Hsp70, and Hsp90, positive Hsp60 expression was independently associated with favorable responses ($p = 0.05$). However, no survival advantage was observed for Hsp60-positive tumors.

Two studies demonstrated the possible utility of serum and blood biomarkers, C-reactive protein (CRP) and lymphocytopenia, in predicting prognosis of MIBC patients treated with BPT [39,40]. Yoshida et al. reported that elevated serum CRP (>0.5 mg/dL) was independently associated with worse CSS (HR 1.8, $p = 0.046$) among 88 MIBC patients undergoing chemoradiation-based BPT [39]. CRP was not associated with chemoradiation response. Joseph et al. reported that lymphocytopenia ($<1.5 \times 10^9$ /L) was significantly associated with worse disease-free survival (HR 3.9, $p = 0.003$) among 74 MIBC patients receiving chemoradiation (52.5 Gy + gemcitabine) [40].

4. Conclusions

Possible roles of the abovementioned biomarkers in predicting chemoradiation response and prognosis on chemoradiation-based BPT in MIBC patients are summarized in Figures 1 and 2, respectively. Higher Ki-67 LI, negative erbB2, higher expression of MRE11, higher AI, higher Bax/Bcl-2 ratio, lower ADC values, negative ERCC1, Uro subtype in the Lund University subtyping model, positive Hsp60, positive EGFR, lower expression of VEGF-related proteins, presence of DDR gene alterations, lower serum CRP, and absence of lymphocytopenia are possible biomarkers to predict favorable clinical outcomes in these patients. Of these biomarkers, Ki-67 LI and MRE11 may be used for selecting BPT or RC because a higher Ki-67 LI and higher MRE11 expression appear to favor BPT rather than RC in terms of post-therapeutic survival. Ki-67 LI and erbB2 may be used for predicting both chemoradiation response and prognosis of patients on BPT. Concurrent use of trastuzumab and CON can overcome chemoradiation resistance conferred by erbB2 overexpression and tumor hypoxia.

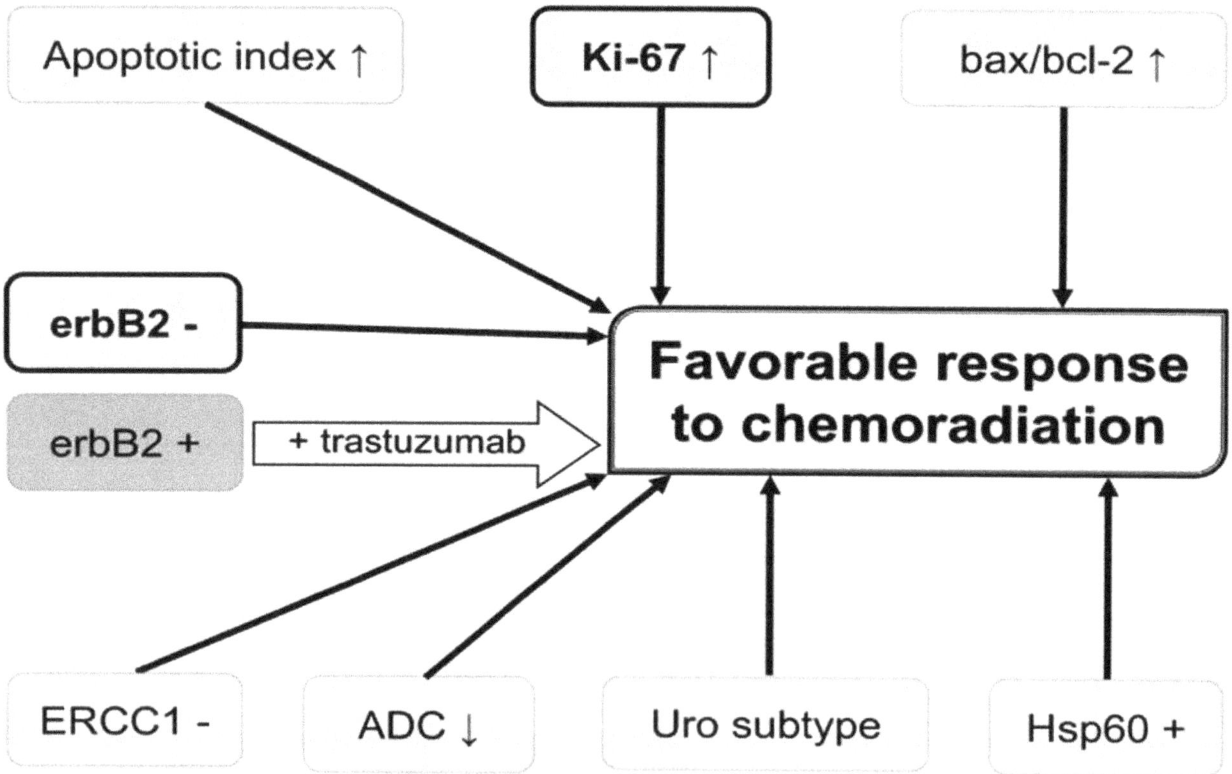

Figure 1. Biomarkers that may be used for predicting and improving the chemoradiation response. Biomarkers in bold letter are also associated with favorable prognosis on bladder preservation therapy. Overexpression of erbB2 is associated with unfavorable chemoradiation response, which can be overcome by trastuzumab. ADC, apparent diffusion coefficient value on diffusion-weighted magnetic resonance imaging; erbB2, erythroblastic leukemia viral oncogene homolog 2; ERCC1, excision repair cross-complementing group 1; Hsp60, heat shock protein 60; Uro subtype, urobasal subtype in the Lund University subtyping model;↑, high value;↓, low value.

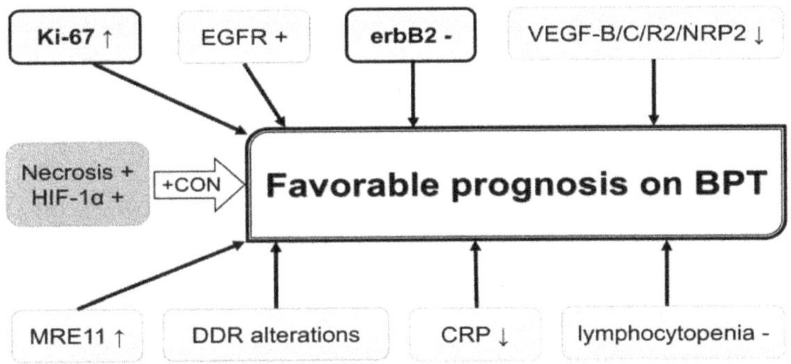

Figure 2. Biomarkers that may be used for predicting and improving prognosis on bladder preservation therapy. Biomarkers in bold letter are also associated with favorable chemoradiation response. Biomarkers in dark shadow are associated with unfavorable clinical outcomes, which can be overcome by CON. BPT, bladder preservation therapy; CON, carbogen and nicotinamide; CRP, C-reactive protein; DDR, DNA damage response; EGFR, epidermal growth factor receptor; erbB2, erythroblastic leukemia viral oncogene homolog 2; HIF-1α, hypoxia-inducible factor-1α; MRE11, meiotic recombination 11; NRP2, neutropilin 2; VEGF, vascular endothelial growth factor;↑, increased expression;↓, decreased expression or low value.

The introduction of immune-oncology drugs (IODs) to daily clinical practices may create a paradigm shift in the management of bladder cancer patients. IODs have the potential to provide long-term survival to a subset of metastatic bladder cancer patients who are considered incurable in the pre-IOD era [55]. Currently, chemoradiation-based BPT is proposed for non-metastatic MIBC patients who desire to retain their bladders and for whom RC is not a treatment option [2]. Hereafter, indications of intensive therapy to the primary site, including chemoradiation and RC, may expand to metastatic MIBC patients for whom long-term survival is expected on IODs. In this respect, identification of biomarkers and development of biomarker panels for comprehensively predicting clinical courses of bladder cancer patients are in increasing demand. In the near future, progress on biomarker research could allow for personalized management of MIBC patients, including those with metastatic disease, eventually providing better prognosis and QOL with BPT and IODs for optimally select patients.

Author Contributions: All authors made substantial contributions to this work; acquisition and interpretation of data by online search, F.K., K.T., and H.F.; draft and supervision of the work, F.K.; revision of the work, F.K., K.T., and H.F. All authors have approved the final version and agree to be personally accountable for the author's own contributions.

Acknowledgments: This work was partly supported by JSPS KAKENHI Grant Number JP 17K11167 (F.K.).

References

1. Siegel, R.L.; Miller, K.D.; Jemal, A. Cancer statistics, 2018. *CA Cancer J. Clin.* **2018**, *68*, 7–30. [CrossRef] [PubMed]
2. Chang, S.S.; Bochner, B.H.; Chou, R.; Dreicer, R.; Kamat, A.M.; Lerner, S.P.; Lotan, Y.; Meeks, J.J.; Michalski, J.M.; Morgan, T.M.; et al. Treatment of Non-Metastatic Muscle-Invasive Bladder Cancer: AUA/ASCO/ASTRO/SUO Guideline. *J. Urol.* **2017**, *198*, 552–559. [CrossRef] [PubMed]
3. Novara, G.; Catto, J.W.; Wilson, T.; Annerstedt, M.; Chan, K.; Murphy, D.G.; Motttrie, A.; Peabody, J.O.; Skinner, E.C.; Wiklund, P.N.; et al. Systematic review and cumulative analysis of perioperative outcomes and complications after robot-assisted radical cystectomy. *Eur. Urol.* **2015**, *67*, 376–401. [CrossRef] [PubMed]
4. Gilbert, S.M.; Wood, D.P.; Dunn, R.L.; Weizer, A.Z.; Lee, C.T.; Montie, J.E.; Wei, J.T. Measuring health-related quality of life outcomes in bladder cancer patients using the Bladder Cancer Index (BCI). *Cancer* **2007**, *109*, 1756–1762. [CrossRef] [PubMed]

5. Koga, F.; Kihara, K. Selective bladder preservation with curative intent for muscle-invasive bladder cancer: A contemporary review. *Int. J. Urol.* **2012**, *19*, 388–401. [CrossRef] [PubMed]
6. Giacalone, N.J.; Shipley, W.U.; Clayman, R.H.; Niemierko, A.; Drumm, M.; Heney, N.M.; Michaelson, M.D.; Lee, R.J.; Saylor, P.J.; Wszolek, M.F.; et al. Long-term Outcomes After Bladder-preserving Tri-modality Therapy for Patients with Muscle-invasive Bladder Cancer: An Updated Analysis of the Massachusetts General Hospital Experience. *Eur. Urol.* **2017**, *71*, 952–960. [CrossRef] [PubMed]
7. Ploussard, G.; Daneshmand, S.; Efstathiou, J.A.; Herr, H.W.; James, N.D.; Rodel, C.M.; Shariat, S.F.; Shipley, W.U.; Sternberg, C.N.; Thalmann, G.N.; et al. Critical analysis of bladder sparing with trimodal therapy in muscle-invasive bladder cancer: A systematic review. *Eur. Urol.* **2014**, *66*, 120–137. [CrossRef] [PubMed]
8. Rodel, C.; Grabenbauer, G.G.; Kuhn, R.; Papadopoulos, T.; Dunst, J.; Meyer, M.; Schrott, K.M.; Sauer, R. Combined-modality treatment and selective organ preservation in invasive bladder cancer: Long-term results. *J. Clin. Oncol.* **2002**, *20*, 3061–3071. [CrossRef] [PubMed]
9. Koga, F.; Numao, N.; Saito, K.; Masuda, H.; Fujii, Y.; Kawakami, S.; Kihara, K. Sensitivity to chemoradiation predicts development of metastasis in muscle-invasive bladder cancer patients. *Urol. Oncol.* **2013**, *31*, 1270–1275. [CrossRef] [PubMed]
10. Coppin, C.M.; Gospodarowicz, M.K.; James, K.; Tannock, I.F.; Zee, B.; Carson, J.; Pater, J.; Sullivan, L.D. Improved local control of invasive bladder cancer by concurrent cisplatin and preoperative or definitive radiation. The National Cancer Institute of Canada Clinical Trials Group. *J. Clin. Oncol.* **1996**, *14*, 2901–2907. [CrossRef] [PubMed]
11. James, N.D.; Hussain, S.A.; Hall, E.; Jenkins, P.; Tremlett, J.; Rawlings, C.; Crundwell, M.; Sizer, B.; Sreenivasan, T.; Hendron, C.; et al. Radiotherapy with or without chemotherapy in muscle-invasive bladder cancer. *N. Engl. J. Med.* **2012**, *366*, 1477–1488. [CrossRef] [PubMed]
12. Choudhury, A.; Swindell, R.; Logue, J.P.; Elliott, P.A.; Livsey, J.E.; Wise, M.; Symonds, P.; Wylie, J.P.; Ramani, V.; Sangar, V.; et al. Phase II study of conformal hypofractionated radiotherapy with concurrent gemcitabine in muscle-invasive bladder cancer. *J. Clin. Oncol.* **2011**, *29*, 733–738. [CrossRef] [PubMed]
13. Muller, A.C.; Diestelhorst, A.; Kuhnt, T.; Kuhn, R.; Fornara, P.; Scholz, H.J.; Dunst, J.; Zietman, A.L. Organ-sparing treatment of advanced bladder cancer: Paclitaxel as a radiosensitizer. *Strahlenther. Onkol.* **2007**, *183*, 177–183. [CrossRef] [PubMed]
14. Iwai, A.; Koga, F.; Fujii, Y.; Masuda, H.; Saito, K.; Numao, N.; Sakura, M.; Kawakami, S.; Kihara, K. Perioperative complications of radical cystectomy after induction chemoradiotherapy in bladder-sparing protocol against muscle-invasive bladder cancer: A single institutional retrospective comparative study with primary radical cystectomy. *Jpn. J. Clin. Oncol.* **2011**, *41*, 1373–1379. [CrossRef] [PubMed]
15. Koga, F.; Kihara, K.; Yoshida, S.; Yokoyama, M.; Saito, K.; Masuda, H.; Fujii, Y.; Kawakami, S. Selective bladder-sparing protocol consisting of induction low-dose chemoradiotherapy plus partial cystectomy with pelvic lymph node dissection against muscle-invasive bladder cancer: Oncological outcomes of the initial 46 patients. *BJU Int.* **2012**, *109*, 860–866. [CrossRef] [PubMed]
16. Koga, F.; Yoshida, S.; Kawakami, S.; Kageyama, Y.; Yokoyama, M.; Saito, K.; Fujii, Y.; Kobayashi, T.; Kihara, K. Low-dose chemoradiotherapy followed by partial or radical cystectomy against muscle-invasive bladder cancer: An intent-to-treat survival analysis. *Urology* **2008**, *72*, 384–388. [CrossRef] [PubMed]
17. Azuma, H.; Inamoto, T.; Takahara, K.; Nomi, H.; Hirano, H.; Ibuki, N.; Uehara, H.; Komura, K.; Minami, K.; Uchimoto, T.; et al. Novel bladder preservation therapy with Osaka Medical College regimen. *J. Urol.* **2015**, *193*, 443–450. [CrossRef] [PubMed]
18. Cahn, D.B.; Handorf, E.A.; Ghiraldi, E.M.; Ristau, B.T.; Geynisman, D.M.; Churilla, T.M.; Horwitz, E.M.; Sobczak, M.L.; Chen, D.Y.T.; Viterbo, R.; et al. Contemporary use trends and survival outcomes in patients undergoing radical cystectomy or bladder-preservation therapy for muscle-invasive bladder cancer. *Cancer* **2017**, *123*, 4337–4345. [CrossRef] [PubMed]
19. Ritch, C.R.; Balise, R.; Prakash, N.S.; Alonzo, D.; Almengo, K.; Alameddine, M.; Venkatramani, V.; Punnen, S.; Parekh, D.J.; Gonzalgo, M.L. Propensity matched comparative analysis of survival following chemoradiation or radical cystectomy for muscle-invasive bladder cancer. *BJU Int.* **2018**, *121*, 745–751. [CrossRef] [PubMed]
20. Kulkarni, G.S.; Hermanns, T.; Wei, Y.; Bhindi, B.; Satkunasivam, R.; Athanasopoulos, P.; Bostrom, P.J.; Kuk, C.; Li, K.; Templeton, A.J.; et al. Propensity Score Analysis of Radical Cystectomy Versus Bladder-Sparing

Trimodal Therapy in the Setting of a Multidisciplinary Bladder Cancer Clinic. *J. Clin. Oncol.* **2017**, *35*, 2299–2305. [CrossRef] [PubMed]

21. Coen, J.J.; Paly, J.J.; Niemierko, A.; Kaufman, D.S.; Heney, N.M.; Spiegel, D.Y.; Efstathiou, J.A.; Zietman, A.L.; Shipley, W.U. Nomograms predicting response to therapy and outcomes after bladder-preserving trimodality therapy for muscle-invasive bladder cancer. *Int. J. Radiat. Oncol. Biol. Phys.* **2013**, *86*, 311–316. [CrossRef] [PubMed]
22. Rodel, C.; Grabenbauer, G.G.; Rodel, F.; Birkenhake, S.; Kuhn, R.; Martus, P.; Zorcher, T.; Fursich, D.; Papadopoulos, T.; Dunst, J.; et al. Apoptosis, p53, bcl-2, and Ki-67 in invasive bladder carcinoma: Possible predictors for response to radiochemotherapy and successful bladder preservation. *Int. J. Radiat. Oncol. Biol. Phys.* **2000**, *46*, 1213–1221. [CrossRef]
23. Matsumoto, H.; Wada, T.; Fukunaga, K.; Yoshihiro, S.; Matsuyama, H.; Naito, K. Bax to Bcl-2 ratio and Ki-67 index are useful predictors of neoadjuvant chemoradiation therapy in bladder cancer. *Jpn. J. Clin. Oncol.* **2004**, *34*, 124–130. [CrossRef] [PubMed]
24. Tanabe, K.; Yoshida, S.; Koga, F.; Inoue, M.; Kobayashi, S.; Ishioka, J.; Tamura, T.; Sugawara, E.; Saito, K.; Akashi, T.; et al. High Ki-67 Expression Predicts Favorable Survival in Muscle-Invasive Bladder Cancer Patients Treated with Chemoradiation-Based Bladder-Sparing Protocol. *Clin. Genitourin. Cancer* **2015**, *13*, e243-51. [CrossRef] [PubMed]
25. Yoshida, S.; Koga, F.; Kobayashi, S.; Ishii, C.; Tanaka, H.; Tanaka, H.; Komai, Y.; Saito, K.; Masuda, H.; Fujii, Y.; et al. Role of diffusion-weighted magnetic resonance imaging in predicting sensitivity to chemoradiotherapy in muscle-invasive bladder cancer. *Int. J. Radiat. Oncol. Biol. Phys.* **2012**, *83*, e21-7. [CrossRef] [PubMed]
26. Chakravarti, A.; Winter, K.; Wu, C.L.; Kaufman, D.; Hammond, E.; Parliament, M.; Tester, W.; Hagan, M.; Grignon, D.; Heney, N.; et al. Expression of the epidermal growth factor receptor and Her-2 are predictors of favorable outcome and reduced complete response rates, respectively, in patients with muscle-invading bladder cancers treated by concurrent radiation and cisplatin-based chemotherapy: A report from the Radiation Therapy Oncology Group. *Int. J. Radiat. Oncol. Biol. Phys.* **2005**, *62*, 309–317. [PubMed]
27. Inoue, M.; Koga, F.; Yoshida, S.; Tamura, T.; Fujii, Y.; Ito, E.; Kihara, K. Significance of ERBB2 overexpression in therapeutic resistance and cancer-specific survival in muscle-invasive bladder cancer patients treated with chemoradiation-based selective bladder-sparing approach. *Int. J. Radiat. Oncol. Biol. Phys.* **2014**, *90*, 303–311. [CrossRef] [PubMed]
28. Michaelson, M.D.; Hu, C.; Pham, H.T.; Dahl, D.M.; Lee-Wu, C.; Swanson, G.P.; Vuky, J.; Lee, R.J.; Souhami, L.; Chang, B.; et al. A Phase 1/2 Trial of a Combination of Paclitaxel and Trastuzumab With Daily Irradiation or Paclitaxel Alone with Daily Irradiation After Transurethral Surgery for Noncystectomy Candidates With Muscle-Invasive Bladder Cancer (Trial NRG Oncology RTOG 0524). *Int. J. Radiat. Oncol. Biol. Phys.* **2017**, *97*, 995–1001. [CrossRef] [PubMed]
29. Kawashima, A.; Nakayama, M.; Kakuta, Y.; Abe, T.; Hatano, K.; Mukai, M.; Nagahara, A.; Nakai, Y.; Oka, D.; Takayama, H.; et al. Excision repair cross-complementing group 1 may predict the efficacy of chemoradiation therapy for muscle-invasive bladder cancer. *Clin. Cancer Res.* **2011**, *17*, 2561–2569. [CrossRef] [PubMed]
30. Tanaka, H.; Yoshida, S.; Koga, F.; Toda, K.; Yoshimura, R.; Nakajima, Y.; Sugawara, E.; Akashi, T.; Waseda, Y.; Inoue, M.; et al. Impact of Immunohistochemistry-Based Subtypes in Muscle-Invasive Bladder Cancer on Response to Chemoradiotherapy. *Int. J. Radiat. Oncol. Biol. Phys.* **2018**. [CrossRef] [PubMed]
31. Urushibara, M.; Kageyama, Y.; Akashi, T.; Otsuka, Y.; Takizawa, T.; Koike, M.; Kihara, K. HSP60 may predict good pathological response to neoadjuvant chemoradiotherapy in bladder cancer. *Jpn. J. Clin. Oncol.* **2007**, *37*, 56–61. [CrossRef] [PubMed]
32. Lautenschlaeger, T.; George, A.; Klimowicz, A.C.; Efstathiou, J.A.; Wu, C.L.; Sandler, H.; Shipley, W.U.; Tester, W.J.; Hagan, M.P.; Magliocco, A.M.; et al. Bladder preservation therapy for muscle-invading bladder cancers on Radiation Therapy Oncology Group trials 8802, *8903*, 9506, and 9706: Vascular endothelial growth factor B overexpression predicts for increased distant metastasis and shorter survival. *Oncologist* **2013**, *18*, 685–686. [CrossRef] [PubMed]
33. Keck, B.; Wach, S.; Taubert, H.; Zeiler, S.; Ott, O.J.; Kunath, F.; Hartmann, A.; Bertz, S.; Weiss, C.; Honscheid, P.; et al. Neuropilin-2 and its ligand VEGF-C predict treatment response after transurethral resection and radiochemotherapy in bladder cancer patients. *Int. J. Cancer* **2015**, *136*, 443–451. [CrossRef] [PubMed]

34. Choudhury, A.; Nelson, L.D.; Teo, M.T.; Chilka, S.; Bhattarai, S.; Johnston, C.F.; Elliott, F.; Lowery, J.; Taylor, C.F.; Churchman, M.; et al. MRE11 expression is predictive of cause-specific survival following radical radiotherapy for muscle-invasive bladder cancer. *Cancer Res.* **2010**, *70*, 7017–7026. [CrossRef] [PubMed]
35. Sakano, S.; Ogawa, S.; Yamamoto, Y.; Nishijima, J.; Miyachika, Y.; Matsumoto, H.; Hara, T.; Matsuyama, H. ERCC1 and XRCC1 expression predicts survival in bladder cancer patients receiving combined trimodality therapy. *Mol. Clin. Oncol.* **2013**, *1*, 403–410. [CrossRef] [PubMed]
36. Desai, N.B.; Scott, S.N.; Zabor, E.C.; Cha, E.K.; Hreiki, J.; Sfakianos, J.P.; Ramirez, R.; Bagrodia, A.; Rosenberg, J.E.; Bajorin, D.F.; et al. Genomic characterization of response to chemoradiation in urothelial bladder cancer. *Cancer* **2016**, *122*, 3715–3723. [CrossRef] [PubMed]
37. Eustace, A.; Irlam, J.J.; Taylor, J.; Denley, H.; Agrawal, S.; Choudhury, A.; Ryder, D.; Ord, J.J.; Harris, A.L.; Rojas, A.M.; et al. Necrosis predicts benefit from hypoxia-modifying therapy in patients with high risk bladder cancer enrolled in a phase III randomised trial. *Radiother. Oncol.* **2013**, *108*, 40–47. [CrossRef] [PubMed]
38. Hunter, B.A.; Eustace, A.; Irlam, J.J.; Valentine, H.R.; Denley, H.; Oguejiofor, K.K.; Swindell, R.; Hoskin, P.J.; Choudhury, A.; West, C.M. Expression of hypoxia-inducible factor-1alpha predicts benefit from hypoxia modification in invasive bladder cancer. *Br. J. Cancer* **2014**, *111*, 437–443. [CrossRef] [PubMed]
39. Yoshida, S.; Saito, K.; Koga, F.; Yokoyama, M.; Kageyama, Y.; Masuda, H.; Kobayashi, T.; Kawakami, S.; Kihara, K. C-reactive protein level predicts prognosis in patients with muscle-invasive bladder cancer treated with chemoradiotherapy. *BJU Int.* **2008**, *101*, 978–981. [CrossRef] [PubMed]
40. Joseph, N.; Dovedi, S.J.; Thompson, C.; Lyons, J.; Kennedy, J.; Elliott, T.; West, C.M.; Choudhury, A. Pre-treatment lymphocytopaenia is an adverse prognostic biomarker in muscle-invasive and advanced bladder cancer. *Ann. Oncol.* **2016**, *27*, 294–299. [CrossRef] [PubMed]
41. Zinkel, S.; Gross, A.; Yang, E. BCL2 family in DNA damage and cell cycle control. *Cell Death Differ.* **2006**, *13*, 1351–1359. [CrossRef] [PubMed]
42. Margulis, V.; Lotan, Y.; Karakiewicz, P.I.; Fradet, Y.; Ashfaq, R.; Capitanio, U.; Montorsi, F.; Bastian, P.J.; Nielsen, M.E.; Muller, S.C.; et al. Multi-institutional validation of the predictive value of Ki-67 labeling index in patients with urinary bladder cancer. *J. Natl. Cancer Inst.* **2009**, *101*, 114–119. [CrossRef] [PubMed]
43. Koh, D.M.; Collins, D.J. Diffusion-weighted MRI in the body: Applications and challenges in oncology. *AJR Am. J. Roentgenol.* **2007**, *188*, 1622–1635. [CrossRef] [PubMed]
44. Mitsudomi, T.; Yatabe, Y. Epidermal growth factor receptor in relation to tumor development: EGFR gene and cancer. *FEBS J.* **2010**, *277*, 301–308. [CrossRef] [PubMed]
45. Harris, A.L. Hypoxia—A key regulatory factor in tumour growth. *Nat. Rev. Cancer* **2002**, *2*, 38–47. [CrossRef] [PubMed]
46. Thompson, L.H. Recognition, signaling, and repair of DNA double-strand breaks produced by ionizing radiation in mammalian cells: The molecular choreography. *Mutat. Res.* **2012**, *751*, 158–246. [CrossRef] [PubMed]
47. Hanawalt, P.C.; Spivak, G. Transcription-coupled DNA repair: Two decades of progress and surprises. *Nat. Rev. Mol. Cell Biol.* **2008**, *9*, 958–970. [CrossRef] [PubMed]
48. Iyer, G.; Balar, A.V.; Milowsky, M.I.; Bochner, B.H.; Dalbagni, G.; Donat, S.M.; Herr, H.W.; Huang, W.C.; Taneja, S.S.; Woods, M.; et al. Multicenter Prospective Phase II Trial of Neoadjuvant Dose-Dense Gemcitabine Plus Cisplatin in Patients with Muscle-Invasive Bladder Cancer. *J. Clin. Oncol.* **2018**, *36*, 1949–1956. [CrossRef] [PubMed]
49. Plimack, E.R.; Dunbrack, R.L.; Brennan, T.A.; Andrake, M.D.; Zhou, Y.; Serebriiskii, I.G.; Slifker, M.; Alpaugh, K.; Dulaimi, E.; Palma, N.; et al. Defects in DNA Repair Genes Predict Response to Neoadjuvant Cisplatin-based Chemotherapy in Muscle-invasive Bladder Cancer. *Eur. Urol.* **2015**, *68*, 959–967. [CrossRef] [PubMed]
50. Teo, M.Y.; Bambury, R.M.; Zabor, E.C.; Jordan, E.; Al-Ahmadie, H.; Boyd, M.E.; Bouvier, N.; Mullane, S.A.; Cha, E.K.; Roper, N.; et al. DNA Damage Response and Repair Gene Alterations Are Associated with Improved Survival in Patients with Platinum-Treated Advanced Urothelial Carcinoma. *Clin. Cancer Res.* **2017**, *23*, 3610–3618. [CrossRef] [PubMed]
51. Hoskin, P.J.; Rojas, A.M.; Bentzen, S.M.; Saunders, M.I. Radiotherapy with concurrent carbogen and nicotinamide in bladder carcinoma. *J. Clin. Oncol.* **2010**, *28*, 4912–4918. [CrossRef] [PubMed]

52. Cancer Genome Atlas Research Network. Comprehensive molecular characterization of urothelial bladder carcinoma. *Nature* **2014**, *507*, 315–322. [CrossRef] [PubMed]

53. Choi, W.; Porten, S.; Kim, S.; Willis, D.; Plimack, E.R.; Hoffman-Censits, J.; Roth, B.; Cheng, T.; Tran, M.; Lee, I.L.; et al. Identification of distinct basal and luminal subtypes of muscle-invasive bladder cancer with different sensitivities to frontline chemotherapy. *Cancer Cell* **2014**, *25*, 152–165. [CrossRef] [PubMed]

54. Sjodahl, G.; Lovgren, K.; Lauss, M.; Patschan, O.; Gudjonsson, S.; Chebil, G.; Aine, M.; Eriksson, P.; Mansson, W.; Lindgren, D.; et al. Toward a molecular pathologic classification of urothelial carcinoma. *Am. J. Pathol.* **2013**, *183*, 681–691. [CrossRef] [PubMed]

55. Bellmunt, J.; de Wit, R.; Vaughn, D.J.; Fradet, Y.; Lee, J.L.; Fong, L.; Vogelzang, N.J.; Climent, M.A.; Petrylak, D.P.; Choueiri, T.K.; et al. Pembrolizumab as Second-Line Therapy for Advanced Urothelial Carcinoma. *N. Engl. J. Med.* **2017**, *376*, 1015–1026. [CrossRef] [PubMed]

Aberrant *N*-Glycosylation Profile of Serum Immunoglobulins is a Diagnostic Biomarker of Urothelial Carcinomas

Toshikazu Tanaka [1], Tohru Yoneyama [2,*], Daisuke Noro [1], Kengo Imanishi [1], Yuta Kojima [1], Shingo Hatakeyama [1], Yuki Tobisawa [1], Kazuyuki Mori [1], Hayato Yamamoto [1], Atsushi Imai [1], Takahiro Yoneyama [1], Yasuhiro Hashimoto [2], Takuya Koie [1], Masakazu Tanaka [3], Shin-Ichiro Nishimura [3], Shizuka Kurauchi [4], Ippei Takahashi [4] and Chikara Ohyama [1,2]

1 Department of Urology, Hirosaki University Graduate School of Medicine, Hirosaki 036-8562, Japan; yosage1205@yahoo.co.jp (T.T.); noro.daisuke@camel.plala.or.jp (D.N.); born_2b_snower@yahoo.co.jp (K.I.); y_kojima0319@yahoo.co.jp (Y.K.); shingoh@hirosaki-u.ac.jp (S.H.); tobisawa@hirosaki-u.ac.jp (Y.T.); moribio@hirosaki-u.ac.jp (K.M.); yamahaya10@yahoo.co.jp (H.Y.); tsushi.imai@gmail.com (A.I.); uroyone@hirosaki-u.ac.jp (T.Y.); goodwin@hirosaki-u.ac.jp (T.K.); coyama@hirosaki-u.ac.jp (C.O.)

2 Department of Advanced Transplant and Regenerative Medicine, Hirosaki University Graduate School of Medicine, Hirosaki 036-8562, Japan; bikkuri@opal.plala.or.jp

3 Graduate School of Life Science, Frontier Research Centre for Advanced Material and Life Science, Hokkaido University, Sapporo 060-0810, Japan; tanaka@soyaku.co.jp (M.T.); shin@sci.hokudai.ac.jp (S.-I.N.)

4 Department of Social Medicine, Hirosaki University Graduate School of Medicine, Hirosaki 036-8562, Japan; k-shizu@hirosaki-u.ac.jp (S.K.); ippei@hirosaki-u.ac.jp (I.T.)

* Correspondence: tohruyon@hirosaki-u.ac.jp

Abstract: The aim of this study to determine whether the aberrant *N*-glycosylated serum immunoglobulins (Igs) can be applied as a diagnostic marker of urothelial carcinoma (UC). Between 2009 and 2016, we randomly obtained serum available from 237 UC and also 96 prostate cancer as other cancer controls from our serum bank and also obtained—from 339 healthy volunteers (HV)—controls obtained from community-dwelling volunteers in Iwaki Health Promotion Project. A total of 32 types of *N*-glycan levels on Igs were determined by high-throughput *N*-glycomics and analyzed by multivariable discriminant analysis. We found five UC-associated aberrant *N*-glycans changes on Igs and also found that asialo-bisecting GlcNAc type *N*-glycan on Igs were significantly accumulated in UC patients. The diagnostic *N*-glycan Score (d*N*GScore) established by combination of five *N*-glycans on Igs discriminated UC patients from HV and prostate cancer (PC) patients with 92.8% sensitivity and 97.2% specificity. The area under the curve (AUC) for of the d*N*GScore was 0.969 for UC detection that was much superior to that of urine cytology (AUC, 0.707) and hematuria (AUC, 0.892). Furthermore, d*N*GScore can detect hematuria and urine cytology negative patients. The d*N*Gscore based on aberrant *N*-glycosylation signatures of Igs were found to be promising diagnostic biomarkers of UCs.

Keywords: diagnostic biomarker; urothelial carcinoma of the bladder; upper urinary tract urothelial carcinoma; *N*-glycomics; immunogloburins; aberrant *N*-glycosylation

---

1. Introduction

Urothelial carcinomas (UCs) are the eighth-most lethal cancer in men in the United States [1]. The majority of UCs originate from bladder, called UC of the bladder (UCB), and between 5% and 10% of UCs originate from the ureter or renal pelvis [2,3], which are collectively called upper urinary tract UCs (UTUCs), with a worse prognosis than that of UCB. The most common symptom is visible- or non-visible hematuria (70–80%) [4,5] and then the standard examinations are performed, involving urine cytology, urinary tract imaging and cystoscopy, which are powerful diagnostic tools for UCs. However, 60% of UTUCs are invasive at time of diagnosis [6,7]. Urine cytology is not reliable in patients with early stage UCs, including UTUC, and it is difficult to visualise small tumors via imaging modalities, such as ultrasound or computed tomography. Several diagnostic urine-based biomarkers are reported such as bladder tumor antigen (BTA), nuclear matrix protein number 22 (NMP22) and UroVysion [8–10]. Although sensitivities can be better for BTA (50–80%), NMP22 (68.5–88.5%) and UroVysion (58–96%) over urine cytology (50–67%), the specificities are quite low. Because those tests are soluble antigen test or cellular assay depending on the amount of tumor cells, they are not suitable for the detection of low-grade and low-stage tumors. Furthermore, the prevalence of urinary markers of only about 30% is not enough to complement urine cytology and other invasive tests. Thus, more sensitive and non-invasive biomarkers, such as serum-based biomarkers, to avoid under-detection in patients at high risk of UCs is required.

Glycosylation is a common post-translational modification that has an important role in various biological functions. Previously, our group demonstrated that high-throughput, comprehensive and quantitative *N*-glycomics based on the glycoblotting method combined with mass spectrometry is a promising way to screen glycans for use as diagnostic and prognostic markers of several cancer [11–15]. Recently, the evaluation of glycosylation profile is an innovative topic in different cancer types, especially in immunotherapeutic targets, as like as PD-L1 [16–18]. Most recently, our group reported that a combination of several serum *N*-glycans (*N*-glycan score, *N*GScore) is a novel serum marker for UCs including UTUC that detected 93% of UC patients and is therefore far more specific than classic urine cytology [19]. We hypothesized that these serum aberrant *N*-glycan change is derived from serum major *N*-glycosylated proteins, such as immunoglobulins (Igs). Although differences in Ig glycosylation are mainly described in immune system-related diseases [20–23], there are several papers describing aberrant glycosylation of IgG in cancer such as prostate cancer, gastric cancer and colorectal cancer [24–27]. In addition, aberrant *N*-glycosylation of immunoglobulins in UC has not been reported elsewhere. Thus, in the present study, we performed *N*-glycomics of serum Igs fractions between healthy volunteers (HVs), prostate cancer (PC) and UCs patients to identify the UC-specific aberrant *N*-glycosylated Igs. Furthermore, for clinical applications, we established a diagnostic *N*GScore (d*N*GScore) based on a combination of five *N*-glycans of Igs associated with detection of UCs.

2. Results

2.1. *Downregulation of Asialo Biantennary Type N-Glycans and Accumulation of Asialo-Bisecting GlcNAc with Core Fucosylated N-Glycan on Igs May Occur as a UC-Associated Aberrant N-Glycosylation of Igs*

SDS-PAGE analysis between whole serum (Figure A1b, lanes 1–4) and Igs fractions (Figure A1b, lanes 5–8) revealed that non-Igs proteins were effectively eliminated from whole serum by Melon Gel chromatography. *N*-glycomics of the Igs fraction (Figure A1a–e) identified 32 types of BOA-labelled *N*-glycans on Igs (Table A1, Figure A1f). Patient characteristics in the non-UC (HV and PC) and UC groups are shown in Table 1. There were no statistically significant differences in age, history of smoking, benign prostatic hyperplasia (BPH) and stone former between both non-UC group and UC group.

To detect UC, we performed multivariable discriminant analysis by inputting UCs event as an explanatory variable and the *N*-glycan level of Igs as objective variables and selected candidate *N*-glycans (complex biantennary type: m/z 1606, 1769, 2074; core fucosylated bisecting GlcNAc type: m/z 2118, 2423) that formed the most sensitive and specific combination for detection of UCs (Figure 1a–c and Table 2).

Table 1. Patients' demographics in each cohort.

	Non-UC [a]		UC [b]	*p* Value a vs. b
	HV *n*, (%)	PC *n*, (%)	*n*, (%)	
Total patients (*n*)	339	96	237	
Sex (Male, %)	122 (36.0)	96 (100)	191 (80.6)	<0.001
Median age (IQR [1])	68.0 (63–73)	74.0 (68–78)	70.0 (62–75)	0.700
Former or current smoker	75 (22.1)	18 (18.8)	71 (29.9)	0.101
Stone former	4 (1.2)	0 (0)	0 (0)	0.184
BPH [2]	7 (2.1)	0 (0)	0 (0)	0.145
HSPC [3]	0 (0)	96 (100)	0 (0)	<0.001
hematuria+	0 (0)	0 (0)	186 (78.5)	<0.001
Urine Cytology Class				
I, II			81 (34.2)	
III			58 (24.5)	
IV			16 (6.7)	
V			82 (34.6)	
Tumor Location of UC				
Bladder			177 (67.6)	
Renal pelvis			27 (11.4)	
Ureter			28 (11.8)	
Multiple			4 (1.7)	
Tumor Grade of UC				
Low grade noninvasive			68 (28.7)	
High grade noninvasive			43 (18.1)	
Muscle invasive			109 (45.9)	
Lymph node stage N1		0 (0.0)	20 (8.4)	0.115
Metastatic disease		4 (4.2)	47 (19.8)	0.010

[1] IQR, Interquartile range; [2] BPH, benign prostatic hyperplasia; [3] HSPC, hormone sensitive prostate cancer; HV: healthy volunteers; PC: prostate cancer. [a] non-urothelial carcinoma, non-UC; [b] urothelial carcinoma, UC.

Table 2. Multivariable discriminant analysis for prediction of UCs.

Variables	Wilks' Lambda	*F* Value	ODF [1]	TDF [2]	*p* Value	Discriminant Function
m/z 1606	0.9742	17.72	1	670	<0.001	0.1925
m/z 1769	0.9707	20.24	1	670	<0.001	0.4932
m/z 2074	0.9377	44.54	1	670	<0.001	0.4941
m/z 2118	0.5894	466.73	1	670	<0.001	-3.2460
m/z 2423	0.9984	1.04	1	670	<0.001	0.6179
				Constant term		-0.4905

[1] ODF, one degree of freedom; [2] TDF, two degrees of freedom.

The asialo biantennary type *N*-glycans (*m/z* 1606 and 2074) on Igs were significantly downregulated in the UC group compared with the levels in the HV and PC groups ($p = 0.0001$). Only the asialo biantennary type *N*-glycan (*m/z* 1769) on Igs was significantly downregulated in the PC group compared with the level in the UC and HV groups ($p = 0.0001$). The monosialyl bisecting GlcNAc with core fucosylated bisecting GlcNAc *N*-glycan (*m/z* 2423) was not significantly changed between UC and HV group, but significantly decreased in PC and UTUC group ($p = 0.0001$). Especially the asialo bisecting GlcNAc with core fucosylated *N*-glycan (*m/z* 2118) on Igs was significantly upregulated in UC group ($p = 0.0001$) but not detectable in HV and PC groups. However, total Igs level in UC patients was significantly lower than HV and PC patients (Figure 2a–d).

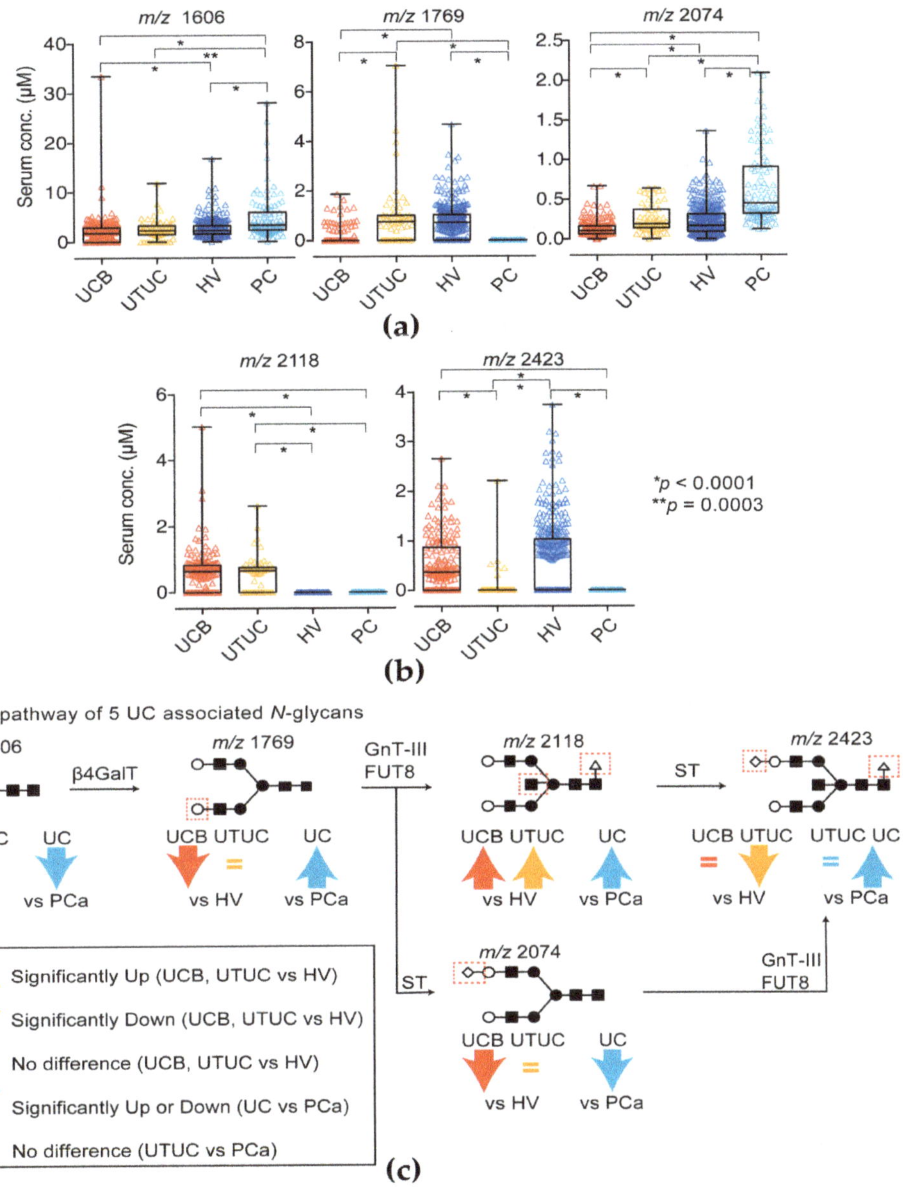

Figure 1. Five UC-associated *N*-glycan levels of immunoglobulins (Igs) fractions. (**a**) Complex biantennary-type *N*-glycan (m/z 1606, 1769 and 2074) levels and (**b**) fucosylated bisecting GlcNAc-type *N*-glycan (m/z 2118 and 2423) of the Ig fractions in the UC, HV and PC groups. The results shown are representative of three independent experiments. Intergroup differences were statistically compared using the Mann–Whitney *U*-test for non-normally distributed models; (**c**) Synthetic pathway of candidate *N*-glycans in the present study. Red up- and downward arrows indicates significantly changed in UC compare with HV group. Cyan up- and downward arrows indicates significantly changed in UC compare with PC group. The equals mark indicates that it did not significantly change. *N*-glycan structures are indicated by monosaccharide symbols: white circles, galactose (Gal); black circles, mannose (Man); black squares, *N*-acetylglucosamine (GlcNAc); black triangle, fucose (Fuc) and black diamonds, sialic acid. β4GalT: β1,4-galactosyltransferase, GnT-III: *N*-acetylglucosaminyltransferase-III, FUT8: fucosyltransferase 8, ST: sialyltransferase.

According to the synthetic pathway of *N*-glycans shown in Figure 1b and the above results, a downregulation of asialo biantennary type *N*-glycans and accumulation of asialo-bisecting GlcNAc with core fucosylated *N*-glycan on Igs may occur as a UC-associated aberrant *N*-glycosylation of Igs.

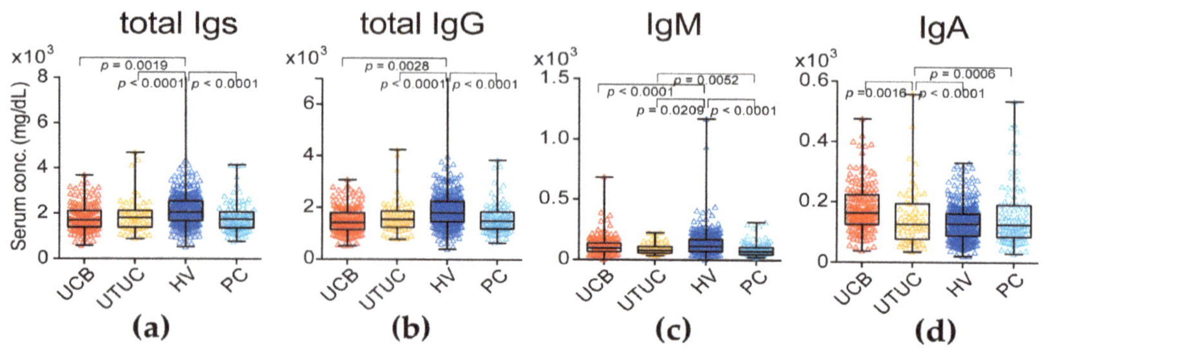

Figure 2. Serum immunoglobulin (Ig) levels in UC (UC of the bladder (UCB) and upper urinary tract UC (UTUC)) patients and healthy volunteers (HVs) and prostate cancer (PC). (**a**) Serum total Igs (sum of IgG1-4, IgM and IgA) levels in the UC, HV and PC groups; (**b**) Serum total IgG (IgG1-4) levels in the UC, HV and PC groups; (**c**) Serum IgM levels in the UC, HV and PC groups; (**d**) Serum IgA levels in the UC, HV and PC groups. The results shown are representative of three independent experiments. Intergroup differences were statistically compared using the Mann–Whitney *U*-test for non-normally distributed models.

2.2. UC Diagnostic N-Glycan Score Based on Aberrant N-Glycosylation of Igs Was Far Superior to Classic Urine Cytology and Hematuria Status

To apply these candidate aberrant *N*-glycosylation profile on Igs for UC detection, we established the UC diagnostic *N*-glycan score (d*N*GScore) that was calculated according to the following formula:

$$\text{d}N\text{GScore} = (\text{serum level of } m/z\ 1606 \times 0.1925) + (\text{serum level of } m/z\ 1769 \times 0.4932) + (\text{serum level of } m/z\ 2074 \times 0.4941) + (\text{serum level of } m/z\ 2118 \times -3.2460) + (\text{serum level of } m/z\ 2423 \times 0.6179) + (-0.4905) \quad (1)$$

The d*N*GScore was significantly lower in the UC (UCB and UTUC) patients than in the non-UC group including HVs and PC (Mann–Whitney *U*-test: $p = 0.0001$, permutation test: $p = 0.001$) (Figure 3a,c). The d*N*GScore of UCB was significantly lower than those of HV (Mann–Whitney *U*-test: $p = 0.0001$, permutation test: $p = 0.012$) and PC (Mann–Whitney *U*-test: $p = 0.0001$, permutation test: $p = 0.0017$) (Figure 3a). The d*N*GScore of UTUC was also significantly lower than those of HV (Mann–Whitney *U*-test: $p = 0.0001$, permutation test: $p = 0.014$) and PC (Mann–Whitney *U*-test: $p = 0.0001$, permutation test: $p = 0.0021$) (Figure 3a). The AUC of d*N*GScore for prediction of UCs (for UCs, 0.969, for UCB, 0.993, for UTUC, 0.907, respectively) was much higher than that of hematuria (AUC, 0.892) and urine cytology (AUC, 0.707) (Figure 3b and Table 3). At the cut-off d*N*GScore (−0.0955 points) for prediction of UCs, the negative predictive value (NPV) was 96.1%, which was much higher than the NPV of urine cytology (75.8%) and hematuria (89.5%). The d*N*GScore was not significantly associated with hematuria status and class of urine cytology (Figure 3d,e), but significantly associated with invasiveness of UCB (Figure 3f).

Table 3. Comparing diagnostic performance of UCs on each test.

Variables	AUC	95% CI	Sensitivity (%)	Specificity (%)	PPV (%)	NPV (%)
Hematuria	0.892	0.861–0.924	78.5	100.0	100.0	89.5
Urine cytology	0.707	0.661–0.753	41.4	100.0	100.0	75.8
d*N*GScore [1] for UC	0.969	0.952–0.986	92.8	97.2	94.8	96.1
d*N*GScore for UCB	0.993	0.982–0.100	98.3	97.2	93.5	99.3
d*N*GScore for UTUC	0.907	0.854–0.959	77.1	97.2	79.7	96.8

[1] d*N*GScore, diagnostic *N*-glycan score.

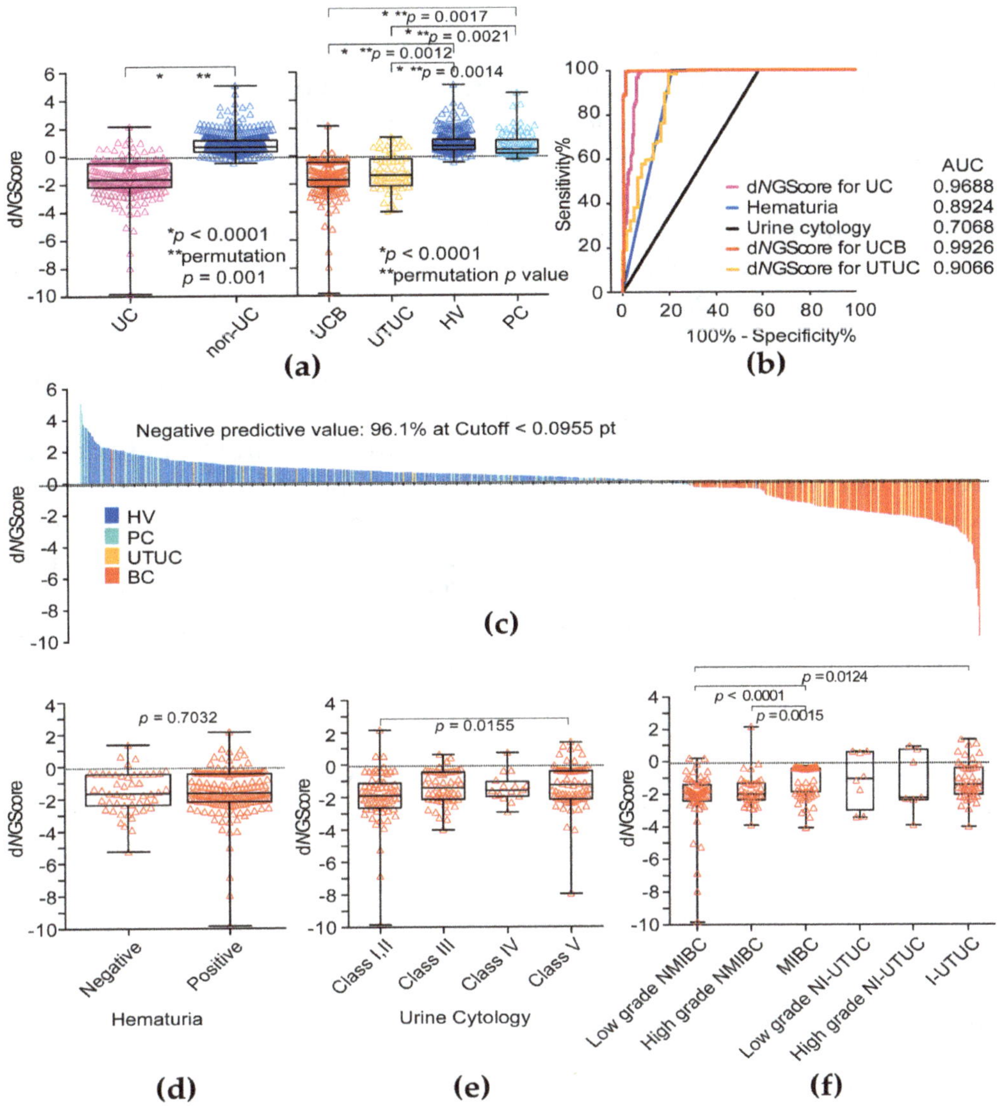

Figure 3. Clinical significance of diagnostic *N*-glycan score. (**a**) The diagnostic *N*-glycan score (d*N*GScore) level was significantly higher in the UC (UCB and UTUC) group than in the HV and PC group; (**b**) ROC curve analysis of d*N*GScore, hematuria and urine cytological results for detection of UC (UCB and UTUC); (**c**) Waterfall plot of d*N*GScore; (**d**) Association between d*N*GScore level and hematuria status; (**e**) Association between d*N*GScore level and urine cytology; (**f**) Association between d*N*GScore level and tumor invasiveness. NMIBC: non-muscle invasive bladder cancer, MIBC: muscle invasive bladder cancer, NI-UTUC: noninvasive UTUC, I-UTUC: invasive UTUC. Intergroup differences were statistically compared using the Mann–Whitney *U*-test for non-normally distributed models and performed permutation test.

3. Discussion

Several studies have shown that differences in serum *N*-glycan profiles between diseased and benign states analyzing high-throughput, comprehensive and quantitative *N*-glycomics may be useful in the diagnosis or prognosis of diseases [11–14,19]. A few studies have investigated the use of serum *N*-glycans as diagnostic markers for UC, including UTUC [13,19]. Although these reports showed that the levels of highly branched sialylated *N*-glycans (m/z 2890, 3560, 3865) were increased in the sera of patients with bladder cancer [13,19], they did not identify carrier proteins of aberrant *N*-glycosylation. Furthermore, these highly branched sialylated *N*-glycans in serum were also significantly upregulated in plural cancer, such as prostate or kidney cancer [11,12]. To identify which carrier protein is aberrantly glycosylated, in the present study, we focused on *N*-glycomics of serum major *N*-glycosylated protein such as Igs. We showed that, in total, five types of *N*-glycans, including bisecting GlcNAc-, biantennary-type *N*-glycans with or without core fucose in serum Igs fractions, were associated with UC detection (Figure 1). According to the biosynthetic pathway of *N*-glycans (Figure 1c), bisecting GlcNAc *N*-glycans were synthesized from biantennary-type *N*-glycan by β1,4-*N*-acetylglucosaminyltransferase (GnT-III) and then modified terminal galactosylation and/or sialylation by galactosyltransferase and sialyltransferase. In this study, we found asialo biantennary- (m/z 1606 and 1769) and monosialyl biantennary-typed *N*-glycan (m/z 2074) and monosialyl bisecting GlcNAc-typed *N*-glycans (m/z 2423) were significantly decreased in UC patients and upregulated only asialo bisecting GlcNAc typed *N*-glycan (m/z 2118) on Igs in UC patients. Thus, we hypothesize asialo biantennary typed *N*-glycan on Igs was transformed to asialo bisecting type *N*-glycan on Igs by GnT-III activity and less sialyltransferase activity in UC patients and resulted in a decrease of biantennary and sialyl bisecting GlcNAc type *N*-glycan on Igs in UC patients. In addition, in the UTUC case, the level of monosialyl bisecting GlcNAc-typed *N*-glycans (m/z 2423) on Igs was significantly lower than that of UCB group. Thus, accumulation of asialo bisecting GlcNAc typed *N*-glycan (m/z 2118) was more of a UTUC-specific phenomenon than that of UCB. This suggests that aberrant *N*-glycosylation profile UTUC was little different from that of UCB. This difference may reflect the difference of tumor environment between bladder and urinary/renal pelvis, and/or may reflect different embryonic background of tumor origin. On the other hand, in PC case, upregulation of monosialyl biantennary-typed *N*-glycan (m/z 2074) and down-regulation of monosialyl bisecting GlcNAc-typed *N*-glycans (m/z 2423) is observed. This suggests that monosialyl biantennary-typed *N*-glycan (m/z 2074) on Igs is significantly accumulated in PC patients and might be the candidate aberrant glycosylation of prostate cancer detection. These aberrant *N*-glycosylation profiles of Igs were different from the whole serum aberrant *N*-glycosylation profiles obtained in previous studies [13,19]. Thus, asialo bisecting type *N*-glycosylated Igs can be applied as a promising UC-specific diagnostic biomarker. To the best of our knowledge, this is the first report to demonstrate the clinical significance of aberrant *N*-glycosylated Igs as diagnostic biomarkers of UCs. It is well known that glycosylation of Igs has a critical role in the development of diseases. Wuhrer et al. reported that asialo bisecting type *N*-glycosylated IgG induced anti-inflammatory response and agalactosyl bisecting type *N*-glycosylated IgG induced pro-inflammatory response in cerebrospinal fluid [20]. Overproduction of aberrantly glycosylated IgA1 has a key role in the development of IgA nephropathy [21]. A recent report suggested that antibody-mediated rejection after kidney transplantation is closely associated with the levels of immunomodulatory sialylated IgG antibodies [22]. Furthermore, Kazuno et al. reported that α2,6-sialylated IgG was significantly decreased in prostate cancer immunoreactions [24]. Rademacher et al. reported that agalactosyl bisecting GlcNAc type *N*-glycoslated IgG was increased in rheumatoid arthritis patient and related autoimmune disease [23]. From these observations, aberrant glycosylated Igs appear to change their glycans because of disease-associated immunoreactions. In a future study, we will examine *N*-glycosylation profile of Igs between benign disease and UC patients to address the UC associated aberrant glycosylation on Igs are part of inflammatory response.

In the present study, the d*N*GScore, combination of 5 *N*-glycans including biantennary and bisecting GlcNAc, clearly discriminate UC from healthy controls and prostate cancer patients with 92.8% sensitivity and 97.2% specificity. Our results also suggested that the level of d*N*GScore was not related to urine cytological classifications and hematuria (Figure 3d,e), which suggested a higher predictive value for urine cytology-negative (<Class IV) cases and hematuria negative cases. In addition, d*N*GScore can discriminate both low- and high-grade non-muscle invasive bladder cancer as well as muscle invasive bladder cancer. This suggests that the d*N*GScore may be useful for early diagnosis of UCB.

The limitations of the present study were its small sample size, retrospective nature, selection bias, lack of independent validation group and non-clinical setting. Therefore, the results obtained in this study have to be regarded as preliminary and need further validation study. Because urine cytological results are not reliable in patients with early stage UCs, including UTUC, a large-scale prospective validation study in a natural cohort of patients with hematuria is required. In addition, the usefulness of regular follow-up for detecting recurrence after surgery remains unclear; furthermore, a large-scale prospective follow-up study after surgery was also needed. In addition, this study did not include patients with benign diseases or infections such as calculi, UTI, cystitis, prostatitis. Despite these limitations, the strength of the present study was that it is the largest to assess the implications of aberrant *N*-glycosyleted Igs for UCs detection. Our findings may be useful for detection of UC patients and identification of patients at urine cytology negative UC. Furthermore, to apply the routine clinical practice, we now developed lectin-sandwich immunoassay system to detect aberrant asialo bisecting GlcNAc type *N*-glycosylated Igs as described previously [28].

4. Materials and Methods

4.1. Serum Samples

The present study was conducted in accordance with the ethical standards of the Declaration of Helsinki and approved by the institutional review board of Hirosaki University School of Medicine ("study about carbohydrate structure change in urological disease"; approval number: 2014-195, approval date: 22 December 2014). Written or verbal informed consent was obtained from all serum donors. Between 2009 and 2016, we randomly selected serum available 237 patients with UC and also 96 patients with prostate cancer as other cancer controls from our serum bank. Serum from any clinical treated patients were excluded. We also obtained from 339 healthy controls selected from community-dwelling volunteers in the health maintenance programme of Iwaki Health Promotion Project [19,29]. All serum samples were collected at the first visit and stored at −80 °C until use. All tumors were staged according to the 2017 tumor-node-metastasis classification, 8th edition [30]. Histological classification of UC was performed according to the World Health Organization 1973 and 2004 grading systems [31]. Urine cytology classification was performed according to guideline of The Paris System working group [32]. Patient demographics are shown in Table 1.

4.2. Purification and Quantification of the Igs Fraction from Serum

Each serum sample (100 μL) was applied to the center of the Zeba™ Spin desalting resin plate (Thermo Fisher Scientific, Waltham, MA, USA) equilibrated with phosphate-buffered saline and centrifuged at 1000× *g* for 2 min. The flow-through was collected as buffer-exchanged serum (100 μL). Purification of Igs fraction performed by using Melon™ Gel Spin Purification Kit (Thermo Fisher Scientific) according to the instructions. Buffer-exchanged serum (100 μL) was applied to the center of the Melon Gel resin equilibrated with purification buffer. After 5 min incubation, the Melon Gel resin was centrifuged at 1000× *g* for 2 min and the flow-through was collected as a purified Igs fraction. A 10-μL aliquot of the Igs fraction was subjected to *N*-glycomics. To confirm the purity of the Igs fraction, the Melon Gel flow-through Igs fraction was subjected to SDS-PAGE and stained with CBB. Igs (total IgG, IgM and IgA) levels of purified Igs fraction were measured by using a Bio-plex Pro Human Isotyping 6-plex kit (Bio-Rad Laboratories, Hercules, CA, USA) according to the instructions.

4.3. Serum N-Glycomics of Igs Performed by Using the Glycoblotting Method and Mass Spectorometric Analysis

N-glycomics was performed as described previously. A 10-μL aliquot of the purified Igs fractions were analyzed using the glycoblotting method [11,12,15,33] on a Sweetblot instrument (System Instruments, Hachioji, Tokyo, Japan). Then, the resulting benzyloxiamine (BOA)-labelled glycans were detected by matrix-assisted laser desorption time-of-flight (MALDI-TOF) mass spectrometry (Ultraflex 3 TOF/TOF mass spectrometer; Bruker Daltonics, Bremen, Germany) (Figure A1a–f). Composition and structures of the glycans were predicted using the GlycoMod Tool (available online:

http://web.expasy.org/glycomod/) (Table A1). Quantitative reproducibility test of each *N*-glycans levels were then evaluated as described previously [19].

4.4. Statistical Analysis

Statistical analyses of clinical data were performed using SPSS v.22.0 (IBM Corporation, Armonk, NY, USA) and GraphPad Prism v.6.03 (GraphPad Software, San Diego, CA, USA). Categorical variables were reported as percentages and compared using the Fisher exact test. Age data were expressed as medians with 25th and 75th quartiles (Q1, Q3). Differences between the groups were statistically compared using the Student *t*-test for normally distributed data or the Mann–Whitney *U*-test for non-normally distributed data. Multivariable discriminant analysis for detection of UCs was performed by inputting UC event as an explanatory variable and *N*-glycan level as an objective variable. The diagnostic *N*-glycan score was calculated by multiplying candidate *N*-glycan levels by each discriminant function value. The diagnostic performance of *N*-glycan scores was evaluated using receiver operating characteristic (ROC) curve analysis developed using the library "rms" in R (available online: http://www.r-project.org/), and statistical differences between area under the curves (AUCs) were calculated using the same programme [34]. In order to assess the significant difference among two group of subjects we implemented a permutation tests and calculate permutation p value [35]. Differences with $p < 0.05$ were considered statistically significant.

5. Conclusions

In conclusion, aberrant *N*-glycosylation profiles of Igs determined by *N*-glycomics may be useful as diagnostic biomarkers for identifying UC patients. Future large-scale prospective validation studies are of vital importance.

Acknowledgments: The authors thank Satomi Sakamoto, Shoko Nagata and Yukie Nishizawa for their invaluable help with patient data management. This work was supported by Grants-in-Aid for Scientific Research (Nos. 15H02563 15K15579, 25220206, 17K11118, 17K11119, 17K16768, 17K16770 and 17K16771) from the Japan Society for the Promotion of Science.

Author Contributions: Toshikazu Tanaka and Tohru Yoneyama performed the bulk of the experiments. Shingo Hatakeyama, Kazuyuki Mori, Yuki Tobisawa, Shizuka Kurauchi and Ippei Takahashi provided serum samples and provided the patients' clinical information from healthy volunteers and urothelial carcinoma and prostate cancer patients. Daisuke Noro, Kengo Imanishi, Yuta Kojima, Shingo Hatakeyama, Hayato Yamamoto, Atsushi Imai, Takahiro Yoneyama, Yasuhiro Hashimoto, Takuya Koie and Chikara Ohyama diagnosed urothelial carcinoma and prostate cancer patients. Masakazu Tanaka and Shin-Ichiro Nishimura performed MALDI-TOF MS analysis. Yasuhiro Hashimoto performed pathological analyses. Chikara Ohyama and Tohru Yoneyama designed all the experiments, interpreted the data and wrote the manuscript.

Abbreviations

UC	Urothelial carcinoma
UCB	Urothelial carcinoma of the bladder
UTUC	Upper urinary tract urothelial carcinoma
HV	Healthy volunteers
PC	Prostate cancer
BPH	Beneign prostatic hyperplasia
HSPC	Hormone sensitive prostate cancer
NMIBC	Nonmuscle invasive bladder cancer
MIBC	Muscle invasive bladder cancer
NI-UTUC	Noninvasive UTUC
I-UTUC	Invasive UTUC
Igs	Immunogloblins
d*N*GScore	Diagnostic *N*-glycan Score

AUC	Area under the curve
ROC	Receiver operating characteristic curves
BTA	Bladder tumor antigen
NMP22	Nuclear matrix protein number 22
IQR	Interquartile range
NPV	Negative predictive value
PPV	Positive predictive value
UTI	Urinary tract infection
MALDI-TOF	Matrix-assisted laser desorption time-of-flight
Man	Mannose
Gal	Galactose
GlcNAc	*N*-acetylglucosamine
Fuc	Fucose
Sia	*N*-acetylneuraminic acid
CBB	Coomassie brilliant blue

Appendix A

Table A1. Thirty-two types of *N*-glycans that showed good quantitative reproducibility in all Igs fraction samples and could be analyzed statistically.

#	*m/z*	Composition
1	1362.5	(Hex)2 + (Man)3(GlcNAc)2
2	1524.5	(Hex)3 + (Man)3(GlcNAc)2
3	1565.5	(Hex)5 + (HexNAc)3
4	1590.6	(HexNAc)2(dHex)1 + (Man)3(GlcNAc)2
5	1606.6	(Hex)1(HexNAc)2 + (Man)3(GlcNAc)2
6	1647.6	(HexNAc)3 + (Man)3(GlcNAc)2
7	1686.6	(Hex)4 + (Man)3(GlcNAc)2
8	1708.6	(Hex)1(HexNAc)1(NeuAc)1 + (Man)3(GlcNAc)2
9	1752.6	(Hex)1(HexNAc)2(dHex)1 + (Man)3(GlcNAc)2
10	1768.6	(Hex)2(HexNAc)2 + (Man)3(GlcNAc)2
11	1793.7	(HexNAc)3(dHex)1 + (Man)3(GlcNAc)2
12	1809.7	(Hex)1(HexNAc)3 + (Man)3(GlcNAc)2
13	1848.6	(Hex)5 + (Man)3(GlcNAc)2
14	1870.7	(Hex)2(HexNAc)1(NeuAc)1 + (Man)3(GlcNAc)2
15	1914.7	(Hex)2(HexNAc)2(dHex)1 + (Man)3(GlcNAc)2
16	1955.7	(Hex)1(HexNAc)3(dHex)1 + (Man)3(GlcNAc)2
17	2010.7	(Hex)6 + (Man)3(GlcNAc)2
18	2032.7	(Hex)3(HexNac)1(NeuAc)1 + (Man)3(GlcNAc)2
19	2057.8	(Hex)1(HexNAc)2(dHex)1(NeuAc)1 + (Man)3(GlcNAc)2
20	2073.8	(Hex)2(HexNAc)2(NeuAc)1 + (Man)3(GlcNAc)2
21	2117.8	(Hex)2(HexNAc)3(dHex)1 + (Man)3(GlcNAc)2
22	2219.8	(Hex)2(HexNAc)2(dHex)1(NeuAc)1 + (Man)3(GlcNAc)2
23	2336.9	(Hex)3(HexNAc)4 + (Man)3(GlcNAc)2
IS	2348.9 [1]	Internal standard (BOA-labeled A2 amide)
24	2378.9	(Hex)2(HexNAc)2(NeuAc)2 + (Man)3(GlcNAc)2
25	2422.9	(Hex)2(HexNAc)3(dHex)1(NeuAc)1 + (Man)3(GlcNAc)2
26	2524.9	(Hex)2(HexNAc)2(dHex)1(NeuAc)2 + (Man)3(GlcNAc)2
27	2727.9	(Hex)2(HexNAc)3(dHex)1(NeuAc)2 + (Man)3(GlcNAc)2
28	2743.9	(Hex)3(HexNAc)3(NeuAc)2 + (Man)3(GlcNAc)2
29	2890.1	(Hex)3(HexNAc)3(dHex)1(NeuAc)2 + (Man)3(GlcNAc)2
30	3049.1	(Hex)3(HexNAc)3(NeuAc)3 + (Man)3(GlcNAc)2
31	3195.2	(Hex)3(HexNAc)3(dHex)1(NeuAc)3 + (Man)3(GlcNAc)2
32	3341.2	(Hex)3 (HexNAc)3 (Deoxyhexose)2 (NeuAc)3 + (Man)3(GlcNAc)2

[1] *m/z* 2348.9 is the internal standard, disialo-galactosylated biantennary *N*-glycan, which contains amidated sialic acid residues (A2 amide glycans). Compositional annotations and putative structures are represented by the following abbreviations. Hex: hexose, HexNAc: *N*-acetylhexosamine, dHex: deoxyhexose.

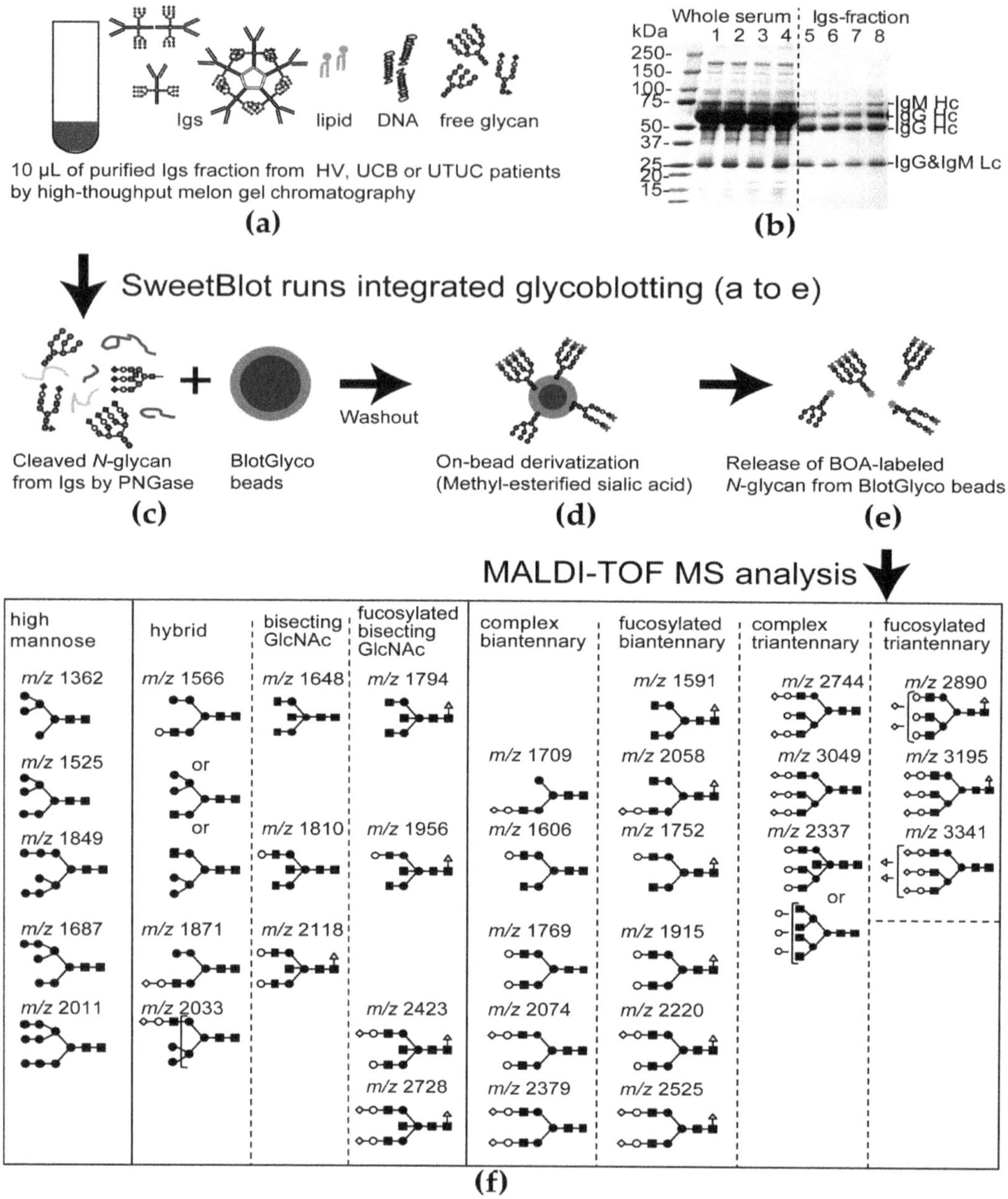

Figure A1. The general protocol for the integrated glycoblotting technique and workflow for glycoblotting-based high-throughput clinical glycan analysis. (**a**) Ten-microliter serum Ig fraction samples were applied to SweetBlot™ (System Instruments, Hachioji, Japan) for glycoblotting; (**b**) Coomassie brilliant blue (CBB)-stained band patterns on a sodium dodecyl sulfate-polyacrylamide gel for representative whole serum and purified Ig fraction samples; (**c**) After enzymatic *N*-glycan cleavage from Ig proteins, the total *N*-glycans released into the digestion mixture were directly mixed with BlotGlyco H beads (Sumitomo Bakelite, Co., Tokyo, Japan) to capture *N*-glycans; (**d**) After the beads were separated from other molecules by washing, sialic acid was methyl esterified; (**e**) These processed *N*-glycans were then labelled with benzyloxyamine (BOA) and released from BlotGlyco H beads; (**f**) Mass spectra of BOA-labelled *N*-glycans from Ig fractions were acquired using an Ultraflex III instrument (Bruker Daltonics, Germany). Total 32 type of *N*-glycans were identified in Igs fraction. Identified *N*-glycan structures are indicated by monosaccharide symbols: white circles, galactose (Gal); black circles, mannose (Man); black squares, *N*-acetylglucosamine (GlcNAc); black triangle, fucose (Fuc) and black diamonds, sialic acid.

References

1. Park, J.C.; Hahn, N.M. Bladder cancer: A disease ripe for major advances. *Clin. Adv. Hematol. Oncol.* **2014**, *12*, 838–845. [PubMed]
2. Munoz, J.J.; Ellison, L.M. Upper tract urothelial neoplasms: Incidence and survival during the last 2 decades. *J. Urol.* **2000**, *164*, 1523–1525. [CrossRef]
3. Siegel, R.; Naishadham, D.; Jemal, A. Cancer statistics, 2012. *CA Cancer J. Clin.* **2012**, *62*, 10–29. [CrossRef] [PubMed]
4. Inman, B.A.; Tran, V.T.; Fradet, Y.; Lacombe, L. Carcinoma of the upper urinary tract: Predictors of survival and competing causes of mortality. *Cancer* **2009**, *115*, 2853–2862. [CrossRef] [PubMed]
5. Cowan, N.C. CT urography for hematuria. *Nat. Rev. Urol.* **2012**, *9*, 218–226. [CrossRef] [PubMed]
6. Babjuk, M.; Bohle, A.; Burger, M.; Capoun, O.; Cohen, D.; Comperat, E.M.; Hernandez, V.; Kaasinen, E.; Palou, J.; Roupret, M.; et al. EAU Guidelines on Non-Muscle-invasive Urothelial Carcinoma of the Bladder: Update 2016. *Eur. Urol.* **2016**, *71*, 447–461. [CrossRef] [PubMed]
7. Margulis, V.; Shariat, S.F.; Matin, S.F.; Kamat, A.M.; Zigeuner, R.; Kikuchi, E.; Lotan, Y.; Weizer, A.; Raman, J.D.; Wood, C.G. Outcomes of radical nephroureterectomy: A series from the Upper Tract Urothelial Carcinoma Collaboration. *Cancer* **2009**, *115*, 1224–1233. [CrossRef] [PubMed]
8. Ramakumar, S.; Bhuiyan, J.; Besse, J.A.; Roberts, S.G.; Wollan, P.C.; Blute, M.L.; O'Kane, D.J. Comparison of screening methods in the detection of bladder cancer. *J. Urol.* **1999**, *161*, 388–394. [CrossRef]
9. Narayan, V.M.; Adejoro, O.; Schwartz, I.; Ziegelmann, M.; Elliott, S.; Konety, B.R. The Prevalence and Impact of Urinary Marker Testing in Patients with Bladder Cancer. *J. Urol.* **2017**. [CrossRef] [PubMed]
10. Gopalakrishna, A.; Longo, T.A.; Fantony, J.J.; Owusu, R.; Foo, W.C.; Dash, R.; Inman, B.A. The diagnostic accuracy of urine-based tests for bladder cancer varies greatly by patient. *BMC Urol.* **2016**, *16*, 30. [CrossRef] [PubMed]
11. Hatakeyama, S.; Amano, M.; Tobisawa, Y.; Yoneyama, T.; Tsuchiya, N.; Habuchi, T.; Nishimura, S.-I.; Ohyama, C. Serum N-Glycan Alteration Associated with Renal Cell Carcinoma Detected by High Throughput Glycan Analysis. *J. Urol.* **2014**, *191*, 805–813. [CrossRef] [PubMed]
12. Ishibashi, Y.; Tobisawa, Y.; Hatakeyama, S.; Ohashi, T.; Tanaka, M.; Narita, S.; Koie, T.; Habuchi, T.; Nishimura, S.-I.; Ohyama, C.; et al. Serum tri- and tetra-antennary *N*-glycan is a potential predictive biomarker for castration-resistant prostate cancer. *Prostate* **2014**, *74*, 1521–1529. [CrossRef] [PubMed]
13. Maho Amano, M.T. *N*- and *O*-glycome analysis of serum and urine from bladder cancer patients using a high-throughput glycoblotting method. *J. Glycom. Lipidom.* **2013**, *3*, 108. [CrossRef]
14. Narita, T.; Hatakeyama, S.; Yoneyama, T.; Narita, S.; Yamashita, S.; Mitsuzuka, K.; Sakurai, T.; Kawamura, S.; Tochigi, T.; Takahashi, I.; et al. Clinical implications of serum *N*-glycan profiling as a diagnostic and prognostic biomarker in germ-cell tumors. *Cancer Med.* **2017**, *6*, 739–748. [CrossRef] [PubMed]
15. Nouso, K.; Amano, M.; Ito, Y.M.; Miyahara, K.; Morimoto, Y.; Kato, H.; Tsutsumi, K.; Tomoda, T.; Yamamoto, N.; Nakamura, S.; et al. Clinical utility of high-throughput glycome analysis in patients with pancreatic cancer. *J. Gastroenterol.* **2013**, *48*, 1171–1179. [CrossRef] [PubMed]
16. Kirwan, A.; Utratna, M.; O'Dwyer, M.E.; Joshi, L.; Kilcoyne, M. Glycosylation-Based Serum Biomarkers for Cancer Diagnostics and Prognostics. *Biomed. Res. Int.* **2015**, *2015*, 490531. [CrossRef] [PubMed]
17. Li, C.W.; Lim, S.O.; Xia, W.; Lee, H.H.; Chan, L.C.; Kuo, C.W.; Khoo, K.H.; Chang, S.S.; Cha, J.H.; Kim, T.; et al. Glycosylation and stabilization of programmed death ligand-1 suppresses T-cell activity. *Nat. Commun.* **2016**, *7*, 12632. [CrossRef] [PubMed]
18. Veillon, L.; Fakih, C.; Abou-El-Hassan, H.; Kobeissy, F.; Mechref, Y. Glycosylation Changes in Brain Cancer. *ACS Chem. Neurosci.* **2017**. [CrossRef] [PubMed]
19. Oikawa, M.; Hatakeyama, S.; Yoneyma, T.; Tobisawa, Y.; Narita, T.; Yamamoto, H.; Hashimoto, Y.; Koie, T.; Narita, S.; Sasaki, A.; et al. Significance of Serum *N*-glycan Profiling as a Diagnostic Biomarker in Urothelial Carcinoma. *Eur. Urol. Focus* **2016**. [CrossRef] [PubMed]
20. Wuhrer, M.; Selman, M.H.; McDonnell, L.A.; Kumpfel, T.; Derfuss, T.; Khademi, M.; Olsson, T.; Hohlfeld, R.; Meinl, E.; Krumbholz, M. Pro-inflammatory pattern of IgG1 Fc glycosylation in multiple sclerosis cerebrospinal fluid. *J. Neuroinflamm.* **2015**, *12*, 235. [CrossRef] [PubMed]

21. Suzuki, Y.; Suzuki, H.; Makita, Y.; Takahata, A.; Takahashi, K.; Muto, M.; Sasaki, Y.; Kelimu, A.; Matsuzaki, K.; Yanagawa, H.; et al. Diagnosis and activity assessment of immunoglobulin A nephropathy: Current perspectives on noninvasive testing with aberrantly glycosylated immunoglobulin A-related biomarkers. *Int. J. Nephrol. Renovasc. Dis.* **2014**, *7*, 409–414. [CrossRef] [PubMed]
22. Malard-Castagnet, S.; Dugast, E.; Degauque, N.; Pallier, A.; Soulillou, J.P.; Cesbron, A.; Giral, M.; Harb, J.; Brouard, S. Sialylation of antibodies in kidney recipients with de novo donor specific antibody, with or without antibody mediated rejection. *Hum. Immunol.* **2015**, *77*, 1076–1083. [CrossRef] [PubMed]
23. Rademacher, T.W.; Parekh, R.B.; Dwek, R.A.; Isenberg, D.; Rook, G.; Axford, J.S.; Roitt, I. The role of IgG glycoforms in the pathogenesis of rheumatoid arthritis. *Springer Semin. Immunopathol.* **1988**, *10*, 231–249. [CrossRef] [PubMed]
24. Kazuno, S.; Furukawa, J.; Shinohara, Y.; Murayama, K.; Fujime, M.; Ueno, T.; Fujimura, T. Glycosylation status of serum immunoglobulin G in patients with prostate diseases. *Cancer Med.* **2016**, *5*, 1137–1146. [CrossRef] [PubMed]
25. Ruhaak, L.R.; Barkauskas, D.A.; Torres, J.; Cooke, C.L.; Wu, L.D.; Stroble, C.; Ozcan, S.; Williams, C.C.; Camorlinga, M.; Rocke, D.M.; et al. The Serum Immunoglobulin G Glycosylation Signature of Gastric Cancer. *EuPA Open Proteom.* **2015**, *6*, 1–9. [CrossRef] [PubMed]
26. Theodoratou, E.; Thaci, K.; Agakov, F.; Timofeeva, M.N.; Stambuk, J.; Pucic-Bakovic, M.; Vuckovic, F.; Orchard, P.; Agakova, A.; Din, F.V.; et al. Glycosylation of plasma IgG in colorectal cancer prognosis. *Sci. Rep.* **2016**, *6*, 28098. [CrossRef] [PubMed]
27. Zhang, D.; Chen, B.; Wang, Y.; Xia, P.; He, C.; Liu, Y.; Zhang, R.; Zhang, M.; Li, Z. Disease-specific IgG Fc *N*-glycosylation as personalized biomarkers to differentiate gastric cancer from benign gastric diseases. *Sci. Rep.* **2016**, *6*, 25957. [CrossRef] [PubMed]
28. Hagiwara, K.; Tobisawa, Y.; Kaya, T.; Kaneko, T.; Hatakeyama, S.; Mori, K.; Hashimoto, Y.; Koie, T.; Suda, Y.; Ohyama, C.; et al. Wisteria floribunda Agglutinin and Its Reactive-Glycan-Carrying Prostate-Specific Antigen as a Novel Diagnostic and Prognostic Marker of Prostate Cancer. *Int. J. Mol. Sci.* **2017**, *18*, 261. [CrossRef] [PubMed]
29. Tanaka, T.; Hatakeyama, S.; Yamamoto, H.; Narita, T.; Hamano, I.; Matsumoto, T.; Soma, O.; Tobisawa, Y.; Yoneyama, T.; Yoneyama, T.; et al. Clinical relevance of aortic calcification in urolithiasis patients. *BMC Urol.* **2017**, *17*, 25. [CrossRef] [PubMed]
30. James, D.B.; Gospodarowicz, M.K.; Wittekind, C. *TNM Classification of Malignant Tumours*, 8th ed.; Wiley-Blackwell: Oxford, UK, 2016; p. 272.
31. Humphrey, P.A.; Moch, H.; Cubilla, A.L.; Ulbright, T.M.; Reuter, V.E. The 2016 WHO Classification of Tumours of the Urinary System and Male Genital Organs-Part B: Prostate and Bladder Tumours. *Eur. Urol.* **2016**, *70*, 106–119. [CrossRef] [PubMed]
32. Barkan, G.A.; Wojcik, E.M.; Nayar, R.; Savic-Prince, S.; Quek, M.L.; Kurtycz, D.F.; Rosenthal, D.L. The Paris System for Reporting Urinary Cytology: The Quest to Develop a Standardized Terminology. *Adv. Anat. Pathol.* **2016**, *23*, 193–201. [CrossRef] [PubMed]
33. Hatakeyama, S.; Amano, M.; Tobisawa, Y.; Yoneyama, T.; Tsushima, M.; Hirose, K.; Yoneyama, T.; Hashimoto, Y.; Koie, T.; Saitoh, H.; et al. Serum *N*-Glycan Profiling Predicts Prognosis in Patients Undergoing Hemodialysis. *Sci. World J.* **2013**, *2013*, 268407. [CrossRef] [PubMed]
34. Harrell, F.E., Jr.; Lee, K.L.; Mark, D.B. Multivariable prognostic models: Issues in developing models, evaluating assumptions and adequacy, and measuring and reducing errors. *Stat. Med.* **1996**, *15*, 361–387. [CrossRef]
35. Christie, D. Resampling with Excel. *Teach. Stat.* **2004**, *26*, 9–14. [CrossRef]

7

Activating Telomerase *TERT* Promoter Mutations and their Application for the Detection of Bladder Cancer

Maria Zvereva [1,2,*], Eduard Pisarev [3], Ismail Hosen [4], Olga Kisil [5], Simon Matskeplishvili [6], Elena Kubareva [7], David Kamalov [6], Alexander Tivtikyan [6], Arnaud Manel [8], Emmanuel Vian [9], Armais Kamalov [6], Thorsten Ecke [10] and Florence Le Calvez-Kelm [2]

1 Chair of Chemistry of Natural Compounds, Department of Chemistry, Lomonosov Moscow State University, 119991 Moscow, Russia
2 International Agency for Research on Cancer (IARC), 69372 Lyon, France; lecalvezf@iarc.fr
3 Faculty of Bioengineering and Bioinformatics, Lomonosov Moscow State University, 119234 Moscow, Russia; profard95@gmail.com
4 Department of Biochemistry and Molecular Biology, Faculty of Biological Sciences, University of Dhaka, Dhaka 1000, Bangladesh; ismail.hosen@du.ac.bd
5 Gause Institute of New Antibiotics, 119021 Moscow, Russia; olvv@mail.ru
6 Medical Research and Education Center, Lomonosov Moscow State University, 119992 Moscow, Russia; simonmats@yahoo.com (S.M.); davidffm@mail.ru (D.K.); aleksandertivtikyan@yandex.ru (A.T.); kamalov@mc.msu.ru (A.K.)
7 Belozersky Institute of Physico-Chemical Biology, Moscow State University, 119992 Moscow, Russia; kubareva@belozersky.msu.ru
8 Le Creusot Hospital, 71200 Le Creusot, France; manelarnaud69@gmail.com
9 Department of Urology, Protestant Clinic of Lyon, 69300 Lyon, France; emmanuel.vian@gmail.com
10 Department of Urology, HELIOS Hospital Bad Saarow, D-15526 Bad Saarow, Germany; thorsten.ecke@helios-gesundheit.de
* Correspondence: mzvereva@chem.msu.ru

Abstract: This review summarizes state-of-the-art knowledge in early-generation and novel urine biomarkers targeting the telomerase pathway for the detection and follow-up of bladder cancer (BC). The limitations of the assays detecting telomerase reactivation are discussed and the potential of transcription-activating mutations in the promoter of the *TERT* gene detected in the urine as promising simple non-invasive BC biomarkers is highlighted. Studies have shown good sensitivity and specificity of the urinary *TERT* promoter mutations in case-control studies and, more recently, in a pilot prospective cohort study, where the marker was detected up to 10 years prior to clinical diagnosis. However, large prospective cohort studies and intervention studies are required to fully validate their robustness and assess their clinical utility. Furthermore, it may be interesting to evaluate whether the clinical performance of urinary *TERT* promoter mutations could increase when combined with other simple urinary biomarkers. Finally, different approaches for assessment of *TERT* promoter mutations in urine samples are presented together with technical challenges, thus highlighting the need of careful technological validation and standardization of laboratory methods prior to translation into clinical practice.

Keywords: bladder cancer; biomarkers; non-invasive detection; telomerase; somatic mutations; *TERT* promoter region

---

1. Introduction

More than 300 thousand new cases of bladder cancer (BC) are diagnosed in the world annually [1]. Currently, the gold standard of BC diagnosis and monitoring is cystoscopy, which is an invasive, painful, and relatively expensive procedure [2]. In the last few years, urine components have attracted the intense focus of investigators aiming to discover novel biomarkers for detection of BC, as urine is in direct contact with potentially malignant urothelium, is easy to obtain, and its testing should potentially be much more cost-effective.

Molecular markers for such analyses can be of different nature (nucleic acids, proteins, small-molecular-weight compounds), but should be directly linked to the cell processes that are altered during neoplastic transformation (for example, avoidance of programmed cell death through disruption of the telomerase pathway). The characterization of molecular genetic alteration changes, associated with the malignant cell transformation, in differentiation or metastatic potential has provided insights into the interplay of these oncogenic processes and the activation of telomerase and its components [3]. This activation is directly related to the disruption of the cell division control system and, therefore, leads to uncontrolled cell growth. It has been widely demonstrated that telomerase activity is enhanced in 85–90% of tumor cell types [4]. There are multiple underlying mechanisms of telomerase activation [5], but genetic alterations in the promoter region of telomerase reverse transcriptase (*TERT*), leading to both increased gene expression and activity of the enzyme, are considered the most frequent. Therefore, they are considered highly promising putative biomarkers of cancer [6]. The process of reactivating the telomerase enzyme includes alterations in the gene promoter of the catalytic subunit of telomerase caused by methylation [7] and somatic mutations [8], both leading to its overexpression.

In this review, we trace the history of the early-generation of urine BC biomarkers identified in the telomerase pathway, discuss the limitations of the detection of related assays, and highlight the potential of transcription-activating mutations in the promoter of the *TERT* gene detected in the urine as promising simple non-invasive biomarkers for the detection of BC and surveillance for its relapse. Mutations in the *TERT* promoter have been shown to occur in many histological tumor types, making these alterations the most frequent somatic abnormalities detected in cancer so far. In BC particularly, they are detected in 60–85% of cases in all stages and grades of the disease. These mutations have been detected in the intracellular and extracellular DNA fragments from urine samples collected both at the time of primary clinical diagnosis of BC and during post-surgical follow-up. Therefore, they represent promising biomarkers to detect and monitor BC [9]. Recent publications reveal an important short-term clinical perspective of the use of *TERT* promoter mutations as BC urinary biomarkers [10,11]. However, additional validations in large prospective cohort studies and interventional studies are necessary to fully assess their clinical performance and utility. Moreover, it is necessary to evaluate whether the sensitivity of the urinary *TERT* promoter mutations in detecting BC is increased when combined with other urinary biomarkers. Finally, careful technological validation and standardization of laboratory methods for assessing *TERT* promoter mutations in urine samples are critical for their clinical implementation.

2. Telomerase Reactivation in Bladder Cancer and Early-Generation of Telomerase Urinary-Based Biomarkers

Telomerase reactivation in BC has been first described in the mid-1990s [12]. Telomerase is an RNA-protein machinery that synthesizes repeating telomeric DNA. Telomeres are special structures at the ends of chromosomes where DNA interacts with specific proteins, shaping the "cap" to protect chromosome ends from degradation and to maintain their integrity [13]. Human telomerase contains a protein component (reverse transcriptase or hTERT) and a matrix RNA constituent (telomerase RNA, hTR), which, together with other proteins, form the active holoenzyme whose function is to extend telomeric DNA with new repeats and, therefore, revert the progressive loss of sequences at the ends of chromosomes associated with incomplete DNA replication [14]. In differentiated human cells, telomeres are typically shortened with every cell division up to a programmed critical length that leads to cell aging and apoptosis. During tumorigenesis, the mechanism leading to critical telomere shortening is counteracted by telomerase activation, thus preventing cell death.

Enhanced through genetic or epigenetic changes, telomerase activity is, therefore, a telltale sign of malignancy [15]. Bladder cancer cells have shorter telomeres than adjacent normal urothelium [12]. Telomerase activity was shown to be high in BC tumor samples but not in the normal epithelium of patients with BC. Therefore, in many early studies, the measurement of telomerase activity as a biomarker of cancer diagnosis was considered. A relatively simple and accurate test called the Telomere Repeat Amplification Protocol (TRAP) was established to determine telomerase activity in cells and tissue samples [16]. The method relies on the amplification and measurement of the total number of telomeric repeats newly synthesized by the telomerase on a telomere-like oligonucleotide. Due to its direct contact to the urothelium, urine provides the most easily accessible reservoir of potential biomarkers to study urological diseases, so the possibility to use the TRAP assay to detect increased levels of telomerase secreted into the urine by bladder cancer cells has been tested. A case-control study involving 134 primary BC cases and 84 controls demonstrated promising performance of the urine TRAP assay with a sensitivity of 90% and specificity of 88% (when telomerase activity is 50 arbitrary enzymatic units (AEU)) in detecting the presence of bladder tumors in men [17]. While other studies reported a high sensitivity (70–90%) compared to the current standard urine cytology, specificity proved to be lower, ranging from 66% to 88% [17–20]. The suboptimal of specificity has been attributed to the inherent telomerase activity in inflammatory or non-urothelial cells present in urine samples [21], which results in a significant variability in telomerase activity in urine of healthy individuals but also in cancer patients. This was observed by the same authors who reported an average value of telomerase activity of 27 AEU (total range of 0–88) in urine of healthy individuals and 112 AEU (total range of 30–382) in bladder cancer patients [17]. Another limitation of this method, which possibly reflects the lack of reproducibility between studies, includes the sensitivity of urine samples to inactivating agents that rapidly reduce the activity of the enzyme, giving rise to the need for strict protocols of handling samples at special conditions between sample collection and processing in order to maintain stability of the RNA-protein complex. Therefore, the lack of standardization of the TRAP assay and difficulties due to the technical requirements limit its use as a clinical biomarker for bladder cancer detection [22]. A recent alternative method to determine telomerase activity in human urine samples using the hybridization chain reaction and dynamic light scattering has been developed for the detection of bladder cancer [23]. Preliminary findings indicate a high specificity in cellular models and in few healthy individuals and patients with malignancies other than bladder cancer [24–26], but this needs to be confirmed in large case-control studies.

Another existing method to analyze telomerase reactivation is the quantitative measurement of the expression level of telomerase subunits TERT and telomerase RNA (TR) using real-time reverse transcription polymerase chain reaction (qRT-PCR). High expressions of these mRNAs have been observed consistently across many different malignancies, suggesting a promising avenue for early cancer detection in body fluids, especially in urine samples of patients with BC [27]. The quantitative analysis of TR and TERT in urine samples had an overall sensitivity of 77.0% and 55.2%, respectively, and a specificity of 72.1% and 85.0%, and determining both TERT mRNA and TR levels turned out to be more sensitive but less specific than urine cytology [28]. More recently, a protocol of combined modified TRAP and qRT-PCR methods to interrogate urine sediments gave encouraging results for the non-invasive detection of BC [29]. However, obstacles remain before urine telomerase activity-based assays can be translated into clinical practice [30]: (1) A high false-positive rate due to the telomerase activity of blood cells or non-urothelial cells in urine, which, despite attempts to sort out positive non-tumor cells, is yet to be solved; (2) an inconsistent correlation between TERT mRNA and telomerase activity in some tissues [31]; (3) a low number of telomerase-positive cells in urine in early stages of BC, and (4) a possible high rate of telomerase or RNA degradation in the urine and serious technical constraints to maintain their stability. Based on the above considerations, it was of clinical interest to search for novel non-telomerase activity-based urinary biomarkers for the detection and surveillance of BC. Nowadays, several urine-based bladder cancer biomarkers have received FDA-approval: (1) The immunoassays based on the detection of the Nuclear matrix protein 22

(NMP22® BC and its improved variant, the NMP22® BladderChek®, Alere, Waltham, MA, USA) [32] and the detection of the complement factor H-related protein (BTA stat® and BTA TRAK®); (2) the immunofluorescence assays based on the detection of the carcinoembryonic antigen and 2 mucins (ImmunoCyt™/uCyt), and (3) the multitarget fluorescence in situ hybridization (FISH) assay based on the detection of aneuploidy of several chromosomal regions (UroVysion) [33]. Other interesting commercially available biomarkers are emerging: The UBC® rapid (IDL, Bromma, Sweden) test to measure soluble fragments of cytokeratins 8 and 18 in urine [34] and the CxBladder test to identify the presence of five mRNAs (MDK, HOXA13, CDC2, IGFBP5, and CXCR2) in the urine [35]. Only few studies compared the performance of telomerase-based assays with FDA-approved tests for BC detection [32,36,37]. The UroVysion assay (FISH) had higher specificity than the TRAP assays and other urine markers; meanwhile, Bravaccini and colleagues showed that the combination of urine cytology and FISH to the TRAP assay had some potential in discriminating patients with bladder cancer from individuals with other urinary symptoms [36]. Another study conducted in a group of workers employed in the production of tires and, therefore, exposed to various potential bladder carcinogens, and in a control group of unexposed subjects showed that the two-step design using the TRAP assay with standard urine cytology and comet assay as the primary screening tool, and then FISH (UroVysion) in TRAP-positive cases increased the accuracy for the detection of BC as compared to the conventional urine cytology [38].

However, based on performance and cost considerations, none of the commercially available urine biomarkers to date are recommended as reliable diagnostic targets both by the European Association of Urology (link to NMIBC guideline https://uroweb.org/guideline/non-muscle-invasive-bladder-cancer/#5; link to MIBC guideline https://uroweb.org/guideline/bladder-cancer-muscle-invasive-and-metastatic/#6) and American Urological Association (link to NMIBC guideline https://www.auanet.org/guidelines/bladder-cancer-non-muscle-invasive-guideline#x2517) for routine BC clinical management or for screening in high-risk populations [39–42]. The absence of urine biomarkers that can be clinically exploited and the fact that the re-activation of telomerase is a crucial mechanism of urothelial carcinogenesis (observed in 99% of urothelial carcinomas) rekindled the interest in further research on other markers indirectly influencing telomerase activation, for example, through recurrent genetic changes that have been identified in the regulatory elements of the *TERT* gene.

3. Urinary *TERT* Promoter Mutations: The Holy Grail of a Biomarker for Bladder Cancer Detection and Surveillance?

3.1. *TERT Promoter Mutations and Biological Significance in Bladder Carcinogenesis*

Since their discovery in 2013 in melanoma samples, mutations in the promoter region of the *TERT* gene have been found to be frequent in several tumor types [43]. Their functional impact has been well-characterized in vitro and associated with the creation of new binding sites to numerous cellular transcription factors, resulting in an increase in *TERT* expression and telomerase reactivation. [44,45]. The introduction of mutations in the *TERT* promoter sequence caused a two- to four-fold increase in promoter activity in reporter cell lines [44]. Thus, detection of such mutations can be seen as an indirect measure of telomerase reactivation and neoplastic transformation of cells.

Two hotspot mutations of the *TERT* promoter have been detected with high frequency in bladder cancer but not in neighboring normal tissues [43,46,47]. These mutations occur at two positions upstream of the transcription starting site, at −124 bp (nucleotide polymorphism G > A, g.1295228 (chr5, 1, 295, 228 assembly GRCh37) or g.1295113 (chr5, 1, 295, 113 assembly GRCh38)) and −146 bp (nucleotide polymorphism G > A, g.1295250 (chr5, 1, 295, 250, assembly GRCh37) or g.1295135 (chr5, 1, 295, 135 assembly GRCh38)) in a GC-rich genome region, which specifies its alternative organization (Figure 1). Reported to be mutually exclusive, somatic mutations in *TERT* promoter occur in 60–80% cases of all stages and grades of BC [40,48–53]. Specifically, Kinde et al. were the first to show that *TERT* promoter mutations occur frequently in low-grade, high-grade papillary tumors and carcinoma in situ lesions [54]. Allory et al. reported a *TERT* promoter mutation frequency of 87% in cell lines and of 83% in bladder tumors, regardless of stages or the risk associated with disease. Mutation frequency was virtually the same for low-risk non-muscle-invading bladder cancer (NMIBC) (73%), high-risk NMIBC (74%), and muscle-invading bladder cancer (MIBC) (53%). These mutations occurred more frequently than any other genomic changes in both NMIBC risk categories. *TERT* promoter mutations were not shown to be associated with age, sex, or smoking [48]. In addition to urothelial carcinomas, these mutations have also been reported in other rare histological variants of primary BC, such as squamous cell carcinoma (SCC) [55], small cell carcinoma [56], adenocarcinoma of non-enteric type [57], and plasmacytoid urothelial carcinoma [58].

Furthermore, it has been shown that the two single nucleotide substitutions C228T and C250T together account for 99% of *TERT* promoter mutations in BC. Of the two-thirds of bladder tumors carrying a *TERT* promoter mutation, Rachakonda P.S. and colleagues observed that the C228T mutation (G > A) was the most frequent change in BC followed by the C250T mutation, identified in 53.5% and 11.6% of all tumors, respectively [53]. Two additional rare nucleotide mutations were C228A (number of tumors, $n = 3$) and 57A > C (T > G) −57 (nucleotide polymorphism A > C, g.1295161 (chr5, 1, 295, 161 assembly GRCh37) or g.1295046 (chr5, 1, 295, 046 assembly GRCh38), ($n = 1$)). Mutations in all positions −57, −124, and −146 were mutually exclusive and resulted in the creation of a new common binding site de novo for transcription factors Ets/TCF. Similar results were obtained by Allory and colleagues [48]. The most frequent mutation was C228T ($n = 65$) followed by C250T ($n = 10$), and two additional rare mutations were C242T/C243T ($n = 2$) and C228A ($n = 1$). All mutations were mutually exclusive.

With regard to their potential as prognostic markers, one study investigated the relation between the disease-specific survival of patients with urothelial cancer and (1) the presence of C228T and C250T mutations in the *TERT* promoter; and (2) the level of TERT mRNA expression in two independent cohorts of previously untreated patients ($n = 35$ and $n = 87$). A significant decline in survival was strongly correlated with increased TERT mRNA level, but not with the presence of mutation in the *TERT* promoter [59]. Interestingly, the authors also demonstrated that the presence of a *TERT* mutation was associated with an increase in TERT mRNA expression level, leading to the enhancement in telomerase activity and telomere elongation. It has been hypothesized that this unexpected effect is due to the alternative functions of the telomerase catalytic subunit [60], and the existence of alternative mechanisms, other than mutations in the *TERT* promoter, such as epigenetic changes, also contribute to telomerase activation.

3.2. Analytical Methods for Detecting Mutations in the TERT Promoter: Comparison of Analytical Performance and Bias

There is a wide range of established analytical approaches for detecting mutations in the *TERT* promoter. However, the detection of these mutations is complicated by the composition and the structure of the *TERT* promoter genomic region, which is characterized by the highly GC-rich sequence and alternative structures of double stranded DNA in the form of G-quadruplexes, as illustrated in Figure 1 [61]. Another challenge is the detection of low-abundance tumor-derived mutations in body fluids. The DNA fragments carrying the tumor-specific alterations can represent a very small fraction of the total DNA. In blood samples, for example, the circulating tumor DNA fraction has been reported to be as low as 0.5% [62]. The analytical sensitivity of the assays is, therefore, critical in such settings. Despite such constraints, many quantitative PCR-based diagnostics described below have been successfully applied to human biological fluids, e.g., whole blood [63], urine (see Table 1), and urine samples of patients with hematuria (Table S4).

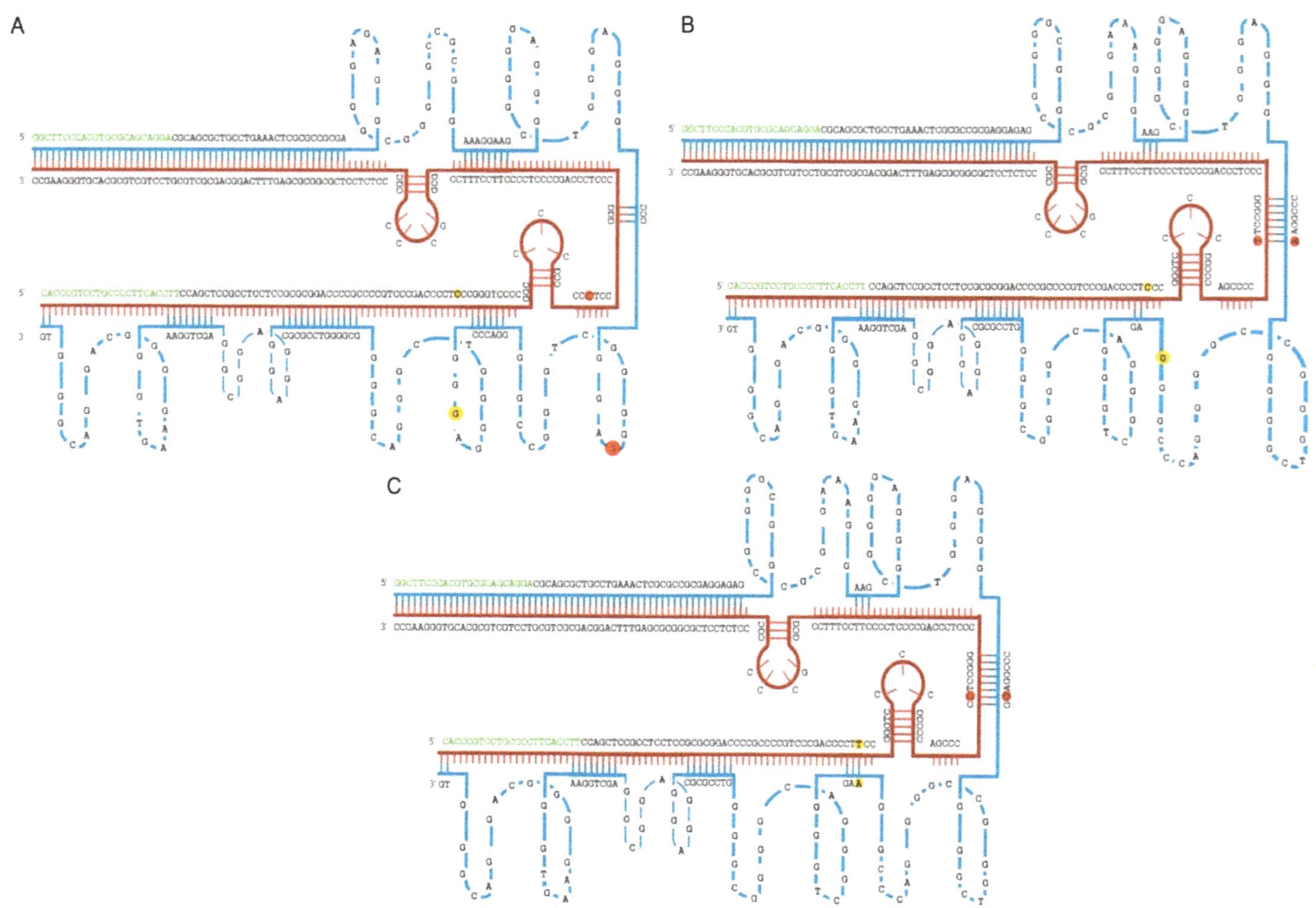

Figure 1. Predicted intramolecular distribution of putative Quadruplex forming G-Rich Sequences (QGRS) in the *TERT* promoter sequence. (**A**) the structure of wild type (WT) DNA; (**B**) only with mutation C228T; (**C**) only with mutation C250T. The two nucleotides at −124 and −146 positions from the ATG start site are highlighted with red and yellow circles respectively. These two hotspots affected by mutations predominantly including C228T and C250T are of the interest for both fundamental research and clinical diagnostics. G-strand and C-strand are marked in blue and claret lines respectively. Regions corresponding to the primers applied to amplify this fragment are marked in green. Despite the close resemblance between all three types of structures they differ substantially. The structures were obtained using online programs "QGRS Mapper" [64] (output data are provided in Tables S1–S3). In this manner both G- and C-strands were analyzed, however only G-strand contains G-quadruplexes. Procedure and software used to calculate and create the structures are described in the Supplementary Materials in more detail.

Currently, the used method for detecting known genetic changes in clinical research is real-time PCR (quantitative PCR and its modifications). Yet, they often lack the sensitivity to detect underrepresented genetic alterations, so-called low mutant allelic fraction (MAF), which are often found diluted with wild-type DNA fragments originating from non-malignant cells or non-mutated cells. Furthermore, the heterogeneous composition of DNA fragments found in 'liquid biopsy' samples may also complicate the analysis. Studies that used real-time PCR to detect *TERT* promoter mutations in tumor and urine samples are shown in Table 1. Successful application of a qPCR-based method known as castPCR was described by Wang and co-workers [61]. In comparison to Sanger-sequencing, castPCR demonstrated dramatically higher sensitivity and specificity in a wide range of tumors of the urinary system (Table 1). The most recent progress with regard to the detection of *TERT* promoter mutations by qPCR has been achieved by Batista and colleagues who demonstrated that their sensitive, urine-based assay called Uromonitor® (Uromonitor Maia, Portugal) based on competitive allele-specific discrimination PCR was capable of detecting trace amounts of *TERT* promoter mutations in urine samples [65].

Next-generation sequencing (NGS) can simultaneously analyze millions of DNA copies. The identification of low-allelic somatic mutations requires ultra-deep sequencing so that the few sequencing reads with the mutant allele can be generated within the pool of wild-type reads. To achieve such high sequencing coverage of the screened genomic region(s), sequencing must be targeted. Traditional NGS-based targeted sequencing is able to detect mutant DNA forms at or higher than 2% allelic fraction against the background of the wild type DNA [66], but recent developments of NGS systems, such as Safe-SeqS [54,67], Tam-Seq [68,69], and CAPP-seq [70], improved threshold limits, the latter reaching an analytical sensitivity of 0.0025% MAF. Avogbe et al. recently developed UroMuTERT, a simple, non-invasive, and sensitive NGS-based assay for the detection of low-level *TERT* promoter mutations. Combined with a specific algorithm developed by the same group, called Needlestack [71], UroMuTERT achieved detection thresholds of 0.8% and 0.5% mutant allelic fraction MAFs for C228T and C250T mutations, respectively [10].

In addition to the next-generation sequencing methods, another platform that can detect low-abundance mutant DNA molecules against a background of the thousand-fold excess of wild-type molecules is droplet-digital PCR (ddPCR). It combines the short hands-on-time and easy laboratory workflows and does not require complex bioinformatic analysis (Table 1), making it highly suitable for implementation into clinical practice.

Figure 1 shows a possible organization of the *TERT* promoter region. This model was generated in the online server "QGRS Mapper" and the particular fragment shown on the picture was described [61] to determine mutations C228T and C250T in upper tract urothelial carcinomas (UTUC) using PCR in conjunction with subsequent Sanger sequencing. All the analytical approaches described above include an amplification step of genomic regions containing −124 and −146 sites from the ATG starting codon, whose length may vary according to primer design. The occurrence of C228T and C250T mutations can distort the double-stranded structure of this region, and the amplification efficiency may also be subject to the ability of primers to anneal and extend template DNA in such complex regions with secondary structures. This could explain the wide ranges of reported sensitivities and specificities.

To develop diagnostic approaches based on the identification of mutations in the promoter region of the *TERT* gene, it will be critical to compare the performance of screening methods and provide harmonized and standardized laboratory procedures.

Table 1. Accuracy and methodological characteristics of tests for detecting the *TERT* promoter mutations in the urine for various neoplasias of the urinary system.

Article	Tumor Type	Method	Number of Patients	Size of Control Group	Sensitivity %	Specificity %	Length of PCR Product	Primers (Sequences Are Presented from 5′ End to End) and Probes
[56]	Small cell carcinoma (SCC)	PCR+ Sanger sequencing	11	3	100	100	163	CAGCGCTGCCTGAAACTC; GTCCTGCCCCTTCACCTT
[61]	Ureter carcinoma (UC)	PCR+ Sanger sequencing	20	0	94	10	193	CACCCGTCCTGCCCCTTCACCTT; GGCTTCCCACGTGCGCAGCAGGA-
	Renal pelvic carcinoma (RPC)		16	0	93.8	25	193	
	UTUC (RPC + UC) C228T	PCR+ Sanger sequencing	10	37	60	97	193	
		castPCR	10	37	90	92	dnp *	dnp
	BC (C228T)	PCR+ Sanger sequencing	36	33	47	100	193	CACCCGTCCTGCCCCTTCACCTT; GGCTTCCCACGTGCGCAGCAGGA
		castPCR	36	33	86	97	dnp	dnp
	UTUC + BC	PCR+ Sanger sequencing	46	70	50	98	193	CACCCGTCCTGCCCCTTCACCTT; GGCTTCCCACGTGCGCAGCAGGA
		castPCR	46	70	89	96	dnp	dnp
[10]	Urothelial cancer (UC) primary	UroMuTERT (NGS)	45	94	86.7	94.7	147	CTTCCAGCTCCGCCTCCTCCGCGCGG; AGCGCTGCCTGAAACTCGCGCC
	Urothelial cancer (UC) recurrence		48	94	87.5	94.7	147	
	UC (Diaguro)		93	94	87.1	94.7	147	
[72]	Urothelial bladder carcinoma	ddPCR	99	376	81.8	83.5	52	C228T: CGGAAAGGAAGGGGAGGG;GTCCCCGGCCCAGC Mut: [6FAM]-CCC+C+T+T+CCGG-[BHQ_1] WT: [HEX]-CCCC+T+C+CGGG-[BHQ_1]
							60	C250T: TGGGAGGGCCCGGAG;GACCCCGCCCCGT Mut: [6FAM]CCC+C+T+T+CCGG[BHQ_1] WT: [HEX]CCCC+T+C+CCGG[BHQ_1]
[55]	Squamous cell carcinoma Benign transurethral bladder biopsy samples	Safe-SeqS	15 0 [i]	94 [ii] 8	80	dnp	125 dnp	1st couple: CACACAGGAAACAGCTAT GACCATGGGCCGCGGAAAGGAAG; CGACGTAAAACGACGGCCAGTNNNNNNN NNNNNNNCGTCCTGCCCCTTCACC ** 2nd couple: CACACAGGAAACAGCTATGAC CATGGCGGAAAGGAAAGGGAG; CGACGTAAAACGACGGCCAGTNNNNNNN NNNNNNNNCCGTCCCGACCCCTC
[73]	NMIBC primary	SNaPshot assay	230	0	69	52	dnp	dnp

Table 1. *Cont.*

Article	Tumor Type	Method	Number of Patients	Size of Control Group	Sensitivity %	Specificity %	Length of PCR Product	Primers (Sequences Are Presented from 5′ End to End) and Probes
[48]	BC (primary)	SNaPshot assay	118	0	62	–	155	AGCGCTGCCTGAAACTCG; CCCTTCACCTTCCAGCTC
	BC (recurrence)		113	0	42	–	155	Probes: for C228T/A T_{23}GGCTGGGAGGGCCCGGA
	BC (recurrence-free samples)		0	218	–	73	155	for C250T T_{39}CTGGGCCGGGGACCCGG
[74]	Renal pelvic carcinoma (RPC)		5	0	60	dnp	193	CACCCGTCCTGCCCCTTCACCTT; GGCTTCCCACGTGCGCAGCAGGA
	UTUC		14	0	29	dnp	193	
	Chromophobe renal cell carcinoma (CRCC)		8	0	13	dnp	193	
	Ureter carcinoma (UC)		9	0	11	dnp	193	
	Clear cell renal cell carcinoma (CCRCC)		96	0	9.3	dnp	193	
	Renal cell carcinoma [iii] (RCC)		109	0	9.2	dnp	193	
[75]	BC early detection	PCR + Illumina sequencing	570	188	57	99.4	126	GGCCGCGGAAAGGAAG; CGTCCTGCCCCTTCACC
	UTUC		56	188	29	99.4		
	BC surveillance		322	188	57	99.4		
[11]	BC	UroMuTERT and ddPCR	30	101	46.7	100	65	C228T: CCCTCCCGGGTCC; CCGCGGAAAGGAAGG; probes: Mut: CCCGGAaGGGGCTG (FAM_lowaBlack); WT: CGGAgGGGGCTGG (HEX_IowaBlack). C250T CTTCACCTTCCAGCTCC, GAGGGCCCGGAGG; probes: Mut: CCCGGaAGGGGTCG (FAM_lowBlack); WT: ACCCGGgAGGGGT (HEX_IowaBlack).
[47]	UTUC	ddPCR	56	50	46.4	96	113	dnp
[76]	BC (supernatant)	NGS	92	0	46	100		NGS-primers: ACCTTCCAGCTCCGCCTCCTCCGCGCGGAC; AGAGGGCGGGGCCGCGGAAAGGAAGGGGAG
	BC (sediment)		92	0	48	100		
	Non-cancer hematuria		0	33				
[57]	Primary bladder adenocarcinoma	Safe-SeqS	14	94 [iv]	28.6	dnp	125	1st couple: CACACAGGAAACAGCTATGAC CATGGGCCGCGGAAAGGAAG; CGACGTAAAACGACGGCCAGTNNNNNNN NNNNNNNCGTCCTGCCCCTTCACC 2nd couple CACACAGGAAACAGCTATGAC CATGGCGGAAAGGAAAGGGAG; CGACGTAAAACGACGGCCAGTNNNNNN NNNNNNNNCCGTCCCGACCCCTC
	Benign transurethral bladder biopsy samples		0	8			dnp	
[53]	Urothelial cell carcinoma	PCR+ Sanger sequencing	327	0	dnp	65.4	343	AGCACCTCGCGGTAGTGG; GGATTCGCGGGCACAGAC

* "dnp"–data not provided; ** "N" is a degenerate base (it can be A, T, G, or C with equal likelihood); [i]. Table fields with "Number of patients 0" correspond to control group or additional control group; [ii]. Peripheral blood; [iii]. In this study, 6 subtypes of RCC tumor were investigated. In the table data only about 2 subtypes (ccRCC and chRCC) are presented. 4 remaining RCC tumors did not harbor *TERT* promoter mutations; [iv]. Peripheral blood.

3.3. Predictive Significance of Determining TERT Promoter Mutations in Urine

The high frequency and the localization of mutations in a small region of the *TERT* promoter provided an extraordinary opportunity for a simple non-invasive assay for early detection or monitoring the recurrence or progression of disease in the patients whose tumors carry one of those variants. This is especially pertinent for the conception of an early detection test as *TERT* promoter mutations have been reported to be early events in the BC tumorigenesis process [54]. Normal urothelium cells and extracellular DNA (also called cell-free DNA or cfDNA) are constantly released into the urine. Malignant transformation of bladder tissue will lead to exfoliated tumor cells and circulating tumor DNA (also called ctDNA) to mix with normal cells and cfDNA in the urine.

TERT promoter mutations (C228T and C250T) have been previously detected in DNA from urinary exfoliated cells (cellDNA) collected prior to diagnosis and during post-surgical follow-up, with sensitivities and specificities varying from 52% to 82% and from 83% to 99%, respectively, in patients with incident or early BC and from 42% to 74% and 73% to 93%, respectively, in patients with recurrent BC [48,54,72,73,75,77]. Two studies reported a sensitivity of 80% using pre-surgery urine cellDNA but no information was provided on the primary or recurrence status [46,50]. The first indication these mutations detected in urine samples during follow-up was associated with recurrence and, therefore, could potentially serve as markers to monitor the disease status that was provided by the study conducted by Kinde et al. [54]. While limited in size, the authors showed that among patients whose tumors harbored *TERT* promoter mutations (n = 11), the same mutations were present in urine collected for follow-up in seven of eight patients with relapse but in none of the six patients without recurrence [54]. In line with these findings, Descotes and colleagues showed that, in particular, the presence of *TERT* mutant DNA forms in post-surgical urine samples was associated with recurrence in 100 patients initially diagnosed with NMIBC [46].

The association held true in a limited subset of patients with negative cystoscopy (n = 6), suggesting that *TERT* promoter mutations in urine could be a promising avenue for early detection of recurrence in patients under surveillance for BC. The same research group also showed that the detection of urinary mutations could be used as a dynamic monitoring of recurrence. This was illustrated in one patient for whom the absence of the initially detected C250T mutation was noted in post-diagnostic serial urine samples for 7 years before being detectable at the time of recurrence confirmed by cystoscopy. However, Allory et al. reported a relatively low specificity for the prediction of recurrence as mutations were detected in 27% of recurrence-free patients under surveillance for BC [48]. The high false-positive rate may reflect a timeline that is suboptimal for follow-up, which, if prolonged, may contribute to increase specificity, as patients with clinically undetectable tumors at the time of a *TERT* promoter mutation positive test may present with clinically detectable tumors later on. More well-powered longitudinal studies with sufficient follow-up durations and serial post-surgery urine samples are required to fully assess the true performance of these biomarkers for the prediction of BC recurrence.

There is growing evidence supporting the utility of urinary *TERT* promoter mutations to detect primary BC. Allory and colleagues first reported a sensitivity of 62% for the detection of primary BC with a specificity of 90% in individuals with hematuria but no bladder tumor [48] (Table 1 and Table S4). Combining urinary *TERT* promoter mutations with other DNA-based markers was also evaluated [72,75]. In a prospective blinded study, urine samples from 475 patients with gross hematuria collected at the time of standard urological examination (flexible cystoscopy and computed tomography urography) were tested for DNA mutation (*TERT* and *FGFR3*) and methylation biomarkers (*SALL3, ONECUT2, CCNA1, BCL2, EOMES,* and *VIM*) to determine whether a urine-based DNA test could replace flexible cystoscopy in the initial assessment of the most common BC symptom, i.e., gross hematuria. Of the 99 (20.8%) patients presenting urothelial bladder tumors, the DNA test had a sensitivity of 97.0% and a specificity of 76.9%. Detection of mutations in the *TERT* promoter showed the highest sensitivity (81.8%), but at the same time, the lowest specificity (83.5%) for individuals with hematuria [72] (Table 1 and Table S4). The *FGFR3* gene is the most frequently mutated gene in NMIBC with a total frequency of 70%. While they are much less frequent than *TERT* promoter mutations, they could still represent a putative interesting combined biomarker for the detection of BC. The added value of their combination with *TERT* promoter mutations for the comprehensive non-invasive detection of BC has to still be demonstrated in independent study. A combined DNA-based biomarker approach was also recently evaluated in a screening study conducted by Springer et al. where they assessed the performance of a multigene panel assay that includes the screening of *TERT* promoter mutations and regions of interest in ten other somatically mutated genes (UROSEEK) for detecting BC 0–18 months prior to clinical diagnosis in high-risk symptomatic patients. The authors reported a sensitivity of 83% and a specificity of 93% for their panel, while *TERT* promoter mutations were detected in 57% of the cases. Specifically, the sensitivity and specificity of the *TERT* promoter mutation in urine samples of individuals with hematuria were 55% and 90%, respectively (Table S4) [75]. In a recent case-control study, Avogbe et al. used their developed single-plex ultrasensitive UroMuTERT assay to test the urinary DNA samples (both cfDNA or cellDNA) of 93 primary and recurrent cases with urothelial cancer and 94 controls, and compare its performance to that of urine cytology for the detection of urothelial cancer [10]. C228T or C250T mutations were detected in urinary cfDNA or cellDNA with 87.1% sensitivity and 94.7% specificity. The UroMuTERT sensitivity was consistent across primary and recurrent cases, and tumor stages and grades, and highest for urinary cfDNA and cellDNA combined. It also significantly outperformed the sensitivity of urine cytology, especially for detection of low-grade early-stage urothelial cancer [10]. In addition, the UroMuTERT single-gene assay demonstrated comparable performance to that of the UroSEEK multiple markers assay (including C228T and C250T) for the detection of primary or early urothelial cancer (sensitivity of 86.7% versus 83%; specificity of 94.7% versus 93%). Therefore, more studies are required to understand whether the observed differences in the detection rate of urinary *TERT* promoter mutations may originate from pre-analytical procedures or from the use of multiple urinary DNA sources versus one or from differences in prevalence of *TERT* promoter mutations in BC across populations. This has important implications as a simple single-gene assay with harmonized and standardized procedures for urine collection and processing might be able to achieve the same clinical performance for the detection of BC as complex multi-gene assays, which are more expensive and clinically less easily implemented.

While most studies conducted so far have focused on the evaluation of urinary cellDNA, there is, in addition to what Avogbe and colleagues reported [10], accumulating evidence that urinary cfDNA could be a reliable alternative source of urinary DNA for non-invasive genomic profiling of BC. While being based on recurrent clinically actionable genomic aberrations rather than on the assessment on *TERT* promoter mutations, a study reported that the use of urinary cfDNA led to higher analytical sensitivity (90%), as well as the use of urinary cellDNA (61%) for the detection of UC tumor-associated alterations [78]. These findings are in line with an initial study from 2007 reporting the superiority of urinary cfDNA over cellDNA for the detection of genetic alterations of patients with urothelial cancer [78,79]. Applied to the detection of the *TERT* promoter mutations, two recent studies highlighted the potential of the marker in urinary cfDNA for the detection of BC [80,81]. Specifically, of 77 patients whose tumor cells carried the 228 G > A/T mutation, the same mutation was detected by ddPCR in urinary cfDNA of 71 individuals (92%) and the mutation was absent in cfDNA of 26 of 27 healthy patients (specificity of 96%). Patients with false-negative results had an early-stage tumor, and increased mutant allelic fraction was found to correlate with increased stages of the disease. Concordant mutational status between tumor tissues and liquid biopsy was obtained in 92% of cases [80]. However, in studies comparing the analytical sensitivity of both forms of urinary DNAs, the results are sparse. Stasik and colleagues demonstrated a better sensitivity in using cellDNA (83%) than in using cfDNA (77%), but, overall, the *TERT* mutation allelic frequencies (MAF) were highly correlated, suggesting little added value in using cfDNA as an alternative source of urinary DNA [2]. This observation is in agreement with the results from Ward et al. who demonstrated an equal ability to detect somatic tumor mutations in cfDNA and cellDNA [82]. Avogbe and co-workers also reported an overall high concordance between cfDNA and cellDNA results but still observed the highest sensitivity for the combined source of DNA (87.1%) as opposed to cfDNA only (81.8%) and cellDNA (83.5%), highlighting the potential utility of combining multiple sources of DNA for the assessment of the marker in rare cases presenting with discordant results between cfDNA and cellDNA [10]. Interestingly, Stastik et al. observed a potential advantage of using urinary cfDNA in leukocyte-rich urines where the mutant allelic fractions of *TERT* promoter mutations were higher in cfDNA than in cellDNA [2].

In order to validate promising biomarkers, expert groups recommend a nested case-control study design within prospective cohorts in which samples collected at enrolment within the targeted population will be tested for the biomarker(s) in asymptomatic individuals who will develop cancer later and those who will not [83,84]. This sort of study was recently conducted by Hosen et al. who investigated the potential of urinary *TERT* promoter mutations as early detection biomarkers for bladder cancer in asymptomatic individuals in a case-control study nested within a longitudinal population-based prospective cohort of 50,045 Iranian individuals (the Golestan Cohort Study). *TERT* promoter mutations were assessed in baseline urine samples (1.9–4.5 mL) from 38 individuals who subsequently developed primary BC and 152 matched controls using the UroMuTERT and droplet digital PCR assays. Sequencing results were obtained for 30 cases and 101 controls. *TERT* promoter mutations were detected in 14 pre-clinical cases (sensitivity 46.67%) and none of the controls (specificity 100.00%). Most notably, the mutations were detectable up to 10 years prior to clinical diagnosis, indicating that detecting pre-clinical BC using cost-effective urinary *TERT* biomarkers may provide a valuable opportunity for BC screening and management [11].

Avogbe and colleagues [10] developed a predictive assay UroMuTERT, based on NGS (single-plex assay) of the hTERT promoter and the certain algorithm for detecting mutations of low-allelic fractions. Mutations in the *TERT* promoter in the urine DNA (cfDNA or cellDNA) showed superior sensitivity and specificity compared to all the methods described above, significantly surpassing the urine cytology especially for detecting early-stage NMIBC, which allowed the authors to propose modifications to the classic diagnostic protocol. The high recurrence rates of bladder cancer require frequent follow-ups involving expensive and invasive cystoscopic examination, thus further increasing the already high initial expenses for the management of bladder cancer [85,86]. The average costs of cystoscopy are around $206, and the cost of non-invasive urine cytology is around $56 [87]. By contrast, the cost of the NGS-based and ddPCR assays for detecting urinary *TERT* promoter mutations in bladder cancer developed by our group [10,11] is about 24€ per sample, and, therefore, has the potential to be easily implemented for cost-effective bladder cancer management strategies.

4. Conclusions

In summary, urinary *TERT* promoter mutations have demonstrated significant potential to be used as reliable, inexpensive, and non-invasive biomarkers for early detection and monitoring of BC. Moreover, urine ddPCR-based assays have been shown to be capable of detecting very low levels of these mutations, cost-effective, and simple to use, and would therefore represent an attractive method for clinical practice. The fact that *TERT* promoter mutations have been identified in urine years prior to the primary clinical diagnosis of BC and in some relapse-free patients under surveillance reflects the early occurrence of the mutations in the primary carcinogenic and in the relapse processes, providing a window of opportunity for early molecular detection and intervention. It may also explain the lack of specificity in some studies with the insufficient duration of follow-up. Therefore, large studies with a long-duration follow-up should further assess the robustness of these biomarkers for both detection and surveillance of BC. In particular, it should be evaluated whether a clinical diagnosis can be made through cystoscopy or urography in asymptomatic individuals or patients under surveillance presenting with a positive urinary *TERT* promoter mutations assay, or they would benefit from regular *TERT* mutation screening until the tumor becomes detectable.

Studies have shown that screening the high-risk population for bladder cancer with robust urinary markers, while not recommended by urological societies at present, could be cost-effective. Should their clinical relevance be demonstrated in individuals at high-risk of developing the disease (i.e., subjects with symptoms, mainly hematuria and/or lower urinary tract symptoms, or subjects with occupational exposure to certain chemicals), this may increase awareness of bladder cancer risk and facilitate the implementation of screening strategies in defined high-risk groups who would benefit from close surveillance with a non-invasive test. Furthermore, early detection of primary or recurrent BC using urinary *TERT* promoter mutations as a primary tool should lead to timely therapeutic intervention and better survival. It should also reduce both the numbers of unnecessary cystoscopy procedures in patients with a *TERT* promoter mutation negative test and the cost of clinical management of suspected BCs. In addition, as it is unlikely that *TERT* promoter mutations in BC could be detected in urine in all BC cases, it would be important to evaluate whether the clinical performance of this promising and already successfully applied biomarker could further increase when combined with existing urinary biomarkers, which alone lacks the sensitivity and specificity for clinical utility.

Finally, the origin of the occurrence of the *TERT* promoter mutations and their correlation to the BC phenotype still have to be elucidated. Future research on the etiologies of mutations occurrence in certain parts of the genome leading to enhanced activity of the *TERT* promoter will result in a new practical understanding of the biology of BC and possibly the development of preventive approaches. With regard to potential therapeutic applications, it is worth noting that the region of the *TERT* promoter that frequently carries *TERT* promoter mutations in BC, which are absent in normal bladder cells, can presumably become the target of anti-cancer therapy, including novel TERT-based immunotherapies, which could be tailored to patients whose tumors harbor these mutations [88,89].

Abbreviations

BC	Bladder cancer
NMIBC	Non-muscle-invasive bladder cancer
MIBC	Muscle-invasive bladder cancer
HTERT	Human telomerase reverse transcriptase
NGS	Next-generation sequencing
ddPCR	Droplet digital polymerase chain reaction

References

1. Antoni, S.; Ferlay, J.; Soerjomataram, I.; Znaor, A.; Jemal, A.; Bray, F. Bladder Cancer Incidence and Mortality: A Global Overview and Recent Trends. *Eur. Urol.* **2017**, *71*, 96–108. [CrossRef] [PubMed]
2. Stasik, Ş.; Salomo, K.; Heberling, U.; Froehner, M.; Sommer, U.; Baretton, G.B.; Ehninger, G.; Wirth, M.P.; Thiede, C.; Fuessel, S. Evaluation of TERT promoter mutations in urinary cell-free DNA and sediment DNA for detection of bladder cancer. *Clin. Biochem.* **2019**, *64*, 60–63. [CrossRef] [PubMed]
3. Hannen, R.; Bartsch, J.W. Essential roles of telomerase reverse transcriptase hTERT in cancer stemness and metastasis. *FEBS Lett.* **2018**, *592*, 2023–2031. [CrossRef] [PubMed]
4. Jafri, M.A.; Ansari, S.A.; Alqahtani, M.H.; Shay, J.W. Roles of telomeres and telomerase in cancer, and advances in telomerase-targeted therapies. *Genome Med.* **2016**, *8*, 69. [CrossRef] [PubMed]
5. Yuan, X.; Larsson, C.; Xu, D. Mechanisms underlying the activation of TERT transcription and telomerase activity in human cancer: Old actors and new players. *Oncogene* **2019**, *38*, 6172–6183. [CrossRef] [PubMed]

6. Leao, R.; Apolonio, J.D.; Lee, D.; Figueiredo, A.; Tabori, U.; Castelo-Branco, P. Mechanisms of human telomerase reverse transcriptase (hTERT) regulation: Clinical impacts in cancer. *J. Biomed. Sci.* **2018**, *25*, 22. [CrossRef] [PubMed]
7. Lee, D.D.; Leao, R.; Komosa, M.; Gallo, M.; Zhang, C.H.; Lipman, T.; Remke, M.; Heidari, A.; Nunes, N.M.; Apolonio, J.D.; et al. DNA hypermethylation within TERT promoter upregulates TERT expression in cancer. *J. Clin. Investig.* **2019**, *129*, 223–229. [CrossRef]
8. Chiba, K.; Lorbeer, F.K.; Shain, A.H.; McSwiggen, D.T.; Schruf, E.; Oh, A.; Ryu, J.; Darzacq, X.; Bastian, B.C.; Hockemeyer, D. Mutations in the promoter of the telomerase gene TERT contribute to tumorigenesis by a two-step mechanism. *Science* **2017**, *357*, 1416–1420. [CrossRef]
9. Gunes, C.; Wezel, F.; Southgate, J.; Bolenz, C. Implications of TERT promoter mutations and telomerase activity in urothelial carcinogenesis. *Nat. Rev. Urol.* **2018**, *15*, 386–393. [CrossRef]
10. Avogbe, P.H.; Manel, A.; Vian, E.; Durand, G.; Forey, N.; Voegele, C.; Zvereva, M.; Hosen, M.I.; Meziani, S.; De Tilly, B.; et al. Urinary TERT promoter mutations as non-invasive biomarkers for the comprehensive detection of urothelial cancer. *EBioMedicine* **2019**, *44*, 431–438. [CrossRef]
11. Hosen, M.I.; Sheikh, M.; Zvereva, M.; Scelo, G.; Forey, N.; Durand, G.; Voegele, C.; Poustchi, H.; Khoshnia, M.; Roshandel, G.; et al. Urinary TERT promoter mutations are detectable up to 10 years prior to clinical diagnosis of bladder cancer: Evidence from the Golestan Cohort Study. *EBioMedicine* **2020**, *53*, 17. [CrossRef] [PubMed]
12. Kamata, S.; Kageyama, Y.; Yonese, J.; Oshima, H. Significant telomere reduction in human superficial transitional cell carcinoma. *Br. J. Urol.* **1996**, *78*, 704–708. [CrossRef] [PubMed]
13. Turner, K.J.; Vasu, V.; Griffin, D.K. Telomere Biology and Human Phenotype. *Cells* **2019**, *8*, 73. [CrossRef]
14. Zvereva, M.I.; Shcherbakova, D.M.; Dontsova, O.A. Telomerase: Structure, functions, and activity regulation. *Biochemistry* **2010**, *75*, 1563–1583. [CrossRef]
15. Schmidt, J.C.; Cech, T.R. Human telomerase: Biogenesis, trafficking, recruitment, and activation. *Genes Dev.* **2015**, *29*, 1095–1105. [CrossRef] [PubMed]
16. Kim, N.W.; Piatyszek, M.A.; Prowse, K.R.; Harley, C.B.; West, M.D.; Ho, P.L.; Coviello, G.M.; Wright, W.E.; Weinrich, S.L.; Shay, J.W. Specific association of human telomerase activity with immortal cells and cancer. *Science* **1994**, *266*, 2011–2015. [CrossRef]
17. Sanchini, M.A.; Gunelli, R.; Nanni, O.; Bravaccini, S.; Fabbri, C.; Sermasi, A.; Bercovich, E.; Ravaioli, A.; Amadori, D.; Calistri, D. Relevance of urine telomerase in the diagnosis of bladder cancer. *JAMA* **2005**, *294*, 2052–2056. [CrossRef]
18. Landman, J.; Chang, Y.; Kavaler, E.; Droller, M.J.; Liu, B.C. Sensitivity and specificity of NMP-22, telomerase, and BTA in the detection of human bladder cancer. *Urology* **1998**, *52*, 398–402. [CrossRef]
19. Kinoshita, H.; Ogawa, O.; Kakehi, Y.; Mishina, M.; Mitsumori, K.; Itoh, N.; Yamada, H.; Terachi, T.; Yoshida, O. Detection of telomerase activity in exfoliated cells in urine from patients with bladder cancer. *J. Natl. Cancer Inst.* **1997**, *89*, 724–730. [CrossRef]
20. Yoshida, K.; Sugino, T.; Tahara, H.; Woodman, A.; Bolodeoku, J.; Nargund, V.; Fellows, G.; Goodison, S.; Tahara, E.; Tarin, D. Telomerase activity in bladder carcinoma and its implication for noninvasive diagnosis by detection of exfoliated cancer cells in urine. *Cancer* **1997**, *79*, 362–369. [CrossRef]
21. Sanchini, M.A.; Bravaccini, S.; Medri, L.; Gunelli, R.; Nanni, O.; Monti, F.; Baccarani, P.C.; Ravaioli, A.; Bercovich, E.; Amadori, D.; et al. Urine telomerase: An important marker in the diagnosis of bladder cancer. *Neoplasia* **2004**, *6*, 234–239. [CrossRef] [PubMed]
22. Sullivan, P.S.; Chan, J.B.; Levin, M.R.; Rao, J. Urine cytology and adjunct markers for detection and surveillance of bladder cancer. *Am. J. Transl. Res.* **2010**, *2*, 412–440. [PubMed]
23. Li, T.; Zou, L.; Zhang, J.; Li, G.; Ling, L. Non-invasive diagnosis of bladder cancer by detecting telomerase activity in human urine using hybridization chain reaction and dynamic light scattering. *Anal. Chim. Acta* **2019**, *13*, 90–97. [CrossRef] [PubMed]
24. Ludlow, A.T.; Robin, J.D.; Sayed, M.; Litterst, C.M.; Shelton, D.N.; Shay, J.W.; Wright, W.E. Quantitative telomerase enzyme activity determination using droplet digital PCR with single cell resolution. *Nucleic Acids Res.* **2014**, *42*, e104. [CrossRef] [PubMed]
25. Vukašinović, A.R.; Kotur-Stevuljević, J.M.; Mlakar, V.; Sopić, M.D.; Cvetković, Z.P.; Petković, M.R.; Spasojević-Kalimanovska, V.V.; Bogavac-Stanojević, N.B.; Ostanek, B. Telomerase stability and evaluation of real-time telomeric repeat amplification protocol. *Scand. J. Clin. Lab. Investig.* **2019**, *79*, 188–193. [CrossRef]

26. Su, D.; Huang, X.; Dong, C.; Ren, J. Quantitative Determination of Telomerase Activity by Combining Fluorescence Correlation Spectroscopy with Telomerase Repeat Amplification Protocol. *Anal. Chem.* **2018**, *90*, 1006–1013. [CrossRef]
27. Müller, M. Telomerase: Its clinical relevance in the diagnosis of bladder cancer. *Oncogene* **2002**, *21*, 650–655. [CrossRef]
28. Weikert, S.; Krause, H.; Wolff, I.; Christoph, F.; Schrader, M.; Emrich, T.; Miller, K.; Müller, M. Quantitative evaluation of telomerase subunits in urine as biomarkers for noninvasive detection of bladder cancer. *Int. J. Cancer* **2005**, *117*, 274–280. [CrossRef]
29. Glukhov, A.I.; Grigorieva, Y.E.; Gordeev, S.A.; Vinarov, A.Z.; Potoldykova, N.V. Development of noninvasive bladder cancer diagnosis on basis of telomerase and it's subunits hTERT and hTR detection. *Biomed. Khim.* **2015**, *61*, 150–160. [CrossRef]
30. Tilki, D.; Burger, M.; Dalbagni, G.; Grossman, H.B.; Hakenberg, O.W.; Palou, J.; Reich, O.; Roupret, M.; Shariat, S.F.; Zlotta, A.R. Urine markers for detection and surveillance of non-muscle-invasive bladder cancer. *Eur. Urol.* **2011**, *60*, 484–492. [CrossRef]
31. Liu, K.; Hodes, R.J.; Weng, N. Cutting edge: Telomerase activation in human T lymphocytes does not require increase in telomerase reverse transcriptase (hTERT) protein but is associated with hTERT phosphorylation and nuclear translocation. *J. Immunol.* **2001**, *166*, 4826–4830. [CrossRef] [PubMed]
32. March-Villalba, J.A.; Panach-Navarrete, J.; Herrero-Cervera, M.J.; Aliño-Pellicer, S.; Martínez-Jabaloyas, J.M. hTERT mRNA expression in urine as a useful diagnostic tool in bladder cancer. Comparison with cytology and NMP22 BladderCheck Test®. *Actas Urológicas Españolas (Engl. Ed.)* **2018**, *42*, 524–530. [CrossRef]
33. Clinton, T.; Lotan, Y. Review of the Clinical Approaches to the Use of Urine-based Tumor Markers in Bladder Cancer. *Rambam Maimonides Med. J.* **2017**, *8*, e0040. [CrossRef] [PubMed]
34. Ecke, T.H.; Weiß, S.; Stephan, C.; Hallmann, S.; Arndt, C.; Barski, D.; Otto, T.; Gerullis, H. UBC(®) Rapid Test-A Urinary Point-of-Care (POC) Assay for Diagnosis of Bladder Cancer with a focus on Non-Muscle Invasive High-Grade Tumors: Results of a Multicenter-Study. *Int. J. Mol. Sci.* **2018**, *19*, 3841. [CrossRef] [PubMed]
35. O'Sullivan, P.; Sharples, K.; Dalphin, M.; Davidson, P.; Gilling, P.; Cambridge, L.; Harvey, J.; Toro, T.; Giles, N.; Luxmanan, C.; et al. A multigene urine test for the detection and stratification of bladder cancer in patients presenting with hematuria. *J. Urol.* **2012**, *188*, 741–747. [CrossRef] [PubMed]
36. Bravaccini, S.; Casadio, V.; Gunelli, R.; Bucchi, L.; Zoli, W.; Amadori, D.; Silvestrini, R.; Calistri, D. Combining cytology, TRAP assay, and FISH analysis for the detection of bladder cancer in symptomatic patients. *Ann. Oncol.* **2011**, *22*, 2294–2298. [CrossRef]
37. Halling, K.C.; King, W.; Sokolova, I.A.; Karnes, R.J.; Meyer, R.G.; Powell, E.L.; Sebo, T.J.; Cheville, J.C.; Clayton, A.C.; Krajnik, K.L.; et al. A comparison of BTA stat, hemoglobin dipstick, telomerase and Vysis UroVysion assays for the detection of urothelial carcinoma in urine. *J. Urol.* **2002**, *167*, 2001–2006. [CrossRef]
38. Cavallo, D.; Casadio, V.; Bravaccini, S.; Iavicoli, S.; Pira, E.; Romano, C.; Fresegna, A.M.; Maiello, R.; Ciervo, A.; Buresti, G.; et al. Assessment of DNA damage and telomerase activity in exfoliated urinary cells as sensitive and noninvasive biomarkers for early diagnosis of bladder cancer in ex-workers of a rubber tyres industry. *Biomed. Res. Int.* **2014**, *2014*, 370907. [CrossRef]
39. Schmitz-Dräger, B.J.; Droller, M.; Lokeshwar, V.B.; Lotan, Y.; Hudson, M.A.; van Rhijn, B.W.; Marberger, M.J.; Fradet, Y.; Hemstreet, G.P.; Malmstrom, P.U.; et al. Molecular markers for bladder cancer screening, early diagnosis, and surveillance: The WHO/ICUD consensus. *Urol. Int.* **2015**, *94*, 1–24. [CrossRef]
40. Larré, S.; Catto, J.W.; Cookson, M.S.; Messing, E.M.; Shariat, S.F.; Soloway, M.S.; Svatek, R.S.; Lotan, Y.; Zlotta, A.R.; Grossman, H.B. Screening for bladder cancer: Rationale, limitations, whom to target, and perspectives. *Eur. Urol.* **2013**, *63*, 1049–1058. [CrossRef]
41. Xylinas, E.; Kluth, L.A.; Rieken, M.; Karakiewicz, P.I.; Lotan, Y.; Shariat, S.F. Urine markers for detection and surveillance of bladder cancer. *Urol. Oncol.* **2014**, *32*, 222–229. [CrossRef] [PubMed]
42. Shegay, P.V.; Zhavoronkov, A.A.; Gaifullin, N.M.; Vorob'ev, N.V.; Alekseev, B.Y.; Popov, S.V.; Garazha, A.V.; Buzdin, A.A.; Kaprin, A.D. Potentialities of MicroRNA Diagnosis in Patients with Bladder Cancer. *Bull. Exp. Biol. Med.* **2017**, *164*, 106–108. [CrossRef] [PubMed]
43. Killela, P.J.; Reitman, Z.J.; Jiao, Y.; Bettegowda, C.; Agrawal, N.; Diaz, L.A., Jr.; Friedman, A.H.; Friedman, H.; Gallia, G.L.; Giovanella, B.C.; et al. TERT promoter mutations occur frequently in gliomas and a subset of tumors derived from cells with low rates of self-renewal. *Proc. Natl. Acad. Sci. USA* **2013**, *110*, 6021–6026. [CrossRef] [PubMed]

44. Horn, S.; Figl, A.; Rachakonda, P.S.; Fischer, C.; Sucker, A.; Gast, A.; Kadel, S.; Moll, I.; Nagore, E.; Hemminki, K.; et al. TERT promoter mutations in familial and sporadic melanoma. *Science* **2013**, *339*, 959–961. [CrossRef]
45. Huang, F.W.; Hodis, E.; Xu, M.J.; Kryukov, G.V.; Chin, L.; Garraway, L.A. Highly recurrent TERT promoter mutations in human melanoma. *Science* **2013**, *339*, 957–959. [CrossRef]
46. Descotes, F.; Kara, N.; Decaussin-Petrucci, M.; Piaton, E.; Geiguer, F.; Rodriguez-Lafrasse, C.; Terrier, J.E.; Lopez, J.; Ruffion, A. Non-invasive prediction of recurrence in bladder cancer by detecting somatic TERT promoter mutations in urine. *Br. J. Cancer* **2017**, *117*, 583–587. [CrossRef]
47. Hayashi, Y.; Fujita, K.; Matsuzaki, K.; Matsushita, M.; Kawamura, N.; Koh, Y.; Nakano, K.; Wang, C.; Ishizuya, Y.; Yamamoto, Y.; et al. Diagnostic potential of TERT promoter and FGFR3 mutations in urinary cell-free DNA in upper tract urothelial carcinoma. *Cancer Sci.* **2019**, *110*, 1771–1779. [CrossRef]
48. Allory, Y.; Beukers, W.; Sagrera, A.; Flandez, M.; Marques, M.; Marquez, M.; van der Keur, K.A.; Dyrskjot, L.; Lurkin, I.; Vermeij, M.; et al. Telomerase reverse transcriptase promoter mutations in bladder cancer: High frequency across stages, detection in urine, and lack of association with outcome. *Eur. Urol.* **2014**, *65*, 360–366. [CrossRef]
49. Eich, M.-L.; Rodriguez Pena, M.D.C.; Springer, S.U.; Taheri, D.; Tregnago, A.C.; Salles, D.C.; Bezerra, S.M.; Cunha, I.W.; Fujita, K.; Ertoy, D.; et al. Incidence and distribution of UroSEEK gene panel in a multi-institutional cohort of bladder urothelial carcinoma. *Mod. Pathol.* **2019**, *32*, 1544–1550. [CrossRef]
50. Hurst, C.; Platt, F.; Knowles, M. Abstract 2240: TERT promoter mutations are highly prevalent in bladder cancer and represent a potential new urinary biomarker. *Cancer Res.* **2014**, *74*, 2240.
51. Kurtis, B.; Zhuge, J.; Ojaimi, C.; Ye, F.; Cai, D.; Zhang, D.; Fallon, J.T.; Zhong, M. Recurrent TERT promoter mutations in urothelial carcinoma and potential clinical applications. *Ann. Diagn. Pathol.* **2016**, *21*, 7–11. [CrossRef] [PubMed]
52. Pietzak, E.J.; Bagrodia, A.; Cha, E.K.; Drill, E.N.; Iyer, G.; Isharwal, S.; Ostrovnaya, I.; Baez, P.; Li, Q.; Berger, M.F.; et al. Next-generation Sequencing of Nonmuscle Invasive Bladder Cancer Reveals Potential Biomarkers and Rational Therapeutic Targets. *Eur. Urol.* **2017**, *72*, 952–959. [CrossRef] [PubMed]
53. Rachakonda, P.S.; Hosen, I.; de Verdier, P.J.; Fallah, M.; Heidenreich, B.; Ryk, C.; Wiklund, N.P.; Steineck, G.; Schadendorf, D.; Hemminki, K.; et al. TERT promoter mutations in bladder cancer affect patient survival and disease recurrence through modification by a common polymorphism. *Proc. Natl. Acad. Sci. USA* **2013**, *110*, 17426–17431. [CrossRef] [PubMed]
54. Kinde, I.; Munari, E.; Faraj, S.F.; Hruban, R.H.; Schoenberg, M.; Bivalacqua, T.; Allaf, M.; Springer, S.; Wang, Y.; Diaz, L.A., Jr.; et al. TERT promoter mutations occur early in urothelial neoplasia and are biomarkers of early disease and disease recurrence in urine. *Cancer Res.* **2013**, *73*, 7162–7167. [CrossRef]
55. Cowan, M.; Springer, S.; Nguyen, D.; Taheri, D.; Guner, G.; Rodriguez, M.A.; Wang, Y.; Kinde, I.; VandenBussche, C.J.; Olson, M.T.; et al. High prevalence of TERT promoter mutations in primary squamous cell carcinoma of the urinary bladder. *Mod. Pathol.* **2016**, *29*, 511–515. [CrossRef]
56. Zheng, X.; Zhuge, J.; Bezerra, S.M.; Faraj, S.F.; Munari, E.; Fallon, J.T., 3rd; Yang, X.J.; Argani, P.; Netto, G.J.; Zhong, M. High frequency of TERT promoter mutation in small cell carcinoma of bladder, but not in small cell carcinoma of other origins. *J. Hematol. Oncol.* **2014**, *7*, 014–0047. [CrossRef]
57. Cowan, M.L.; Springer, S.; Nguyen, D.; Taheri, D.; Guner, G.; Mendoza Rodriguez, M.A.; Wang, Y.; Kinde, I.; Del Carmen Rodriguez Pena, M.; VandenBussche, C.J.; et al. Detection of TERT promoter mutations in primary adenocarcinoma of the urinary bladder. *Hum. Pathol.* **2016**, *53*, 8–13. [CrossRef]
58. Palsgrove, D.N.; Taheri, D.; Springer, S.U.; Cowan, M.; Guner, G.; Mendoza Rodriguez, M.A.; Rodriguez Pena, M.D.C.; Wang, Y.; Kinde, I.; Ricardo, B.F.P.; et al. Targeted sequencing of plasmacytoid urothelial carcinoma reveals frequent TERT promoter mutations. *Hum. Pathol.* **2019**, *85*, 1–9. [CrossRef]
59. Borah, S.; Xi, L.; Zaug, A.J.; Powell, N.M.; Dancik, G.M.; Cohen, S.B.; Costello, J.C.; Theodorescu, D.; Cech, T.R. Cancer. TERT promoter mutations and telomerase reactivation in urothelial cancer. *Science* **2015**, *347*, 1006–1010. [CrossRef]
60. Ségal-Bendirdjian, E.; Geli, V. Non-canonical Roles of Telomerase: Unraveling the Imbroglio. *Front. Cell Dev. Biol.* **2019**, *7*, 332. [CrossRef]
61. Wang, K.; Liu, T.; Ge, N.; Liu, L.; Yuan, X.; Liu, J.; Kong, F.; Wang, C.; Ren, H.; Yan, K.; et al. TERT promoter mutations are associated with distant metastases in upper tract urothelial carcinomas and serve as urinary biomarkers detected by a sensitive castPCR. *Oncotarget* **2014**, *5*, 12428–12439. [CrossRef] [PubMed]

62. Bettegowda, C.; Sausen, M.; Leary, R.J.; Kinde, I.; Wang, Y.; Agrawal, N.; Bartlett, B.R.; Wang, H.; Luber, B.; Alani, R.M.; et al. Detection of Circulating Tumor DNA in Early- and Late-Stage Human Malignancies. *Sci. Transl. Med.* **2014**, *6*, 224ra24. [CrossRef] [PubMed]
63. Srisuwan, W.; Tatu, T. A Simple Whole-Blood Polymerase Chain Reaction without DNA Extraction for Thalassemia Diagnosis. *Hemoglobin* **2018**, *42*, 178–183. [CrossRef]
64. Kikin, O.; D'Antonio, L.; Bagga, P.S. QGRS Mapper: A web-based server for predicting G-quadruplexes in nucleotide sequences. *Nucl. Acids Res.* **2006**, *34*, W676–W682. [CrossRef]
65. Batista, R.; Vinagre, J.; Prazeres, H.; Sampaio, C.; Peralta, P.; Conceição, P.; Sismeiro, A.; Leão, R.; Gomes, A.; Furriel, F.; et al. Validation of a Novel, Sensitive, and Specific Urine-Based Test for Recurrence Surveillance of Patients With Non-Muscle-Invasive Bladder Cancer in a Comprehensive Multicenter Study. *Front. Genet.* **2019**, *10*, 1237. [CrossRef] [PubMed]
66. Siravegna, G.; Marsoni, S.; Siena, S.; Bardelli, A. Integrating liquid biopsies into the management of cancer. *Nat. Rev. Clin. Oncol.* **2017**, *14*, 531–548. [CrossRef] [PubMed]
67. Kinde, I.; Wu, J.; Papadopoulos, N.; Kinzler, K.W.; Vogelstein, B. Detection and quantification of rare mutations with massively parallel sequencing. *Proc. Natl. Acad. Sci. USA* **2011**, *108*, 9530–9535. [CrossRef]
68. Forshew, T.; Murtaza, M.; Parkinson, C.; Gale, D.; Tsui, D.W.Y.; Kaper, F.; Dawson, S.-J.; Piskorz, A.M.; Jimenez-Linan, M.; Bentley, D.; et al. Noninvasive Identification and Monitoring of Cancer Mutations by Targeted Deep Sequencing of Plasma DNA. *Sci. Transl. Med.* **2012**, *4*, 136ra68. [CrossRef]
69. Gale, D.; Lawson, A.R.J.; Howarth, K.; Madi, M.; Durham, B.; Smalley, S.; Calaway, J.; Blais, S.; Jones, G.; Clark, J.; et al. Development of a highly sensitive liquid biopsy platform to detect clinically-relevant cancer mutations at low allele fractions in cell-free DNA. *PLoS ONE* **2018**, *13*, e0194630. [CrossRef]
70. Newman, A.M.; Bratman, S.V.; To, J.; Wynne, J.F.; Eclov, N.C.; Modlin, L.A.; Liu, C.L.; Neal, J.W.; Wakelee, H.A.; Merritt, R.E.; et al. An ultrasensitive method for quantitating circulating tumor DNA with broad patient coverage. *Nat. Med.* **2014**, *20*, 548–554. [CrossRef]
71. Delhomme, T.M.; Avogbe, P.H.; Gabriel, A.A.G.; Alcala, N.; Leblay, N.; Voegele, C.; Vallée, M.; Chopard, P.; Chabrier, A.; Abedi-Ardekani, B.; et al. Needlestack: An ultra-sensitive variant caller for multi-sample next generation sequencing data. *NAR Genom. Bioinform.* **2020**, *2*, 20. [CrossRef] [PubMed]
72. Dahmcke, C.M.; Steven, K.E.; Larsen, L.K.; Poulsen, A.L.; Abdul-Al, A.; Dahl, C.; Guldberg, P. A Prospective Blinded Evaluation of Urine-DNA Testing for Detection of Urothelial Bladder Carcinoma in Patients with Gross Hematuria. *Eur. Urol.* **2016**, *70*, 916–919. [CrossRef] [PubMed]
73. Critelli, R.; Fasanelli, F.; Oderda, M.; Polidoro, S.; Assumma, M.B.; Viberti, C.; Preto, M.; Gontero, P.; Cucchiarale, G.; Lurkin, I.; et al. Detection of multiple mutations in urinary exfoliated cells from male bladder cancer patients at diagnosis and during follow-up. *Oncotarget* **2016**, *7*, 67435–67448. [CrossRef] [PubMed]
74. Wang, K.; Liu, T.; Liu, L.; Liu, J.; Liu, C.; Wang, C.; Ge, N.; Ren, H.; Yan, K.; Hu, S.; et al. TERT promoter mutations in renal cell carcinomas and upper tract urothelial carcinomas. *Oncotarget* **2014**, *5*, 1829–1836. [CrossRef]
75. Springer, S.U.; Chen, C.-H.; Rodriguez Pena, M.D.C.; Li, L.; Douville, C.; Wang, Y.; Cohen, J.D.; Taheri, D.; Silliman, N.; Schaefer, J.; et al. Non-invasive detection of urothelial cancer through the analysis of driver gene mutations and aneuploidy. *eLife* **2018**, *7*, e32143. [CrossRef]
76. Ou, Z.; Li, K.; Yang, T.; Dai, Y.; Chandra, M.; Ning, J.; Wang, Y.; Xu, R.; Gao, T.; Xie, Y.; et al. Detection of bladder cancer using urinary cell-free DNA and cellular DNA. *Clin. Transl. Med.* **2020**, *9*, 4. [CrossRef]
77. Ward, D.G.; Baxter, L.; Gordon, N.S.; Ott, S.; Savage, R.S.; Beggs, A.D.; James, J.D.; Lickiss, J.; Green, S.; Wallis, Y.; et al. Multiplex PCR and Next Generation Sequencing for the Non-Invasive Detection of Bladder Cancer. *PLoS ONE* **2016**, *11*, e0149756. [CrossRef]
78. Togneri, F.S.; Ward, D.G.; Foster, J.M.; Devall, A.J.; Wojtowicz, P.; Alyas, S.; Vasques, F.R.; Oumie, A.; James, N.D.; Cheng, K.K.; et al. Genomic complexity of urothelial bladder cancer revealed in urinary cfDNA. *Eur. J. Hum. Genet.* **2016**, *24*, 1167–1174. [CrossRef]
79. Szarvas, T.; Kovalszky, I.; Bedi, K.; Szendroi, A.; Majoros, A.; Riesz, P.; Fule, T.; Laszlo, V.; Kiss, A.; Romics, I. Deletion analysis of tumor and urinary DNA to detect bladder cancer: Urine supernatant versus urine sediment. *Oncol Rep.* **2007**, *18*, 405–409. [CrossRef]
80. Russo, I.J.; Ju, Y.; Gordon, N.S.; Zeegers, M.P.; Cheng, K.K.; James, N.D.; Bryan, R.T.; Ward, D.G. Toward Personalised Liquid Biopsies for Urothelial Carcinoma: Characterisation of ddPCR and Urinary cfDNA for the Detection of the TERT 228 G > A/T Mutation. *Bladder Cancer* **2018**, *4*, 41–48. [CrossRef]

81. Hayashi, Y.; Fujita, K.; Matsuzaki, K.; Eich, M.L.; Tomiyama, E.; Matsushita, M.; Koh, Y.; Nakano, K.; Wang, C.; Ishizuya, Y.; et al. Clinical Significance of Hotspot Mutation Analysis of Urinary Cell-Free DNA in Urothelial Bladder Cancer. *Front. Oncol.* **2020**, *10*, 755. [CrossRef] [PubMed]
82. Ward, D.G.; Gordon, N.S.; Boucher, R.H.; Pirrie, S.J.; Baxter, L.; Ott, S.; Silcock, L.; Whalley, C.M.; Stockton, J.D.; Beggs, A.D.; et al. Targeted deep sequencing of urothelial bladder cancers and associated urinary DNA: A 23-gene panel with utility for non-invasive diagnosis and risk stratification. *BJU Int.* **2019**, *124*, 532–544. [CrossRef] [PubMed]
83. Pepe, M.S.; Etzioni, R.; Feng, Z.; Potter, J.D.; Thompson, M.L.; Thornquist, M.; Winget, M.; Yasui, Y. Phases of biomarker development for early detection of cancer. *J. Natl. Cancer Inst.* **2001**, *93*, 1054–1061. [CrossRef] [PubMed]
84. Pesch, B.; Brüning, T.; Johnen, G.; Casjens, S.; Bonberg, N.; Taeger, D.; Müller, A.; Weber, D.G.; Behrens, T. Biomarker research with prospective study designs for the early detection of cancer. *Biochim. Biophys. Acta* **2014**, *5*, 874–883. [CrossRef] [PubMed]
85. Svatek, R.S.; Hollenbeck, B.K.; Holmäng, S.; Lee, R.; Kim, S.P.; Stenzl, A.; Lotan, Y. The economics of bladder cancer: Costs and considerations of caring for this disease. *Eur. Urol.* **2014**, *66*, 253–262. [CrossRef] [PubMed]
86. Leal, J.; Luengo-Fernandez, R.; Sullivan, R.; Witjes, J.A. Economic Burden of Bladder Cancer Across the European Union. *Eur. Urol.* **2016**, *69*, 438–447. [CrossRef] [PubMed]
87. Lotan, Y.; Svatek, R.S.; Sagalowsky, A.I. Should we screen for bladder cancer in a high-risk population?: A cost per life-year saved analysis. *Cancer* **2006**, *107*, 982–990. [CrossRef]
88. Zanetti, M. A second chance for telomerase reverse transcriptase in anticancer immunotherapy. *Nat. Rev. Clin. Oncol.* **2017**, *14*, 115–128. [CrossRef]
89. Carrozza, F.; Santoni, M.; Piva, F.; Cheng, L.; Lopez-Beltran, A.; Scarpelli, M.; Montironi, R.; Battelli, N.; Tamberi, S. Emerging immunotherapeutic strategies targeting telomerases in genitourinary tumors. *Crit. Rev. Oncol. Hematol.* **2018**, *131*, 1–6. [CrossRef]

Specificity of the Metallothionein-1 Response by Cadmium-Exposed Normal Human Urothelial Cells

Rhiannon V. McNeill [1,†], Andrew S. Mason [1], Mark E. Hodson [2], James W.F. Catto [3] and Jennifer Southgate [1,*]

1 Jack Birch Unit for Molecular Carcinogenesis, Department of Biology, York Biomedical Research Institute, University of York, York YO10 5DD, UK; rvm8828@gmail.com (R.V.M.); andrew.mason@york.ac.uk (A.S.M.)
2 Department of Environment and Geography, University of York, York YO10 5DD, UK; mark.hodson@york.ac.uk
3 Academic Urology Unit, University of Sheffield, Sheffield S10 2TN, UK; j.catto@sheffield.ac.uk
* Correspondence: j.southgate@york.ac.uk
† Current address: Department of Psychiatry, Psychosomatic Medicine, and Psychotherapy, University Hospital of Frankfurt, 60590 Frankfurt, Germany.

Abstract: Occupational and environmental exposure to cadmium is associated with the development of urothelial cancer. The metallothionein (MT) family of genes encodes proteins that sequester metal ions and modulate physiological processes, including zinc homeostasis. Little is known about the selectivity of expression of the different MT isoforms. Here, we examined the effect of cadmium exposure on MT gene and isoform expression by normal human urothelial (NHU) cell cultures. Baseline and cadmium-induced MT gene expression was characterized by next-generation sequencing and RT-PCR; protein expression was assessed by Western blotting using isoform-specific antibodies. Expression of the zinc transporter-1 (*SLC30A1*) gene was also assessed. NHU cells displayed transcription of *MT-2A*, but neither *MT-3* nor *MT-4* genes. Most striking was a highly inducer-specific expression of MT-1 genes, with cadmium inducing transcription of *MT-1A*, *MT-1G*, *MT-1H*, and *MT-1M*. Whereas *MT-1G* was also induced by zinc and nickel ions and *MT-1H* by iron, both *MT-1*A and *MT-1M* were highly cadmium-specific, which was confirmed for protein using isoform-specific antibodies. Protein but not transcript endured post-exposure, probably reflecting sequestration. *SLC30A1* transcription was also affected by cadmium ion exposure, potentially reflecting perturbation of intracellular zinc homeostasis. We conclude that human urothelium displays a highly inductive profile of MT-1 gene expression, with two isoforms identified as highly specific to cadmium, providing candidate transcript and long-lived protein biomarkers of cadmium exposure.

Keywords: Metallothionein; urothelium; urothelial cancer; cadmium exposure; zinc transporter

1. Introduction

Occupational and environmental exposure to cadmium has increased as a result of the burning of fossil fuels and widespread use of the "heavy" metal in anthropological activities, such as battery production, electroplating, smelting, and soldering (reviewed [1]). Cadmium ions accumulate in the body in an almost irreversible manner [2], as the metal cannot be metabolized to a less toxic species [3] and has a low excretion rate [4]. This low excretion rate is thought to be due to intracellular sequestration of cadmium ions by metal-binding proteins [5–7]. An association between cadmium exposure and bladder (urothelial) carcinogenesis has been reported, with higher cadmium concentrations demonstrated in the blood [8] and urine [9–11] of patients with bladder cancer. In vitro research supports these correlative studies, with malignant transformation of the immortalized RWPE-1, TLR1215, 16HBE, and UROtsa cell lines reported after extended chronic cadmium exposure [12–15]. The bladder stores concentrated urine prior to voiding, meaning that the urothelial lining of the bladder (which functions as one of the tightest epithelial barriers [16]) is potentially exposed to excreted xenobiotics [16–18]. It is currently not known whether exposure to urinary cadmium is limited by the presence of an intact urinary barrier.

The metallothioneins (MTs) are a superfamily of low-molecular weight (~6 kDa), cysteine-rich proteins that are induced by and bind a range of metal ions, including cadmium [19,20]. Through this sequestration of metal ions MTs are considered to play a primary role in metal detoxification [21,22], but also metal (e.g., zinc) homeostasis [23–25] and the scavenging of reactive oxygen species (ROS) [26,27]. MT involvement in the bodily response to cadmium exposure has been well-documented, with numerous studies demonstrating cadmium-induced MT expression both in vitro [28–34] and in vivo [35,36].

Direct binding of MT protein to cadmium ions [37,38] results in a MT-cadmium complex that is highly resistant to degradation [5–7]. In humans, four main MT subfamilies exist (MT-1, MT-2/2A, MT-3, and MT-4), with MT-1 consisting of nine isoforms (-A, -B, -E, -F, -G, -H, -L, -M, and -X) [39] each encoded on individual genes. It is predicted that the individual MT isoforms have distinct properties including structure [40,41], tissue- and inducer-specific expression [22,34,42–47], induction rate [48], translational efficiency [41], and degradation rate [49,50]. Cadmium is reported to be the most potent inducer of MT expression [51]. This offers the potential that individual MT isoforms may be utilized as specific biomarkers of human exposure to cadmium, although it remains unclear which isoform(s) are responsible for cadmium sequestration. This lack of discrimination is largely due to the high homology between isoforms and the lack of discriminatory reagents, with no validated antibodies able to distinguish MT-1 and MT-2 subfamilies, nor the different MT-1 isoforms [41,52].

MTs are reported to work cooperatively with zinc transporters to regulate cellular zinc homeostasis, potentially by modulating cellular zinc ion concentration [39], although the exact mechanisms are unknown. Thus, a possible consequence of exposure to cadmium ions may be altered cellular zinc homeostasis. Cadmium and zinc possess highly similar properties, and it has been shown that cadmium can substitute for zinc in biological systems [53]. This can disrupt the normal functioning of various biological pathways [54,55], thus indirectly influencing processes involved in carcinogenesis such as cell proliferation and metastasis [56].

Our aims were to investigate MT isoform expression and specificity of induction in human urothelium under baseline and cadmium-exposed conditions, using a well-characterized normal human urothelial (NHU) cell culture system that includes polarized differentiated NHU cell sheets possessing tight barrier function [57,58]. Prior to cadmium exposure, cellular growth assays were performed to assess cytotoxicity. Next, we exposed NHU cells to a variety of potential MT inducers, including reactive oxygen species (ROS) [59,60], essential metals [44,61–66], and heavy metals [67–70] to define the specificity of response. Previously unpublished MT-1 isoform-specific antibodies were used to discriminate between MT-1 isoform proteins. Lastly, we determined whether transcription of the free zinc efflux regulator zinc transporter-1 (*SLC30A1*) [71] was altered as a consequence of cadmium exposure. The results revealed that MT isoform expression was inducer-specific, and that abundance of both *MT-1A* and *MT-1M* transcript and protein was highly cadmium-specific, highlighting their potential as biomarkers of exposure. Cadmium was able to penetrate an intact urothelial barrier and effected transcriptional upregulation of *SLC30A1*, indicating a potential route for cadmium uptake and possible subsequent substitution in zinc homeostatic mechanisms.

2. Results

2.1. *Influence of Cadmium on NHU Cell Culture Growth and Uptake of Cadmium across an Intact Urothelial Barrier*

Exposure of nondifferentiated NHU cells to cadmium revealed that cell growth was unaffected by concentrations ≤ 10 μM $CdCl_2$ whilst exposure to 20 μM $CdCl_2$ resulted in distinct cytotoxicity (Figure 1A). Replication in a second independent cell line confirmed that exposure to 10 μM $CdCl_2$

did not affect NHU cell growth (Figure 1B); this concentration was therefore selected for further experiments. When differentiated NHU cell cultures (three independent cell lines) were grown on permeable membranes in triplicate and exposed apically to 10 μM $CdCl_2$ for 72 h, no effect was seen on barrier function (control versus cadmium-exposed transepithelial electrical resistance (TEER) of 3.24 ± 0.48 kΩ.cm^2 versus 3.17 ± 0.52 kΩ.cm^2, mean ± SEM; $p = 0.93$; Table S1). The barrier was retained during $CdCl_2$ exposures of at least seven days, over which time the TEER increased in the cadmium-exposed culture to 1.8-fold over control. Analysis of cell lysates by inductively coupled plasma optical emission spectroscopy (ICP-OES) revealed an intracellular cadmium concentration of 0.94 μM in lysates from cadmium-exposed cultures compared to 0.08 μM for control cultures.

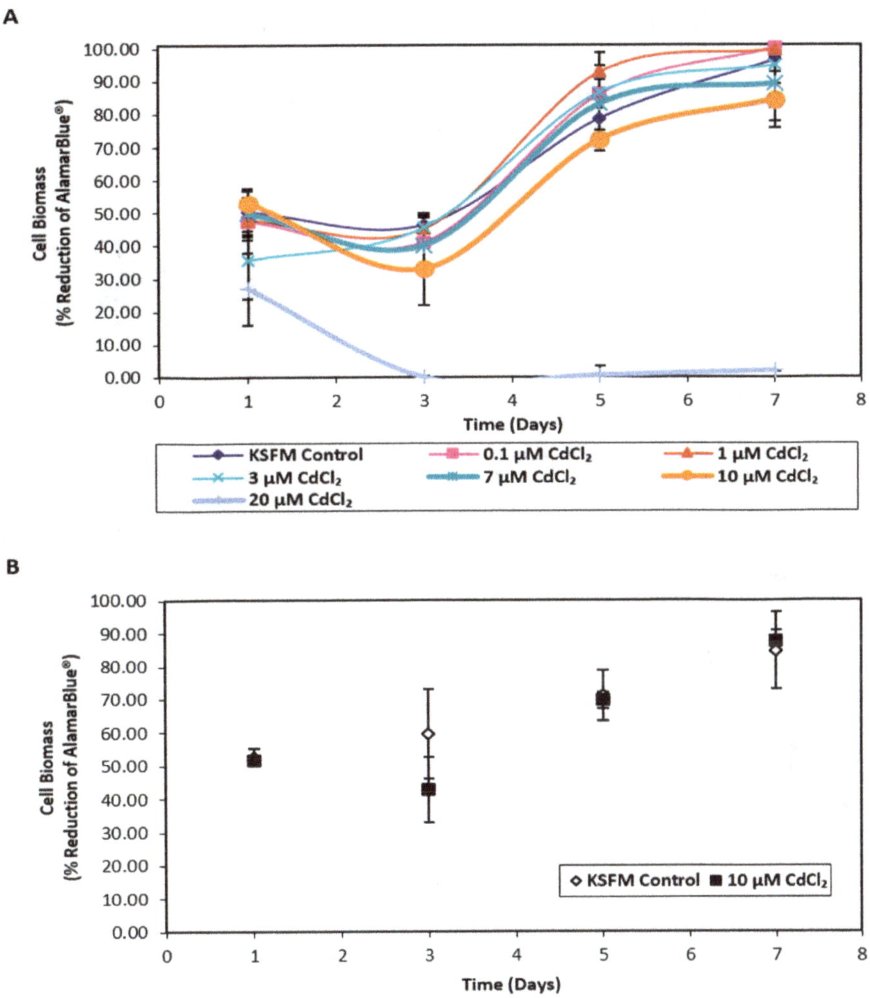

Figure 1. Biomass growth assays for in vitro normal human urothelial (NHU) cell cultures exposed to cadmium. AlamarBlue® assays were performed over 7 days on NHU cell cultures seeded at 6×10^4 cells/cm^2. (**A**) NHU cells were exposed to a range of cadmium concentrations from 0 to 20 μM (n = 1 independent cell line). Each data point represents mean percentage reduction in AlamarBlue® ± S.D. from three replicate cultures. (**B**) NHU cells were exposed to 10 μM $CdCl_2$ for up to 7 days. Data points represent mean percentage reduction in AlamarBlue® ± S.D. from two independent NHU cell lines, each performed in triplicate.

2.2. *Baseline and Cadmium-Induced MT Transcription in NHU Cells*

NHU cells maintained in culture in nondifferentiated and differentiated states were examined for baseline expression of MT genes. Analysis by mRNA-seq of nondifferentiated NHU cells revealed high expression of *MT-1E* and *MT-1X* and low expression of *MT-1A*, *MT-1B*, *MT-1F*, and *MT-1G*; there was no detection of *MT-1H* or *MT-1M* transcripts (Figure 2A). *MT-2A* expression was three times greater than all the MT-1 genes combined. No expression was detected for *MT-3* or *MT-4*. In almost all cases where MT gene expression was detected in nondifferentiated NHU cells, the expression was reduced in the differentiated state. This was most striking for *MT-2A* ($\log_2$FC = 4.2; q = 4.08 × 10^{-3}) and *MT-1E* ($\log_2$FC = 1.5; q = 4.0 × 10^{-4}), although between-donor variation prohibited statistical significance for many genes with lower expression. The apparent exception was *MT-1X*, where the average expression increased in the differentiated state. However, this was inconsistent between donors, and the differential expression was nonsignificant. Interestingly, *MT-1L* (which generates a transcript with a premature stop codon [72]) was expressed at similar abundance to *MT-1E* in the nondifferentiated cells, but with a much greater downregulation in the differentiated state ($\log_2$FC = 5.4; q = 8.4 × 10^{-4}). Previous reports of a truncation-rescuing polymorphism [73] was not identified in these donors, so while *MT-1L* is unlikely to form a functional protein, it may play a role in MT-1 transcript regulation. Expression was detected for *SLC30A1* in both nondifferentiated and differentiated states (Figure 2A), but there was no significant differentiation-associated change in expression.

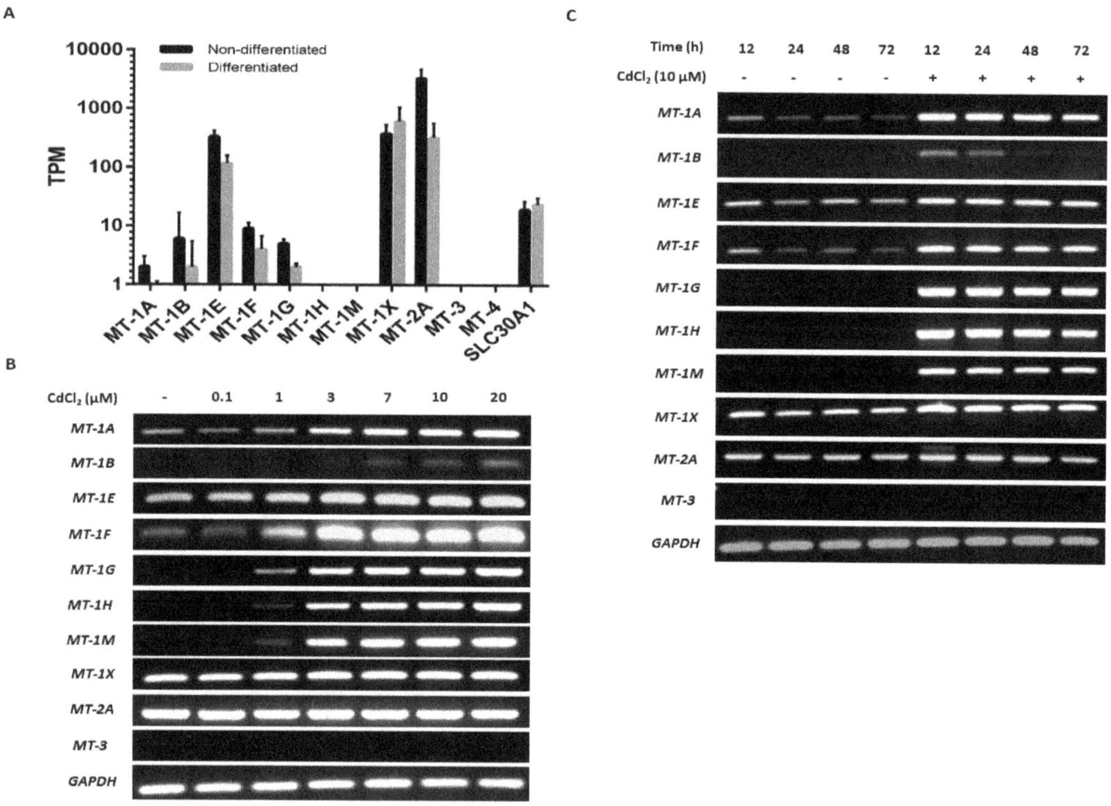

Figure 2. Baseline and cadmium-induced MT transcript expression by NHU cells in vitro. (**A**) Next-generation sequencing data showing baseline MT isoform transcription in nondifferentiated and differentiated NHU cells (*n* = 3 independent cell lines; standard deviation is shown). (**B**,**C**) MT gene expression in NHU cells assessed by RT-PCR. The total cDNA input was 1 μg and PCR reaction products were removed after 25 cycles; *GAPDH* was included as input control. See Table 1 for primer sequences and product sizes. Note that medium was changed at time T = 0 only and there was no renewal of cadmium over the period. The figure shows results representative of *n* = 3 independent NHU cell lines. Additional PCR controls included genomic DNA as a positive control and a no-template (H_2O) negative control; RT negative samples confirmed absence of genomic contamination. In (**B**), the result of exposing nondifferentiated NHU cells to different concentrations of cadmium (0–20 μM) for 72 h on MT gene expression is shown. In (**C**), MT gene expression is shown in differentiated NHU cell cultures following exposure to 10 μM $CdCl_2$ for up to 72 h.

RT-PCR results supported the NGS data, although the variability in transcript detection in nondifferentiated NHU cells indicated a potentially inducible state (Figure 2B). Differentiated NHU cell cultures revealed a more consistent baseline expression of several MT-1 genes, particularly *MT-1X* (Figure 2C).

Exposure to cadmium ions caused a massive induction of all eight MT-1 genes (*MT-1A, MT-1B, MT-1E, MT-1F, MT-1G, MT-1H, MT-1M,* and *MT-1X*) within 12 h of initial exposure, as demonstrated by the RT-PCR results, with expression receding over time (Figure 2B,C). Whereas expression of *MT-1* transcripts was mostly lost after 48 h of continuous cadmium exposure in nondifferentiated cell cultures (Figure 2B with independent cell line repeats in supplementary Figures S1 and S2), MT-1 subfamily transcript expression was still detectable in differentiated cell cultures after 72 h exposure (Figure 2C; with independent repeats in supplementary Figures S3 and S4).

Irrespective of differentiation state and the presence or absence of cadmium, *MT-2A* transcript expression was constitutively high, whilst *MT-3* and *MT-4* transcripts were invariably absent. Based on this, the *MT-2A, MT-3,* and *MT-4* genes were not further studied. By contrast, the strong induction of the *MT-1A, -1G, -1H,* and *-1M* paralogs, which was consistent following cadmium exposure in three independent NHU cell lines, was further investigated for specificity. As the RT-PCR results demonstrated a striking on/off transcriptional response of these MT-1 isoforms to cadmium exposure, it was decided to continue with this approach, as quantitative PCR would not have added anything to the data.

2.3. *Specificity of Cadmium-Induced MT Transcription*

NHU cell cultures were exposed to a variety of candidate MT inducers identified from the literature.

ROS is reported as a by-product of cadmium exposure [59], and therefore we sought to determine the effects of ROS on transcription of MT-1 genes. The ROS-inducing agent sulforaphane ($C_6H_{11}NOS_2$) and ROS-inhibitor ascorbic acid ($C_6H_8O_6$) were titrated against transcription of the ROS-sensitive heme oxygenase-1 (*HMOX1*) gene [74,75] to infer intracellular ROS activity (Figure 3A,B, respectively). Induction of expression of the four MT-1 genes in response to cadmium exposure was unaffected by 25 μg/mL ascorbic acid used to inhibit ROS, suggesting that ROS was not responsible (Figure 3C). This conclusion was supported by the failure of 5 μM sulforaphane to induce MT-1 expression (replicate in supplementary material, Figure S5).

Differential induction of MT-1 paralogs was examined in response to other metal ions, both essential and carcinogenic (replicates in supplementary material, Figures S6 and S7). Both zinc and nickel exposure induced *MT-1G* transcription, whereas *MT-1H* transcript expression was only minimally induced by zinc, and nickel had no effect. *MT-1A* transcription was constitutively low under all conditions apart from cadmium exposure, which increased expression, and *MT-1M* transcription was highly induced by exposure to cadmium alone.

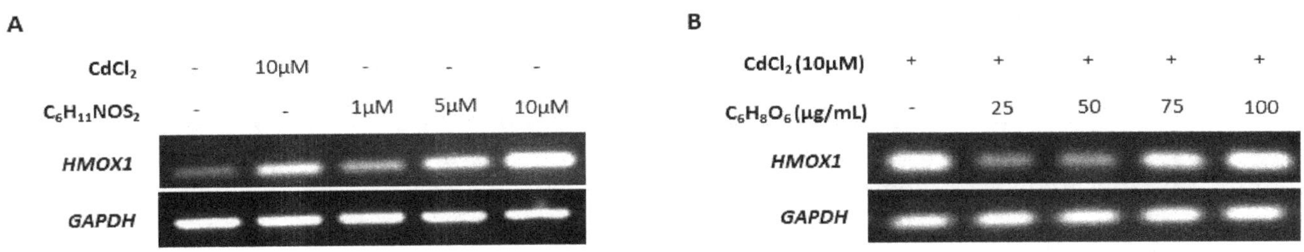

Figure 3. *Cont.*

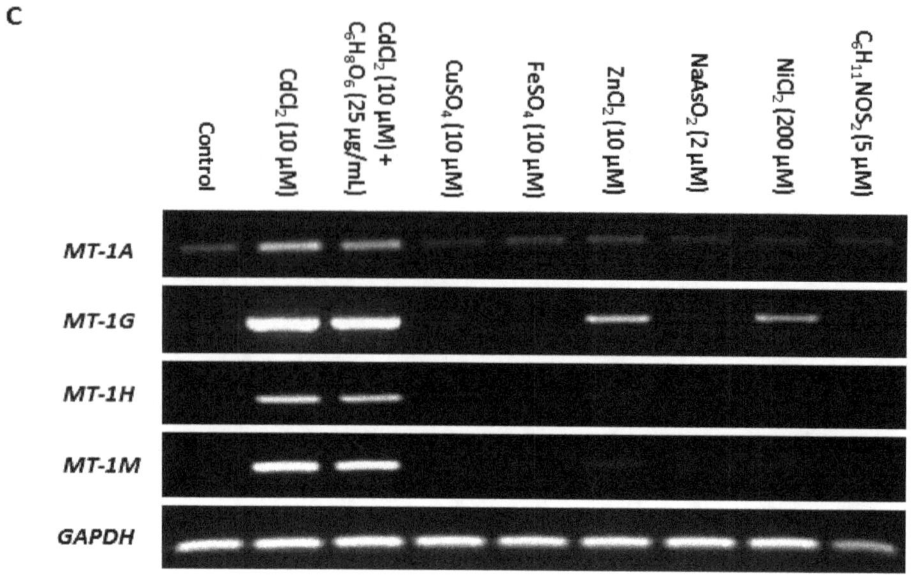

Figure 3. Specificity of metallothionein (MT) transcription induction by cadmium. MT gene expression was assessed by RT-PCR in NHU cells exposed to a variety of candidate inducers. The total cDNA input was 1 µg and PCR reaction products were removed after 25 cycles; *GAPDH* was included as input control. Note that medium was changed at time T = 0 only and there was no renewal of treatments over the period. Additional PCR controls included genomic DNA as a positive control and a no-template (H_2O) negative control; RT negative samples confirmed absence of genomic contamination. In (**A**), nondifferentiated NHU cell cultures were treated with a range of concentrations of sulforaphane ($C_6H_{11}NOS_2$) for 12 h, and the effect on transcription of the ROS-sensitive gene *HMOX1* assessed in comparison to exposure to 10 µM $CdCl_2$ (n = 1 independent cell line). The concentration of $C_6H_{11}NOS_2$ that induced transcription of *HMOX1* to a comparable extent to cadmium was selected. In (**B**), nondifferentiated NHU cell cultures were treated with a range of concentrations of ascorbic acid ($C_6H_8O_6$) for 12 h in combination with 10 µM $CdCl_2$ and the effect on *HMOX1* transcription assessed. The concentration of $C_6H_8O_6$ that caused the biggest decrease in *HMOX1* transcription was selected. In (**C**), NHU cell cultures (n = 2 independent cell lines) were exposed to a range of candidate regulators and transcript expression was assessed for the MT-1 genes shown above to be most sensitive to cadmium induction (from Figure 2B,C). Candidate inducers tested were cadmium (10 µM $CdCl_2$), cadmium combined with ascorbic acid (10 µM $CdCl_2$ + 25 µg/mL $C_6H_8O_6$), copper (10 µM $CuSO_4$), iron (10 µM $FeSO_4$), zinc (10 µM $ZnCl_2$), arsenite (2 µM $NaAsO_2$), nickel (200 µM $NiCl_2$), and sulforaphane (5 µM $C_6H_{11}NOS_2$). Essential metals were applied at equivalent concentrations to cadmium. Arsenite and nickel were both used at their highest noncytotoxic concentrations based on initial titration experiments (not shown).

2.4. Immunoblotting With Isoform-Specific Antibodies

To examine if the observed induction of MT-1 gene expression translated to protein, antibodies specific to the MT-1A and MT-1M isoforms were used to perform Western blotting. Control nondifferentiated NHU cells lacked MT-1A and MT-1M protein expression (Figure 4A). Cadmium exposure caused induction of both MT-1A and MT-1M proteins after 72 h (replicate in supplementary material, Figure S8). Both proteins were also induced in cadmium-exposed differentiated NHU cells (Figure 4B; replicated in supplementary material, Figure S9).

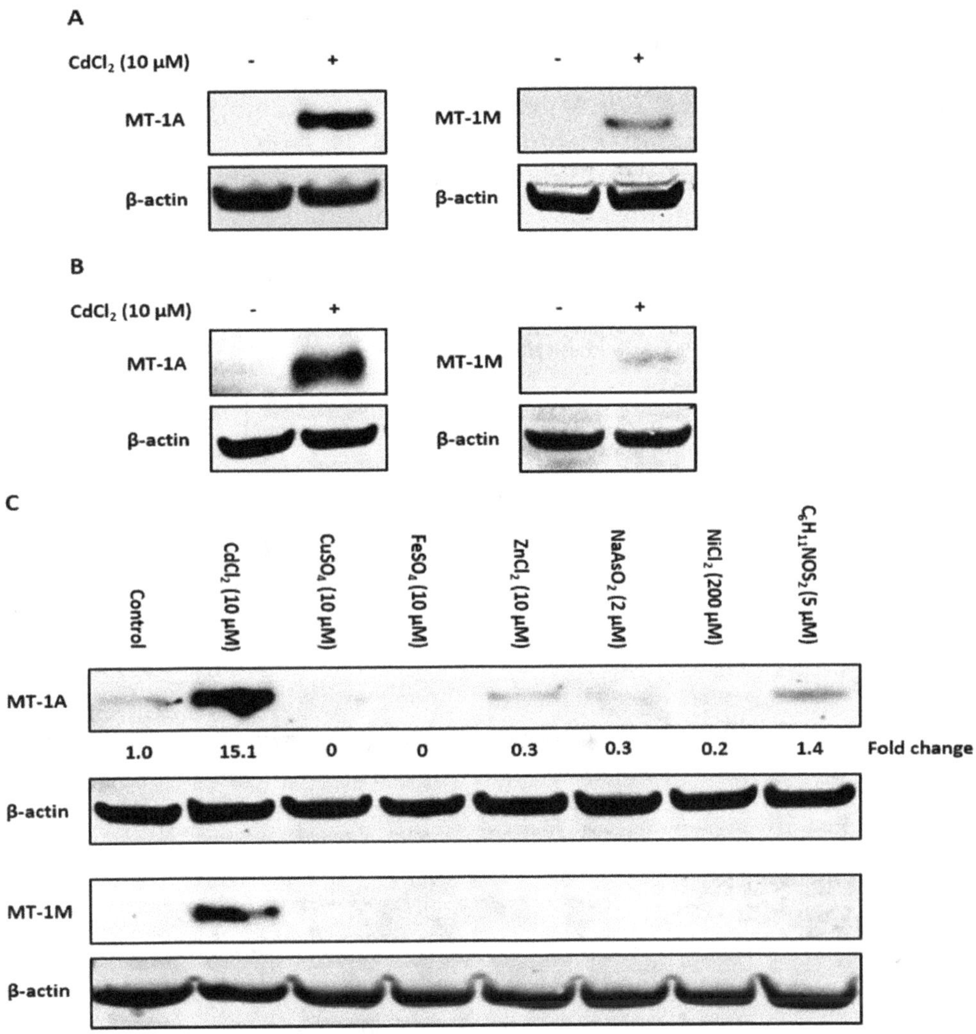

Figure 4. Western blot detection of cadmium-induced MT-1A and MT-1M expression in NHU cells using subtype-specific antibodies. MT-1A and MT-1M protein induction was observed by Western blotting of NHU cells exposed to 10 μM $CdCl_2$ for 72 h. Total protein input was 20 μg per track, with β-actin expression used to verify equal protein loading. Figures show western blots probed with MT-1A and MT-1M isoform-specific antibodies in (**A**) nondifferentiated and (**B**) differentiated NHU cell cultures exposed to cadmium for 72 h (representative blots shown from $n = 3$ independent cell lines). In (B), differentiated barrier formation was confirmed by TEER (see Figure 3B). (**C**) Western blot showing specificity of MT-1A and MT-1M protein induction (representative of $n = 2$ independent cell lines tested). Proliferating NHU cells were exposed to a range of potential inducers for 72 h and protein expression assessed. The candidate inducers tested were cadmium (10 μM $CdCl_2$), copper (10 μM $CuSO_4$), iron (10 μM $FeSO_4$), zinc (10 μM $ZnCl_2$), arsenite (2 μM $NaAsO_2$), nickel (200 μM $NiCl_2$), and sulforaphane (5 μM $C_6H_{11}NOS_2$). MT-1A protein expression is reported as fold-change relative to unexposed control cells.

The specificity of MT-1A and MT-1M protein induction was examined in response to the wider range of candidate inducers. Western blotting revealed that the MT-1M isoform was induced only by cadmium exposure, supporting the RT-PCR results (Figure 4C; replicated in supplementary material, Figure S10). MT-1A protein expression was highly induced by cadmium exposure, although low protein expression was observed under other conditions. As assessed by densitometry, only cadmium was capable of increasing MT-1A protein expression over control, resulting in a ~6-fold increase in MT-1A protein expression (Figure 4D).

2.5. Upregulation of Zinc Transporter-1 (SLC30A1) Transcription in Cadmium-Exposed NHU Cells

RT-PCR of both nondifferentiated and differentiated NHU cells revealed that cadmium exposure resulted in increased *SLC30A1* gene transcription compared to unexposed controls (Figure 5A; replicated in supplementary material, Figure S11). After cessation of exposure, *SLC30A1* transcript expression receded over time, and this decrease was observed to occur most rapidly in nondifferentiated (after 24 h; Figure 3B) compared to differentiated (after 11 days; Figure 5C) cell cultures.

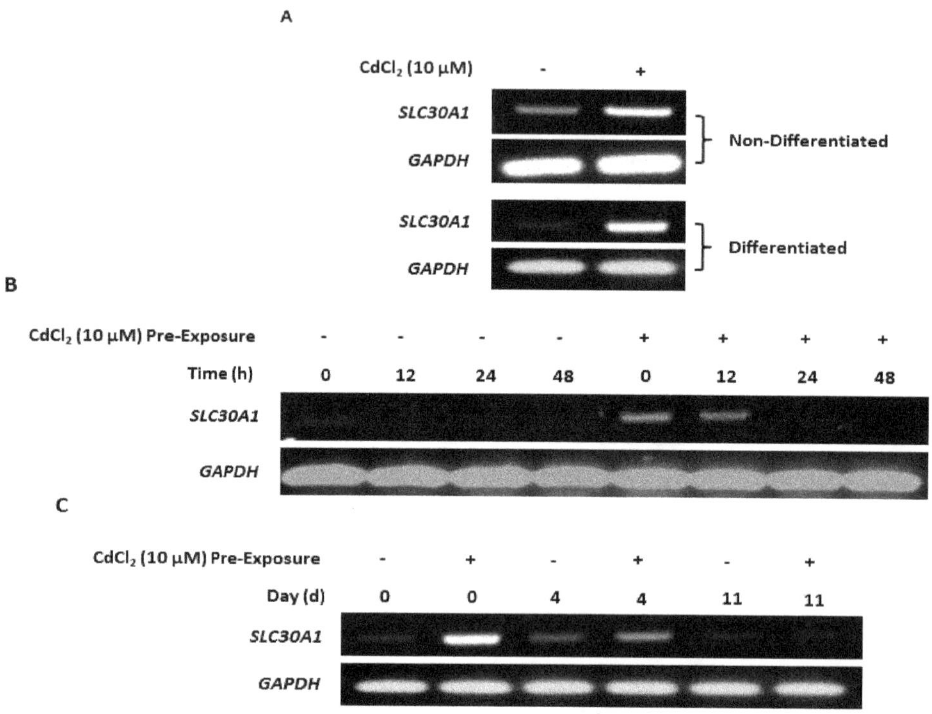

Figure 5. Cadmium induction of zinc transporter-1 (*SLC30A1*) gene transcription. *SLC30A1* gene transcript expression was assessed by RT-PCR, with PCR reaction products removed after 25 cycles. PCR controls included genomic DNA as a positive control and a no-template (H_2O) negative control. Total cDNA input was 1 μg with *GAPDH* used as an input loading control; RT-ve samples confirmed the absence of genomic contamination. For differentiated NHU cells, differentiation was confirmed by assessment of TEER as >1000 $\Omega.cm^2$ (see supplementary materials, Table S1). (**A**) NHU cells in nondifferentiated and differentiated states were maintained in control medium or with 10 μM $CdCl_2$ for up to 72 h. Note that medium was changed at time T = 0 and there was no renewal of the cadmium over the period. The figure shows representative results from n = 3 (nondifferentiated) and n = 1 (differentiated) independent NHU cell lines. (**B**) RT-PCR of NHU cells in a nondifferentiated state maintained in standard medium (control) or with 10 μM $CdCl_2$ for up to 24 h prior to the experiment ('pre-exposure'), whereupon cadmium was removed from the medium (time point 0) and culture continued for a further 48 h. (**C**) RT-PCR of NHU cells in a differentiated state maintained in standard medium (control) or with 10 μM $CdCl_2$ for up to 3 days prior to the experiment ('pre-exposure'), whereupon cadmium was removed from the medium (time point 0) and culture continued for up to 11 days.

3. Discussion

To the best of the authors' knowledge, this is the first study to investigate if cadmium exposure affects urothelial tight barrier function. Previous studies have examined the effect of cadmium exposure on renal [76] and bronchial [77] epithelia, with both studies reporting a decrease or complete collapse of barrier function. By contrast, the results from this study showed that urothelial barrier function was retained and even tightened. This may reflect the type of epithelium being tested, as urothelial cells are known to form one of the tightest epithelial barriers in the human body and thus may be unique in their resistance to cadmium. Although cadmium did not compromise urothelial barrier function, our results found that apical exposure induced expression of MT-1 isoforms in underlying NHU cells and using ICP-OES, cadmium was directly detected in differentiated urothelial cell sheets. Taken together, these results indicate that the urothelium remains intact and may even mount a protective response to cadmium in terms of tight junction tightening, yet the heavy metal is still able to penetrate the urothelial barrier.

Also for the first time, we describe specific MT gene expression by normal human urothelium. Our results are consistent with previous reports in other tissues that MT-1 is the inducible subfamily [22,40,78] whereas *MT-2A* is the most widely expressed isoform, accounting for up to 50 % total MT expression in humans [6,79]. In agreement with the consensus that MT-3 is neural-restricted [80], we found no baseline expression and no agents that could induce *MT-3* transcription in urothelial cells. As an anomaly, one group has previously suggested a link between heavy metal exposure, MT-3 induction, and urothelial carcinogenesis based on high MT-3 expression in malignant bladder cancer [81]. This group further supported their findings using in vitro studies in cadmium-transformed UROtsa cells [82,83]. However, we were not able to replicate those findings in our normal cell system.

Of the MT-1 gene family, transcription of *MT-1F* and *MT-1G* has previously been described as constitutive in human umbilical vein epithelial cells (HUVEC) under baseline conditions [42]. Both these genes exhibited low basal but inducible expression in NHU cells, therefore it cannot be certain whether the expression differences between tissues are constitutive, or perhaps due to inducers present in the culture medium. Whereas we found the majority of MT-1 gene paralogs to be inducible by cadmium exposure, transcript expression was transient, presumably due to sequestration leaving fewer free cadmium ions to maintain induction. By contrast, expression of MT-1 proteins was more stable and in line with the sequestering nature of the formed MT-cadmium complex. Previously, MT-1 protein isoform detection has been performed using mass spectrometry [41], but the demonstrated availability of specific antibodies now opens the door to detection using immunochemical approaches.

Exposure of proliferating NHU cell cultures to a range of divalent metal ions revealed differential and inducer-specific induction of MT-1 isoforms. For example, zinc ions induced strong transcription of *MT-1G*, but not *MT-1A* genes, whereas nickel ions caused *MT-1G* expression exclusively. Inducer-specific expression of MT-1 genes has been noted in other cell types [34,44–47], supporting the hypothesis that individual isoforms have very selective metal ion sequestering functions [5,6,22,39,40,84]. Western blotting revealed that cadmium was the most potent inducer of MT-1A protein expression, whereas MT-1M protein expression was highly specific to cadmium, revealing the potential of both as biomarkers of cadmium exposure. Neither arsenic nor nickel induced MT-1A or MT-1M protein expression, further demonstrating the specificity of MT-1 isoforms to differentiate between different nongenotoxic carcinogenic metals [85,86].

Alongside a pathophysiological role in sequestering carcinogenic metals, the MTs are considered to contribute to the normal homeostasis of zinc, which as a cofactor involved in many key cellular processes [56] is under tight control. MT sequestration and zinc transporter efflux coordinated by a common transcription factor *MTF-1* [87] is thought to regulate the availability of zinc [88–91]. Changes in intracellular zinc concentration have been associated with tumor growth and progression [92]. The displacement of zinc from the proteome by cadmium may affect the intracellular concentration and/or availability of zinc ions and can substitute and destabilize the functional sites of zinc-containing proteins, such as zinc-finger transcription factors, changing the character and/or rendering them nonfunctional [54,55].

Preliminary investigation into the effect of cadmium exposure on zinc homeostasis in normal urothelial cells revealed an upregulation of the zinc transporter-1 (*SLC30A1*) gene transcript in nondifferentiated NHU cells. *SLC30A1* upregulation was also observed in cadmium-exposed differentiated NHU cell sheets possessing a functional barrier, further suggesting that cadmium can penetrate an intact urothelial barrier. Our results agree with a previous study using the human hepatic HepG2 cell line, which demonstrated increased *SLC30A1* protein expression and localization at the cell membrane after acute cadmium exposure [93]. A later study showed cadmium exposure resulted in a 93% increase in the intracellular labile zinc concentration, suggesting a large displacement of zinc ions from the proteome, possibly due to substitution by cadmium [94].

MT expression is often seen as a 'double-edged sword', as on the one hand it functions to protect the cell, but by the same mechanisms can also facilitate malignant events [6,22,95,96]. MTs may contribute to cell survival by increasing resistance to ROS-induced apoptosis [97] and increasing cellular proliferation [32]. Cadmium exposure can result in inhibition of DNA repair [98], which coupled with increased cellular protection via cadmium-induced MT expression, increases the probability of deleterious cells surviving and passing on defects to their progeny [96]. The ability of MT to counteract ROS could also play a role in chemotherapy resistance, and high expression of MT has been correlated with treatment resistance in bladder cancer [99,100]. Specifically, after radical surgery and adjuvant chemotherapy 100% patients with high tumor MT expression progressed within nine months, whereas in patients with low MT expression only 65% had progressed after five years [101].

Our study supports a concordant induction of MT isoforms and *SLC30A1* transcription in response to cadmium exposure. Whereas this does not directly contradict hypotheses that cadmium exposure increases cellular zinc concentration or that cellular zinc homeostasis is maintained through the cooperative regulation of MT and zinc transporters [39], it does proffer a more direct relationship with cadmium responsible for regulating *SLC30A1* expression. This may reveal new insight as to the role of cadmium in (bladder) cancer, where previously reported *SLC30A1* and MT changes may reflect increased concentrations of intracellular cadmium rather than zinc. Our demonstration of differential MT-1 gene paralog induction by zinc and cadmium should help design future (e.g., knockout) experiments to clarify the respective roles. Further experiments might also directly quantify intracellular zinc in NHU cells after cadmium exposure and determine the consequences of cadmium on zinc homeostasis and dysregulated cadmium-substituted proteins.

4. Materials and Methods

4.1. NHU Cell Culture and Exposure to Cadmium and Other Agents

Normal human urothelial (NHU) cells were obtained from the ureter/renal pelvis of patients undergoing urological surgery, and maintained in vitro as nonimmortalized cell lines, as detailed elsewhere [57,102]. For routine culture, NHU cells were grown as adherent monolayers on Primaria™ plasticware (BD Biosciences, Wokingham, UK) in low calcium [0.09 mM] keratinocyte serum-free medium (KSFM) containing bovine pituitary extract and recombinant epidermal growth factor (Fisher Scientific UK Ltd, Loughborough, UK) supplemented with 30 ng/mL cholera toxin (KSFMc). NHU cell lines were subcultured by trypsinization at just-confluence and used in experiments between passages 3–5.

For cadmium exposure, medium was replaced with fresh medium containing 10 μM cadmium chloride ($CdCl_2$). This concentration was selected after preliminary titration for toxicity (Figure 1A,B). For other treatment agents, concentrations were selected following initial titration and target gene expression assessment (Figure 3A,B).

Nonimmortalized NHU cell lines retain the capacity to differentiate to form a functional tight barrier epithelium [58]. Differentiation was induced by switching NHU cells into medium supplemented with 5% adult bovine serum for 5 days before subculture onto semipermeable ThinCert™ (Greiner Bio-One Ltd., Stonehouse, UK) membranes with 0.4-μm pore size. After 24 h, the exogenous calcium (Ca^{2+}) concentration was increased to 2 mM (near physiological) and cultures were maintained for a further 7–9 days to develop a tight barrier. For cadmium exposure of differentiated NHU cell cultures, medium was removed from the apical chamber after establishment of a barrier >1000 $\Omega.cm^2$

(see below) and replaced with fresh medium supplemented with 10 μM $CdCl_2$, in order to mimic apical exposure. RNA and protein were then harvested from these membranes for further analysis.

4.2. Measurement of Transepithelial Electrical Resistance

The barrier function of differentiated NHU cell sheets was assessed in triplicate cultures by measuring the transepithelial electrical resistance (TEER) using an EVOM™ voltohmmeter (World Precision Instruments, Hertfordshire, UK), as described [103]. A blank (no cell) membrane measurement was subtracted from each TEER reading.

4.3. MT Transcript Abundance Quantification by Next-Generation Sequencing

mRNA-seq data for three donor-matched NHU cultured nondifferentiated and differentiated samples were previously generated by our group [104]. Sequencing reads were 'pseudoaligned' to the Ensembl v.91 human transcriptome (GRCh38.p10) using kallisto v0.44.0 [105] and relative gene abundance was calculated as transcripts per million (TPM) following gene-level aggregation with tximport v1.8.0 [106]. Differentiation-associated expression changes in the MT gene family were detected by a differential expression analysis conducted by sleuth [107] accounting for matched-donor samples. Differentially-expressed genes are reported with their $\log_2$ transformed fold change ($\log_2$FC) and 'q' value (Benjamini–Hochberg correction).

4.4. Reverse Transcriptase-Polymerase Chain Reaction (RT-PCR)

RT-PCR was performed to observe actual patterns of MT isoform induction (rather than relative change). RNA was extracted from cells using TRIzol® (Fisher Scientific UK Ltd., Loughborough, UK) and treated with a DNA-free™ kit (Ambion, supplied by Fisher Scientific UK Ltd., Loughborough, UK). cDNA synthesis was performed on 1 μg RNA with random hexamers and the SuperScript®II First-Strand Synthesis System (Fisher Scientific UK Ltd., Loughborough, UK). PCR primers were designed specifically to detect all known splice variants for each MT-1 isoform gene, with GAPDH used as the internal transcript control [108]. Primer sequences and optimized PCR conditions are provided in Table 1. PCR was carried out in a T100 thermal cycler (Bio-Rad Services UK Ltd., Hemel Hempstead Hertfordshire, UK) using 25 reaction cycles. Controls consisted of genomic DNA (gDNA as template positive control), water (no template control), and no reverse transcriptase (gDNA negative control). PCR products were separated on 2 % (*w*/*v*) agarose gels, stained using SYBR® Safe DNA gel stain (Invitrogen supplied by Fisher Scientific UK Ltd., Loughborough, UK) and visualized on a Gene Genius Gel Imaging System (Syngene, Cambridge, UK).

Table 1. Details of primers used for experiments.

Target Gene	Forward or Reverse	Sequence (5′–3′)	Product Size (bp)
GAPDH	Forward	CAAGGTCATCCATGACAACTTTG	90
GAPDH	Reverse	GGGCCATCCACAGTCTTCTG	90
HMOX1	Forward	CCAGCAACAAAGTGCAAGATTC	102
HMOX1	Reverse	GTGTAAGGACCCATCGGAGAAG	102
MT-1A	Forward	CTCGAAATGGACCCCAACT	219
MT-1A	Reverse	ATATCTTCGAGCAGGGCTGTC	219
MT-1B	Forward	GGAACTCCAGGCTTGTCTTGG	77
MT-1B	Reverse	TTGCAGGAGGTACATTTG	77
MT-1E	Forward	TGCGCCGGCTCCTGCAAGTC	118
MT-1E	Reverse	ATGCCCCTTTGCAGACGCAGC	118

Table 1. *Cont.*

Target Gene	Forward or Reverse	Sequence (5′–3′)	Product Size (bp)
MT-1F	Forward	CCTGCACCTGCGCTGGTTCC	110
MT-1F	Reverse	ACAGCCCTGGGCACACTTGC	110
MT-1G	Forward	CTTCTCGCTTGGGAACTCTA	309
MT-1G	Reverse	AGGGGTCAAGATTGTAGCAAA	309
MT-1H	Forward	CCTCTTCTCTTCTCGCTTGG	317
MT-1H	Reverse	GCAAATGAGTCGGAGTTGTAG	317
MT-1M	Forward	CTAGCAGTCGCTCCATTTATCG	180
MT-1M	Reverse	CAGCTGCAGTTCTCCAACGT	180
MT-1X	Forward	GGACCCAACTGCTCCTGCTC	151
MT-1X	Reverse	TTTGCAGATGCAGCCCTGGGC	151
MT-2A	Forward	CCGACTCTAGCCGCCTCTT	259
MT-2A	Reverse	GTGGAAGTCGCGTTCTTTACA	259
MT-3	Forward	AGTGCGAGGGATGCAAATG	98
MT-3	Reverse	GCCTTTGCACACACAGTCCTT	98
SLC30A1	Forward	GCATCAGTTTATGAGGCTGGTCCT	352
SLC30A1	Reverse	CAGGCTGAATGGTAGTAGCGTGAA	352

4.5. Western Blotting

NHU cell cultures were lysed into electrophoresis sample buffer containing protease inhibitors and sonicated. Twenty micrograms of protein was resolved on 4–12% Bis-Tris NuPage™ polyacrylamide gels (Invitrogen) in 2-(N-morphilino) ethanesulfonic acid (MES) buffer and electro-transferred onto polyvinylfluoride membranes (Millipore). Membranes were blocked with Odyssey® blocking buffer (LI-COR Biotechnology OK Ltd., Cambridge, UK), incubated with primary antibodies for 16 h at 4 °C and bound antibody detected using Alexa Fluor® 680-conjugated anti-mouse secondary antibody (Invitrogen, Invitrogen supplied by Fisher Scientific UK Ltd., Loughborough, UK) or an IRDye 800-conjugated anti-rabbit secondary antibody (Tebu-Bio, Peterborough, UK). Antibody binding was visualized using an Odyssey® Sa Infrared Imaging System (LI-COR®). Protein quantification was performed using Odyssey® Image Studio™ software v5.0 (LI-COR®). Details of antibodies are given Tables 2 and 3.

Table 2. Details of primary antibodies used for experiments.

Antigen	Clone	Host	Supplier	Dilution	Molecular Weight (kDa)
Beta-actin	A5441	Mouse	Sigma Aldrich	1:10 000 (WB)	42
MT-1A	B01P	Mouse	Abnova	1:750 (WB)	6
MT-1M	17281-AP	Rabbit	ProteinTech	1 µg/mL (WB)	6

Table 3. Details of secondary antibodies used for experiments.

Antigen	Conjugate	Host	Supplier	Application
Anti-mouse IgG	Alexa 680	Goat	Life Technologies	WB
Anti-rabbit IgG	Alexa 800	Goat	Life Technologies	WB

5. Conclusions

MT-1 isoform expression has been characterized in normal human urothelium for the first time, and a unique expression profile described with the use of isoform-specific antibodies. Individual MT-1 genes demonstrated inducer-specific expression and two paralogs with cadmium-specific or -selective induction were identified as candidate biomarkers of cadmium exposure. With the potential for cadmium to interfere and substitute in the homeostatic regulation of zinc, new approaches are proposed for understanding cadmium-induced nongenotoxic carcinogenesis.

Author Contributions: Conceptualization, R.V.M., M.H., J.W.F.C., and J.S.; Methodology, R.V.M., M.H, A.S.M., and J.W.F.C.; Software, R.V.M. and A.S.M.; Validation, R.V.M. and J.S.; Formal Analysis, R.V.M. and A.S.M.; Investigation, R.V.M.; Resources, M.H., J.W.F.C., and J.S.; Data Curation, R.V.M. and J.S.; Writing—Original Draft Preparation, R.V.M.; Writing—Review and Editing, A.S.M, J.W.F.C., and J.S..; Visualization, R.V.M. and J.S.; Supervision, J.S.; Project Administration, R.V.M. and J.S.; Funding Acquisition, J.W.F.C and J.S.

Abbreviations

HMOX1	Heme oxygenase-1
MT	Metallothionein
NHU	Normal human urothelial
SLC30A1	Solute carrier family A member 1
TEER	Trans-epithelial electrical resistance

References

1. Tchounwou, P.B.; Yedjou, C.G.; Patlolla, A.K.; Sutton, D.J. Heavy Metals Toxicity and the Environment. *EXS* **2012**, *101*, 133–164.
2. Feki-Tounsi, M.; Hamza-Chaffai, A. Cadmium as a possible cause of bladder cancer: A review of accumulated evidence. *Environ. Sci. Pollut. Res.* **2014**, *21*, 10561–10573. [CrossRef] [PubMed]
3. Waalkes, M.P. Cadmium carcinogenesis. *Mutat. Res.* **2003**, *533*, 107–120. [CrossRef] [PubMed]
4. Agency for Toxic Substances and Disease Registry Toxicological Profile for Cadmium. Available online: https://www.atsdr.cdc.gov/toxprofiles/tp.asp?id=48&tid=15 (accessed on 14 September 2016).
5. Coyle, P.; Philcox, J.C.; Carey, L.C.; Rofe, A.M. Metallothionein: The multipurpose protein. *Cell. Mol. Life Sci.* **2002**, *59*, 627–647. [CrossRef] [PubMed]
6. Sigel, A.; Sigel, H.; Sigel, R.K.O. *Metallothioneins and Related Chelators*; Metal Ions in Life Sciences; RSC Publishing: Cambridge, UK, 2009; Volume 5.
7. Klaassen, C.D.; Choudhuri, S.; McKim, J.M.; Lehman-McKeeman, L.D.; Kershaw, W.C. In vitro and in vivo studies on the degradation of metallothionein. *Environ. Health Perspect.* **1994**, *102*, 141–146. [PubMed]
8. Kellen, E.; Zeegers, M.P.; Hond, E.D.; Buntinx, F. Blood cadmium may be associated with bladder carcinogenesis: The Belgian case-control study on bladder cancer. *Cancer Detect. Prev.* **2007**, *31*, 77–82. [CrossRef] [PubMed]
9. Wolf, C.; Strenziok, R.; Kyriakopoulos, A. Elevated metallothionein-bound cadmium concentrations in urine from bladder carcinoma patients, investigated by size exclusion chromatography-inductively coupled plasma mass spectrometry. *Anal. Chim. Acta* **2009**, *631*, 218–222. [CrossRef]
10. Feki-Tounsi, M.; Olmedo, P.; Gil, F.; Khlifi, R.; Mhiri, M.-N.; Rebai, A.; Hamza-Chaffai, A. Cadmium in blood of Tunisian men and risk of bladder cancer: Interactions with arsenic exposure and smoking. *Environ. Sci. Pollut. Res. Int.* **2013**, *20*, 7204–7213. [CrossRef] [PubMed]
11. Chang, C.-H.; Liu, C.-S.; Liu, H.-J.; Huang, C.-P.; Huang, C.-Y.; Hsu, H.-T.; Liou, S.-H.; Chung, C.-J. Association between levels of urinary heavy metals and increased risk of urothelial carcinoma. *Int. J. Urol.* **2016**, *23*, 233–239. [CrossRef]

12. Achanzar, W.E.; Diwan, B.A.; Liu, J.; Quader, S.T.; Webber, M.M.; Waalkes, M.P. Cadmium-induced Malignant Transformation of Human Prostate Epithelial Cells. *Cancer Res.* **2001**, *61*, 455–458.
13. Takiguchi, M.; Achanzar, W.E.; Qu, W.; Li, G.; Waalkes, M.P. Effects of cadmium on DNA-(Cytosine-5) methyltransferase activity and DNA methylation status during cadmium-induced cellular transformation. *Exp. Cell Res.* **2003**, *286*, 355–365. [CrossRef]
14. Lei, Y.-X.; Wei, L.; Wang, M.; Wu, G.-R.; Li, M. Malignant transformation and abnormal expression of eukaryotic initiation factor in bronchial epithelial cells induced by cadmium chloride. *Biomed. Environ. Sci.* **2008**, *21*, 332–338. [CrossRef]
15. Sens, D.A.; Park, S.; Gurel, V.; Sens, M.A.; Garrett, S.H.; Somji, S. Inorganic Cadmium- and Arsenite-Induced Malignant Transformation of Human Bladder Urothelial Cells. *Toxicol. Sci.* **2004**, *79*, 56–63. [CrossRef] [PubMed]
16. Kreft, M.E.; Hudoklin, S.; Jezernik, K.; Romih, R. Formation and maintenance of blood–urine barrier in urothelium. *Protoplasma* **2010**, *246*, 3–14. [CrossRef] [PubMed]
17. Caldwell, J.; Gardner, I.; Swales, N. An Introduction to Drug Disposition: The Basic Principles of Absorption, Distribution, Metabolism, and Excretion. *Toxicol. Pathol.* **1995**, *23*, 102–114. [CrossRef] [PubMed]
18. Krause, M.; Rak-Raszewska, A.; Pietilä, I.; Quaggin, S.E.; Vainio, S. Signaling during Kidney Development. *Cells* **2015**, *4*, 112–132. [CrossRef]
19. Margoshes, M.; Vallee, B.L. A Cadmium Protein from Equine Kidney Cortex. *J. Am. Chem. Soc.* **1957**, *79*, 4813–4814. [CrossRef]
20. Kägi, J.H.; Schäffer, A. Biochemistry of metallothionein. *Biochemistry* **1988**, *27*, 8509–8515. [CrossRef]
21. Hunt, C.T.; Boulanger, Y.; Fesik, S.W.; Armitage, I.M. NMR analysis of the structure and metal sequestering properties of metallothioneins. *Environ. Health Perspect.* **1984**, *54*, 135–145. [CrossRef] [PubMed]
22. Capdevila, M.; Bofill, R.; Palacios, Ò.; Atrian, S. State-of-the-art of metallothioneins at the beginning of the 21st century. *Coord. Chem. Rev.* **2012**, *256*, 46–62. [CrossRef]
23. Dalton, T.; Fu, K.; Palmiter, R.D.; Andrews, G.K. Transgenic mice that overexpress metallothionein-I resist dietary zinc deficiency. *J. Nutr.* **1996**, *126*, 825–833. [CrossRef]
24. Kelly, E.J.; Quaife, C.J.; Froelick, G.J.; Palmiter, R.D. Metallothionein I and II protect against zinc deficiency and zinc toxicity in mice. *J. Nutr.* **1996**, *126*, 1782–1790.
25. Lee, D.K.; Geiser, J.; Dufner-Beattie, J.; Andrews, G.K. Pancreatic metallothionein-I may play a role in zinc homeostasis during maternal dietary zinc deficiency in mice. *J. Nutr.* **2003**, *133*, 45–50. [CrossRef]
26. Penkowa, M.; Cáceres, M.; Borup, R.; Nielsen, F.C.; Poulsen, C.B.; Quintana, A.; Molinero, A.; Carrasco, J.; Florit, S.; Giralt, M.; et al. Novel roles for metallothionein-I + II (MT-I + II) in defense responses, neurogenesis, and tissue restoration after traumatic brain injury: Insights from global gene expression profiling in wild-type and MT-I + II knockout mice. *J. Neurosci. Res.* **2006**, *84*, 1452–1474. [CrossRef] [PubMed]
27. Lazo, J.S.; Kondo, Y.; Dellapiazza, D.; Michalska, A.E.; Choo, K.H.; Pitt, B.R. Enhanced sensitivity to oxidative stress in cultured embryonic cells from transgenic mice deficient in metallothionein I and II genes. *J. Biol. Chem.* **1995**, *270*, 5506–5510. [CrossRef] [PubMed]
28. Karin, M.; Haslinger, A.; Holtgreve, H.; Richards, R.I.; Krauter, P.; Westphal, H.M.; Beato, M. Characterization of DNA sequences through which cadmium and glucocorticoid hormones induce human metallothionein-IIA gene. *Nature* **1984**, *308*, 513–519. [CrossRef]
29. Schulkens, I.A.; Castricum, K.C.M.; Weijers, E.M.; Koolwijk, P.; Griffioen, A.W.; Thijssen, V.L. Expression, regulation and function of human metallothioneins in endothelial cells. *J. Vasc. Res.* **2014**, *51*, 231–238. [CrossRef] [PubMed]
30. Yap, X.; Tan, H.-Y.; Huang, J.; Lai, Y.; Yip, G.W.-C.; Tan, P.-H.; Bay, B.-H. Over-expression of metallothionein predicts chemoresistance in breast cancer. *J. Pathol.* **2009**, *217*, 563–570. [CrossRef]
31. Liu, Z.-M.; van Hasselt, C.A.; Song, F.-Z.; Vlantis, A.C.; Cherian, M.G.; Koropatnick, J.; Chen, G.G. Expression of functional metallothionein isoforms in papillary thyroid cancer. *Mol. Cell. Endocrinol.* **2009**, *302*, 92–98. [CrossRef]
32. Ioachim, E.E.; Charchanti, A.V.; Stavropoulos, N.E.; Athanassiou, E.D.; Michael, M.C.; Agnantis, N.J. Localization of metallothionein in urothelial carcinoma of the human urinary bladder: An immunohistochemical study including correlation with HLA-DR antigen, p53, and proliferation indices. *Anticancer Res.* **2001**, *21*, 1757–1761. [PubMed]

33. Jin, R.; Chow, V.T.-K.; Tan, P.-H.; Dheen, S.T.; Duan, W.; Bay, B.-H. Metallothionein 2A expression is associated with cell proliferation in breast cancer. *Carcinogenesis* **2002**, *23*, 81–86. [CrossRef] [PubMed]
34. Varshney, U.; Jahroudi, N.; Foster, R.; Gedamu, L. Structure, organization, and regulation of human metallothionein IF gene: Differential and cell-type-specific expression in response to heavy metals and glucocorticoids. *Mol. Cell. Biol.* **1986**, *6*, 26–37. [CrossRef] [PubMed]
35. Boonprasert, K.; Ruengweerayut, R.; Aunpad, R.; Satarug, S.; Na-Bangchang, K. Expression of metallothionein isoforms in peripheral blood leukocytes from Thai population residing in cadmium-contaminated areas. *Environ. Toxicol. Pharmacol.* **2012**, *34*, 935–940. [CrossRef] [PubMed]
36. Mita, M.; Satoh, M.; Shimada, A.; Okajima, M.; Azuma, S.; Suzuki, J.S.; Sakabe, K.; Hara, S.; Himeno, S. Metallothionein is a crucial protective factor against Helicobacter pylori-induced gastric erosive lesions in a mouse model. *Am. J. Physiol. Gastrointest. Liver Physiol.* **2008**, *294*, G877–G884. [CrossRef]
37. Kägi, J.H.; Kojima, Y. Chemistry and biochemistry of metallothionein. *Exp. Suppl.* **1987**, *52*, 25–61.
38. Irvine, G.W.; Pinter, T.B.J.; Stillman, M.J. Defining the metal binding pathways of human metallothionein 1a: Balancing zinc availability and cadmium seclusion. *Metallomics* **2016**, *8*, 71–81. [CrossRef] [PubMed]
39. Kimura, T.; Kambe, T. The Functions of Metallothionein and ZIP and ZnT Transporters: An Overview and Perspective. *Int. J. Mol. Sci.* **2016**, *17*, 336. [CrossRef]
40. Miles, A.T.; Hawksworth, G.M.; Beattie, J.H.; Rodilla, V. Induction, Regulation, Degradation, and Biological Significance of Mammalian Metallothioneins. *Crit. Rev. Biochem. Mol. Biol.* **2000**, *35*, 35–70. [CrossRef]
41. Mehus, A.A.; Muhonen, W.W.; Garrett, S.H.; Somji, S.; Sens, D.A.; Shabb, J.B. Quantitation of Human Metallothionein Isoforms: A Family of Small, Highly Conserved, Cysteine-rich Proteins. *Mol. Cell. Proteom.* **2014**, *13*, 1020–1033. [CrossRef]
42. Conway, D.E.; Lee, S.; Eskin, S.G.; Shah, A.K.; Jo, H.; McIntire, L.V. Endothelial metallothionein expression and intracellular free zinc levels are regulated by shear stress. *Am. J. Physiol. Cell. Physiol.* **2010**, *299*, C1461–C1467. [CrossRef]
43. Jahroudi, N.; Foster, R.; Price-Haughey, J.; Beitel, G.; Gedamu, L. Cell-type specific and differential regulation of the human metallothionein genes. Correlation with DNA methylation and chromatin structure. *J. Biol. Chem.* **1990**, *265*, 6506–6511.
44. Miura, N.; Koizumi, S. Heavy metal responses of the human metallothionein isoform genes. *J. Pharm. Soc. Jpn.* **2007**, *127*, 665–673. [CrossRef]
45. Richards, R.I.; Heguy, A.; Karin, M. Structural and functional analysis of the human metallothionein-IA gene: Differential induction by metal ions and glucocorticoids. *Cell* **1984**, *37*, 263–272. [CrossRef]
46. Selvaraj, A.; Balamurugan, K.; Yepiskoposyan, H.; Zhou, H.; Egli, D.; Georgiev, O.; Thiele, D.J.; Schaffner, W. Metal-responsive transcription factor (MTF-1) handles both extremes, copper load and copper starvation, by activating different genes. *Genes Dev.* **2005**, *19*, 891–896. [CrossRef] [PubMed]
47. Sims, H.I.; Chirn, G.-W.; Marr, M.T. Single nucleotide in the MTF-1 binding site can determine metal-specific transcription activation. *PNAS* **2012**, *109*, 16516–16521. [CrossRef] [PubMed]
48. Sadhu, C.; Gedamu, L. Regulation of human metallothionein (MT) genes. Differential expression of MTI-F, MTI-G, and MTII-A genes in the hepatoblastoma cell line (HepG2). *J. Biol. Chem.* **1988**, *263*, 2679–2684.
49. Lehman-McKeeman, L.D.; Andrews, G.K.; Klaassen, C.D. Mechanisms of regulation of rat hepatic metallothionein-I and metallothionein-II levels following administration of zinc. *Toxicol. Appl. Pharmacol.* **1988**, *92*, 1–9. [CrossRef]
50. Klaassen, C.D.; Lehman-McKeeman, L.D. Regulation of the isoforms of metallothionein. *Biol. Trace Elem. Res.* **1989**, *21*, 119–129. [CrossRef]
51. Kim, J.-H.; Wang, S.-Y.; Kim, I.-C.; Ki, J.-S.; Raisuddin, S.; Lee, J.-S.; Han, K.-N. Cloning of a river pufferfish (Takifugu obscurus) metallothionein cDNA and study of its induction profile in cadmium-exposed fish. *Chemosphere* **2008**, *71*, 1251–1259. [CrossRef]
52. Jasani, B.; Schmid, K.W. Significance of metallothionein overexpression in human tumours. *Histopathology* **1997**, *31*, 131–136. [CrossRef]
53. Chaney, R.L. Cadmium and Zinc. In *Trace Elements in Soils*; Wiley: New York, NY, USA, 2010; pp. 409–440.
54. Malgieri, G.; Zaccaro, L.; Leone, M.; Bucci, E.; Esposito, S.; Baglivo, I.; Del Gatto, A.; Russo, L.; Scandurra, R.; Pedone, P.V.; et al. Zinc to cadmium replacement in the A. thaliana SUPERMAN Cys_2 His_2 zinc finger induces structural rearrangements of typical DNA base determinant positions. *Biopolymers* **2011**, *95*, 801–810. [PubMed]

55. Tang, L.; Qiu, R.; Tang, Y.; Wang, S. Cadmium–zinc exchange and their binary relationship in the structure of Zn-related proteins: A mini review. *Metallomics* **2014**, *6*, 1313–1323. [CrossRef] [PubMed]
56. Jeong, J.; Eide, D.J. The SLC39 family of zinc transporters. *Mol. Asp. Med.* **2013**, *34*, 612–619. [CrossRef] [PubMed]
57. Southgate, J.; Hutton, K.A.; Thomas, D.F.; Trejdosiewicz, L.K. Normal human urothelial cells in vitro: Proliferation and induction of stratification. *Lab. Investig.* **1994**, *71*, 583–594. [PubMed]
58. Cross, W.R.; Eardley, I.; Leese, H.J.; Southgate, J. A biomimetic tissue from cultured normal human urothelial cells: Analysis of physiological function. *Am. J. Physiol. Renal Physiol.* **2005**, *289*, F459–F468. [CrossRef]
59. Wang, Y.; Fang, J.; Leonard, S.S.; Rao, K.M.K. Cadmium inhibits the electron transfer chain and induces reactive oxygen species. *Free Radic. Biol. Med.* **2004**, *36*, 1434–1443. [CrossRef]
60. Heyno, E.; Klose, C.; Krieger-Liszkay, A. Origin of cadmium-induced reactive oxygen species production: Mitochondrial electron transfer versus plasma membrane NADPH oxidase. *New Phytol.* **2008**, *179*, 687–699. [CrossRef]
61. Durnam, D.M.; Palmiter, R.D. Induction of metallothionein-I mRNA in cultured cells by heavy metals and iodoacetate: Evidence for gratuitous inducers. *Mol. Cell. Biol.* **1984**, *4*, 484–491. [CrossRef]
62. Alam, J.; Smith, A. Heme-hemopexin-mediated induction of metallothionein gene expression. *J. Biol. Chem.* **1992**, *267*, 16379–16384.
63. Baird, S.K.; Kurz, T.; Brunk, U.T. Metallothionein protects against oxidative stress-induced lysosomal destabilization. *Biochem. J.* **2006**, *394*, 275–283. [CrossRef]
64. Palmiter, R.D. Regulation of metallothionein genes by heavy metals appears to be mediated by a zinc-sensitive inhibitor that interacts with a constitutively active transcription factor, MTF-1. *Proc. Natl. Acad. Sci. USA* **1994**, *91*, 1219–1223. [CrossRef] [PubMed]
65. Kheradmand, F.; Nourmohammadi, I.; Modarressi, M.H.; Firoozrai, M.; Ahmadi Faghih, M.A. Differential Gene-Expression of Metallothionein 1M and 1G in Response to Zinc in Sertoli TM4 Cells. *Iran Biomed. J.* **2010**, *14*, 9–15. [PubMed]
66. Chu, A.; Foster, M.; Ward, S.; Zaman, K.; Hancock, D.; Petocz, P.; Samman, S. Zinc-induced upregulation of metallothionein (MT)-2A is predicted by gene expression of zinc transporters in healthy adults. *Genes Nutr.* **2015**, *10*, 44. [CrossRef] [PubMed]
67. Chen, L.; Ma, L.; Bai, Q.; Zhu, X.; Zhang, J.; Wei, Q.; Li, D.; Gao, C.; Li, J.; Zhang, Z.; et al. Heavy metal-induced metallothionein expression is regulated by specific protein phosphatase 2A complexes. *J. Biol. Chem.* **2014**, *289*, 22413–22426. [CrossRef] [PubMed]
68. Heuchel, R.; Radtke, F.; Georgiev, O.; Stark, G.; Aguet, M.; Schaffner, W. The transcription factor MTF-1 is essential for basal and heavy metal-induced metallothionein gene expression. *EMBO J.* **1994**, *13*, 2870–2875. [CrossRef]
69. Zhou, X.D.; Sens, D.A.; Sens, M.A.; Namburi, V.B.R.K.; Singh, R.K.; Garrett, S.H.; Somji, S. Metallothionein-1 and -2 Expression in Cadmium- or Arsenic-Derived Human Malignant Urothelial Cells and Tumor Heterotransplants and as a Prognostic Indicator in Human Bladder Cancer. *Toxicol. Sci.* **2006**, *91*, 467–475. [CrossRef]
70. Irvine, G.W.; Stillman, M.J. Topographical analysis of As-induced folding of α-MT1a. *Biochem. Biophys. Res. Commun.* **2013**, *441*, 208–213. [CrossRef]
71. McMahon, R.J.; Cousins, R.J. Regulation of the zinc transporter ZnT-1 by dietary zinc. *Proc. Natl. Acad. Sci. USA* **1998**, *95*, 4841–4846. [CrossRef]
72. Holloway, A.F.; Stennard, F.A.; West, A.K. Human metallothionein gene MT1L mRNA is present in several human tissues but is unlikely to produce a metallothionein protein. *FEBS Lett.* **1997**, *404*, 41–44. [CrossRef]
73. Hahn, Y.; Lee, B. Human-specific nonsense mutations identified by genome sequence comparisons. *Hum. Genet.* **2006**, *119*, 169–178. [CrossRef]
74. Ryter, S.W.; Choi, A.M.K. Heme oxygenase-1: Redox regulation of a stress protein in lung and cell culture models. *Antioxid. Redox Signal.* **2005**, *7*, 80–91. [CrossRef]
75. Sarma, S.N.; Kim, Y.-J.; Song, M.; Ryu, J.-C. Induction of apoptosis in human leukemia cells through the production of reactive oxygen species and activation of HMOX1 and Noxa by benzene, toluene, and o-xylene. *Toxicology* **2011**, *280*, 109–117. [CrossRef]
76. Faurskov, B.; Bjerregaard, H.F. Effect of cadmium on active ion transport and cytotoxicity in cultured renal epithelial cells (A6). *Toxicol. In Vitro* **1997**, *11*, 717–722. [CrossRef]

77. Cao, X.; Lin, H.; Muskhelishvili, L.; Latendresse, J.; Richter, P.; Heflich, R.H. Tight junction disruption by cadmium in an in vitro human airway tissue model. *Respir. Res.* **2015**, *16*, 30. [CrossRef]
78. Thirumoorthy, N.; Manisenthil Kumar, K.-T.; Shyam Sundar, A.; Panayappan, L.; Chatterjee, M. Metallothionein: An overview. *World J. Gastroenterol.* **2007**, *13*, 993–996. [CrossRef]
79. Raudenska, M.; Gumulec, J.; Podlaha, O.; Sztalmachova, M.; Babula, P.; Eckschlager, T.; Adam, V.; Kizek, R.; Masarik, M. Metallothionein polymorphisms in pathological processes. *Metallomics* **2013**, *6*, 55–68. [CrossRef] [PubMed]
80. Palmiter, R.D.; Findley, S.D.; Whitmore, T.E.; Durnam, D.M. MT-III, a brain-specific member of the metallothionein gene family. *Proc. Natl. Acad. Sci. USA* **1992**, *89*, 6333–6337. [CrossRef] [PubMed]
81. Sens, M.A.; Somji, S.; Lamm, D.L.; Garrett, S.H.; Slovinsky, F.; Todd, J.H.; Sens, D.A. Metallothionein isoform 3 as a potential biomarker for human bladder cancer. *Environ. Health Perspect.* **2000**, *108*, 413–418. [CrossRef] [PubMed]
82. Zhou, X.D.; Sens, M.A.; Garrett, S.H.; Somji, S.; Park, S.; Gurel, V.; Sens, D.A. Enhanced expression of metallothionein isoform 3 protein in tumor heterotransplants derived from As^{+3}- and Cd^{+2}-transformed human urothelial cells. *Toxicol. Sci.* **2006**, *93*, 322–330. [CrossRef] [PubMed]
83. Somji, S.; Garrett, S.H.; Toni, C.; Zhou, X.D.; Zheng, Y.; Ajjimaporn, A.; Sens, M.A.; Sens, D.A. Differences in the epigenetic regulation of MT-3 gene expression between parental and Cd^{+2} or As^{+3} transformed human urothelial cells. *Cancer Cell Int.* **2011**, *11*, 2. [CrossRef]
84. Brazão-Silva, M.T.; Rodriguez, M.F.S.; Eisenberg, A.L.A.; Dias, F.L.; de Castro, L.M.; Nunes, F.D.; Faria, P.R.; Cardoso, S.V.; Loyola, A.M.; de Sousa, S.C.O.M. Metallothionein gene expression is altered in oral cancer and may predict metastasis and patient outcomes. *Histopathology* **2015**, *67*, 358–367. [CrossRef] [PubMed]
85. International Agency for Research on Cancer Beryllium, cadmium, mercury, and exposures in the glass manufacturing industry. In *IARC Monographs on the Evaluation of the Carcinogenic Risks to Humans*; IARC: Lyon, France, 1993; Volume 58.
86. Salnikow, K.; An, W.G.; Melillo, G.; Blagosklonny, M.V.; Costa, M. Nickel-induced transformation shifts the balance between HIF-1 and p53 transcription factors. *Carcinogenesis* **1999**, *20*, 1819–1823. [CrossRef]
87. Günther, V.; Lindert, U.; Schaffner, W. The taste of heavy metals: Gene regulation by MTF-1. *Biochim. Biophys. Acta (BBA) Mol. Cell Res.* **2012**, *1823*, 1416–1425. [CrossRef] [PubMed]
88. Kimura, T.; Itoh, N.; Andrews, G.K. Mechanisms of Heavy Metal Sensing by Metal Response Element-binding Transcription Factor-1. *J. Health Sci.* **2009**, *55*, 484–494. [CrossRef]
89. Otsuka, F. Molecular Mechanism of the Metallothionein Gene Expression Mediated by Metal-Responsive Transcription Factor 1. *J. Health Sci.* **2001**, *47*, 513–519. [CrossRef]
90. Langmade, S.J.; Ravindra, R.; Daniels, P.J.; Andrews, G.K. The transcription factor MTF-1 mediates metal regulation of the mouse ZnT1 gene. *J. Biol. Chem.* **2000**, *275*, 34803–34809. [CrossRef] [PubMed]
91. Guo, L.; Lichten, L.A.; Ryu, M.-S.; Liuzzi, J.P.; Wang, F.; Cousins, R.J. STAT5-glucocorticoid receptor interaction and MTF-1 regulate the expression of ZnT2 (Slc30a2) in pancreatic acinar cells. *Proc. Natl. Acad. Sci. USA* **2010**, *107*, 2818–2823. [CrossRef]
92. Bafaro, E.; Liu, Y.; Xu, Y.; Dempski, R.E. The emerging role of zinc transporters in cellular homeostasis and cancer. *Signal Transduct. Target. Ther.* **2017**, *2*, 17029. [CrossRef]
93. Urani, C.; Melchioretto, P.; Gribaldo, L. Regulation of metallothioneins and ZnT-1 transporter expression in human hepatoma cells HepG2 exposed to zinc and cadmium. *Toxicol. In Vitro* **2010**, *24*, 370–374. [CrossRef]
94. Urani, C.; Melchioretto, P.; Bruschi, M.; Fabbri, M.; Sacco, M.G.; Gribaldo, L. Impact of Cadmium on Intracellular Zinc Levels in HepG2 Cells: Quantitative Evaluations and Molecular Effects, Impact of Cadmium on Intracellular Zinc Levels in HepG2 Cells: Quantitative Evaluations and Molecular Effects. *BioMed Res. Int. BioMed Res. Int.* **2015**, *2015*, e949514.
95. Pedersen, M.Ø.; Larsen, A.; Stoltenberg, M.; Penkowa, M. The role of metallothionein in oncogenesis and cancer prognosis. *Prog. Histochem. Cytochem.* **2009**, *44*, 29–64. [CrossRef] [PubMed]
96. Hart, B.A.; Potts, R.J.; Watkin, R.D. Cadmium adaptation in the lung—A double-edged sword? *Toxicology* **2001**, *160*, 65–70. [CrossRef]
97. Eneman, J.D.; Potts, R.J.; Osier, M.; Shukla, G.S.; Lee, C.H.; Chiu, J.-F.; Hart, B.A. Suppressed oxidant-induced apoptosis in cadmium adapted alveolar epithelial cells and its potential involvement in cadmium carcinogenesis. *Toxicology* **2000**, *147*, 215–228. [CrossRef]

98. Potts, R.J.; Bespalov, I.A.; Wallace, S.S.; Melamede, R.J.; Hart, B.A. Inhibition of oxidative DNA repair in cadmium-adapted alveolar epithelial cells and the potential involvement of metallothionein. *Toxicology* **2001**, *161*, 25–38. [CrossRef]
99. Satoh, M.; Kloth, D.M.; Kadhim, S.A.; Chin, J.L.; Naganuma, A.; Imura, N.; Cherian, M.G. Modulation of Both Cisplatin Nephrotoxicity and Drug Resistance in Murine Bladder Tumor by Controlling Metallothionein Synthesis. *Cancer Res.* **1993**, *53*, 1829–1832.
100. Wülfing, C.; van Ahlen, H.; Eltze, E.; Piechota, H.; Hertle, L.; Schmid, K.-W. Metallothionein in bladder cancer: Correlation of overexpression with poor outcome after chemotherapy. *World J. Urol.* **2007**, *25*, 199–205. [CrossRef] [PubMed]
101. Yamasaki, Y.; Smith, C.; Weisz, D.; van Huizen, I.; Xuan, J.; Moussa, M.; Stitt, L.; Hideki, S.; Cherian, M.G.; Izawa, J.I. Metallothionein expression as prognostic factor for transitional cell carcinoma of bladder. *Urology* **2006**, *67*, 530–535. [CrossRef] [PubMed]
102. Southgate, J.; Masters, J.R.W.; Trejdosiewicz, L.K. Culture of Human Urothelium. In *Culture of Epithelial Cells*; John Wiley & Sons, Inc.: New York, NY, USA, 2002; pp. 381–399. ISBN 978-0-471-22120-3.
103. Rubenwolf, P.; Southgate, J. Permeability of differentiated human urothelium in vitro. *Methods Mol. Biol.* **2011**, *763*, 207–222.
104. Fishwick, C.; Higgins, J.; Percival-Alwyn, L.; Hustler, A.; Pearson, J.; Bastkowski, S.; Moxon, S.; Swarbreck, D.; Greenman, C.D.; Southgate, J. Heterarchy of transcription factors driving basal and luminal cell phenotypes in human urothelium. *Cell Death Differ.* **2017**, *24*, 809–818. [CrossRef] [PubMed]
105. Bray, N.L.; Pimentel, H.; Melsted, P.; Pachter, L. Near-optimal probabilistic RNA-seq quantification. *Nat. Biotechnol.* **2016**, *34*, 525–527. [CrossRef] [PubMed]
106. Soneson, C.; Love, M.I.; Robinson, M.D. Differential analyses for RNA-seq: Transcript-level estimates improve gene-level inferences. *F1000Research* **2015**, *4*, 1521. [CrossRef] [PubMed]
107. Pimentel, H.; Bray, N.L.; Puente, S.; Melsted, P.; Pachter, L. Differential analysis of RNA-seq incorporating quantification uncertainty. *Nat. Methods* **2017**, *14*, 687–690. [CrossRef] [PubMed]
108. Lobban, E.D.; Smith, B.A.; Hall, G.D.; Harnden, P.; Roberts, P.; Selby, P.J.; Trejdosiewicz, L.K.; Southgate, J. Uroplakin gene expression by normal and neoplastic human urothelium. *Am. J. Pathol.* **1998**, *153*, 1957–1967. [CrossRef]

9

Urinary MicroRNAs as Potential Markers for Non-Invasive Diagnosis of Bladder Cancer

Kati Erdmann [1,2,†], Karsten Salomo [1,†], Anna Klimova [2,3], Ulrike Heberling [1], Andrea Lohse-Fischer [1], Romy Fuehrer [1], Christian Thomas [1], Ingo Roeder [2,3], Michael Froehner [1], Manfred P. Wirth [1] and Susanne Fuessel [1,*]

1 Department of Urology, Technische Universität Dresden, 01307 Dresden, Germany; kati.erdmann@uniklinikum-dresden.de (K.E.); karsten.salomo@googlemail.com (K.S.); ulrike.heberling@uniklinikum-dresden.de (U.H.); andrea.lohse-fischer@uniklinikum-dresden.de (A.L.-F.); romy.fuehrer@uniklinikum-dresden.de (R.F.); christian.thomas@uniklinikum-dresden.de (C.T.); michael.froehner@ediacon.de (M.F.); manfred.wirth@uniklinikum-dresden.de (M.P.W.)

2 National Center for Tumor Diseases (NCT), 01307 Dresden, Germany; anna.klimova@nct-dresden.de (A.K.); ingo.roeder@tu-dresden.de (I.R.)

3 Institute for Medical Informatics and Biometrics, Technische Universität Dresden, 01307 Dresden, Germany

* Correspondence: susanne.fuessel@uniklinikum-dresden.de

† These authors contributed equally to this work.

Abstract: Currently, voided urine cytology (VUC) serves as the gold standard for the detection of bladder cancer (BCa) in urine. Despite its high specificity, VUC has shortcomings in terms of sensitivity. Therefore, alternative biomarkers are being searched, which might overcome these disadvantages as a useful adjunct to VUC. The aim of this study was to evaluate the diagnostic potential of the urinary levels of selected microRNAs (miRs), which might represent such alternative biomarkers due to their BCa-specific expression. Expression levels of nine BCa-associated microRNAs (miR-21, -96, -125b, -126, -145, -183, -205, -210, -221) were assessed by quantitative PCR in urine sediments from 104 patients with primary BCa and 46 control subjects. Receiver operating characteristic (ROC) curve analyses revealed a diagnostic potential for miR-96, -125b, -126, -145, -183, and -221 with area under the curve (AUC) values between 0.605 and 0.772. The combination of the four best candidates resulted in sensitivity, specificity, positive and negative predictive values (NPV), and accuracy of 73.1%, 95.7%, 97.4%, 61.1%, and 80.0%, respectively. Combined with VUC, sensitivity and NPV could be increased by nearly 8%, each surpassing the performance of VUC alone. The present findings suggested a diagnostic potential of miR-125b, -145, -183, and -221 in combination with VUC for non-invasive detection of BCa in urine.

Keywords: miRNA; quantitative PCR; tumor marker; urothelial carcinoma; voided urine cytology

1. Introduction

Bladder cancer (BCa) was the 10th most common malignancy worldwide with 550,000 new cases and an estimated 200,000 deaths in 2018 [1,2]. The highest BCa incidence rates in the world were reported for Southern and Western Europe and North America. In men, who are four times more frequently affected than women, BCa ranks sixth of all newly diagnosed cancers and is the ninth most deadly cancer worldwide [2]. Initial BCa diagnostic steps include voided urine cytology (VUC), as the current standard for non-invasive BCa detection, and cystoscopy, an invasive procedure. Tissue specimens obtained during transurethral resection of the bladder (TUR-B) undergo histopathological examination for assessment of the putative tumor grade and stage [3]. The same approach is used for regular follow-up after treatment to detect BCa recurrence and progression. Among other factors, these life-long, frequent, and cost-intensive surveillance procedures make BCa one of the most expensive tumor entities [4,5].

VUC is an observer-dependent method and characterized by a high specificity of 78–100%. While it displays a moderate sensitivity of 34–84% for high-grade tumors, its sensitivity for low-grade tumors is very low at 12–26% [6]. Even though several alternative biomarker-based tests for non-invasive BCa detection in urine exist, none of them is recommended for routine use in clinical practice due to their inadequate performance [3,7]. The sensitivity of most alternative BCa tests is higher compared to VUC, but their specificity is not able to reach that of VUC so far [8,9]. Therefore, the search for cost-efficient, highly specific, and sensitive biomarkers for non-invasive BCa diagnosis, screening, and follow-up, which eventually allow reducing the number of invasive, inconvenient, and expensive cystoscopies, is ongoing.

Numerous studies have been aimed at the identification of mRNA expression signatures in tumor tissues and tumor-derived urine specimens that reflect the presence and aggressiveness of BCa and additionally characterize the most powerful predictive biomarker combinations [10–12]. In recent years, microRNAs (miRNAs or miRs) emerged as potential diagnostic and prognostic biomarkers due to their tissue- and tumor-specific expression. miRNAs are small, endogenous, non-coding RNAs that function as post-transcriptional regulators of specific target genes via mRNA degradation or inhibition of the translation [13,14]. As regulators of many cellular processes such as differentiation, proliferation, apoptosis or cell cycle control, miRNAs also play an important role in different deregulated, pathological pathways such as tumor onset and progression, making them promising candidates as tumor markers [13–15].

BCa-associated miRNA signatures were investigated by microarray, next-generation sequencing (NGS), and quantitative PCR (qPCR) analyses in malignant and non-malignant bladder tissue specimens, as well as in urine samples from BCa patients and control subjects. Several promising miRNA candidates showing a differential expression and/or an association with BCa aggressiveness emerged from these studies [16–20]. Additionally, the proven involvement of many of these miRNAs in tumor-related pathways deems them worthy of evaluation as potential biomarkers for diagnosis of BCa [21]. On the basis of a literature search comprising single reports, systematic reviews, and meta-analyses, nine miRNAs fulfilling the abovementioned criteria were selected for an independent validation study as putative biomarkers for non-invasive BCa detection in urine specimens: miR-21, -96, -125b, -126, -145, -183, -205, -210, and -221 [22–32] (for details, see also Supplementary Table S1). Using urine sediments from BCa patients and control subjects, the expression levels of these miRNAs determined by qPCR were assessed individually and in combination with regard to their diagnostic potential. In order to determine a potential diagnostic improvement, their diagnostic performance was also evaluated as an adjunct to VUC.

2. Results

2.1. Characteristics of BCa Patients and Control Subjects

A total of 104 patients with histologically-proven BCa at TUR-B were included in the present study (Table 1). This cohort consisted of 83 male and 21 female patients with a median age of 70 years (range 50 to 85 years). The relative distribution of pTa, pT1, pTis, and ≥pT2 tumors was 48.1%, 21.2%, 14.4%, and 16.3%. Since all of the 15 pTis tumors occurred concomitantly with other tumors, the most severe tumor stage was coded. In doing so, patients with non-muscle-invasive BCa (NMIBC; pTa and pT1) and concomitant pTis were allocated to the pTis group (10 of the 15 pTis cases; 9.6% of all BCa). The remaining five patients with muscle-invasive BCa (MIBC) and concomitant pTis were allocated to the group ≥pT2, resulting in a total of 22 patients with MIBC with or without concomitant pTis (21.1% of all BCa). Multifocal tumors occurred in 32 patients (30.8%).

Table 1. Demographic, clinical, and histopathological characteristics of the BCa patients (n = 104). The table shows the absolute and relative distribution of gender, age, and clinicopathological parameters.

Parameter	Category	Number (n)	Percentage (%)
gender	male	83	79.8
	female	21	20.2
age [1] (years)	≤70.0	54	51.9
	>70.0	50	48.1
tumor stage	pTa	50	48.1
	pT1	22	21.2
	pTis	15	14.4
	pTis only	*0*	*0.0*
	pTis + pTa	*3*	*2.9*
	pTis + pT1	*7*	*6.7*
	pTis + ≥ pT2a	*5*	*4.8*
	≥ pT2a	17	16.3
tumor grade (WHO 1973)	G1	14	13.5
	G2	52	50.0
	G3	38	36.5
tumor grade (WHO 2004) multifocality	low-grade	17	16.3
	high-grade	87	83.7
	unifocal	72	69.2
	multifocal	32	30.8
voided urine cytology	positive	80	76.9
	negative	24	23.1

[1] Age was dichotomized at the median (70.0 years).

Using the WHO grading system from 1973, 13.5% G1, 50.0% G2, and 36.5% G3 BCa were reported. According to the WHO grading system from 2004, 83.7% of the BCa patients displayed high-grade tumors, whereas only 16.3% had low-grade tumors.

Moreover, the control group consisted of eight subjects, who underwent a TUR-B without histopathological evidence of BCa and 38 patients with urolithiasis (Table 2).

Table 2. Demographic, clinical, and histopathological characteristics of the control subjects. The control group was comprised of 46 subjects in total, whereupon eight patients were histopathologically negative for BCa at TUR-B and 38 patients had urolithiasis. The table shows the absolute and relative distribution of gender, age and clinicopathological parameters.

Parameter	Category	Number (n)	Percentage (%)
gender	male	30	65.2
	female	16	34.8
age [1] (years)	<64.5	23	50.0
	≥64.5	23	50.0
diagnosis	BCa-negative TUR-B	8	17.4
	urolithiasis	38	82.6
voided urine cytology	positive	0	0.0
	negative	46	100.0

[1] Age was dichotomized at the median (64.5 years).

2.2. Correlations between the Analyzed miRNAs

Relative expression levels of the selected miRNAs (determined by qPCR and normalized to the geometric mean of the reference RNAs RNU44 and RNU48) were analyzed in detail in BCa-derived and control urine sediments. Some of the analyzed miRNAs showed significant correlations with each other as assessed by the pairwise calculation of Spearman's rank correlation coefficients. Most prominent significant positive correlations ($p < 0.01$) were observed between the miRNAs miR-21, -125b, -205, -210, and -221 with correlation coefficients between 0.566 (miR-210 vs. miR-221) and 0.825 (miR-125b vs. miR-221). Significant positive correlations ($p < 0.01$) were also seen between miR-96 and miR-183 ($r_s = 0.557$), miR-96 and miR-126 ($r_s = 0.311$), and miR-126 and miR-183 ($r_s = 0.483$). Finally, miR-145 correlated negatively ($p < 0.01$) with miR-205 ($r_s = -0.433$) and miR-210 ($r_s = -0.483$).

2.3. Associations of Urinary miRNA Transcript Levels and Histopathological Features

The expression levels of miR-125b ($r_s = -0.434$, $p < 0.01$) and miR-205 ($r_s = -0.206$, $p < 0.05$) in the tumor-derived urine samples decreased with increasing tumor stage, whereas those of miR-96 and miR-183 showed a weak positive correlation with tumor stage ($r_s = 0.238$ and 0.246, $p < 0.05$). A weak, but significant negative correlation ($p < 0.01$) with tumor grade according to the WHO classification from 1973 was detected for miR-125b, miR-205, and miR-210 (r_s between −0.309 and −0.334), whereas miR-145 displayed a weak, but significant positive correlation with tumor grade ($r_s = 0.266$, $p < 0.01$). A similar trend of dependence on tumor grade assessed according to the WHO classification from 2004 could only be observed for miR-125b and -210. The inverse relationships between the miR-125b expression levels in urine and tumor stage, as well as with tumor grade are exemplarily shown in Figure 1. Significant differences in relative miR-125b levels were found between the controls and all tumor stages, as well as between pTa tumors and higher tumor stages. Moreover, relative miR-125b levels differed significantly between the controls and G2/G3 or high-grade BCa, as well as between G1 and G2/G3 or low-grade and high-grade tumors (Figure 1). None of the miRNAs displayed substantial alterations between urine samples from patients with unifocal and multifocal BCa.

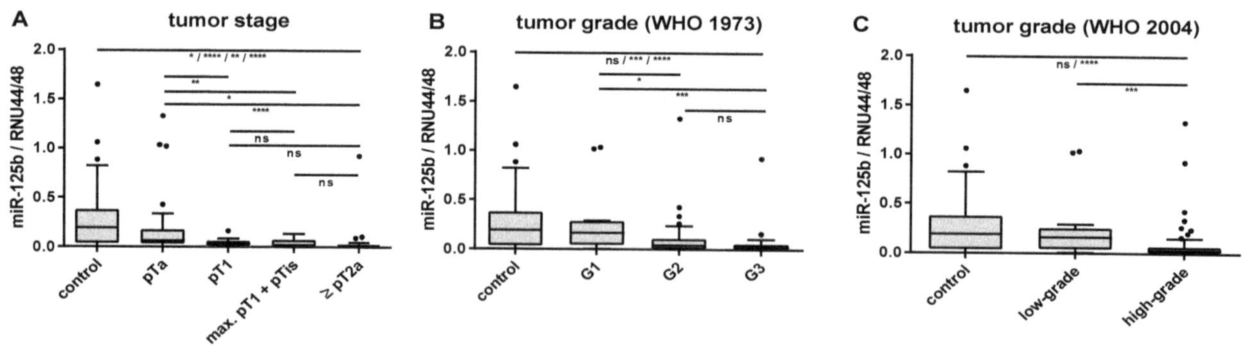

Figure 1. Dependence of the relative miR-125b expression levels (normalized to the geometric mean of the reference RNAs RNU44 and RNU48) in urine sediments on histopathological factors. The relationships between urinary miR-125b expression levels and tumor stage (**A**), as well as tumor grade according to the WHO classifications from 1973 (**B**) and from 2004 (**C**) are shown. Differences were tested by the Mann–Whitney U test. ns, not significant; * $p < 0.05$; ** $p < 0.01$; *** $p < 0.001$; **** $p < 0.0001$.

2.4. Evaluation of the Single miRNAs as Potential Markers for BCa Detection

Next, the relative miRNA expression levels were compared between the urine samples from the eight control patients without histopathological evidence of BCa at TUR-B and from the 38 controls patients with urolithiasis. None of the nine analyzed miRNAs showed significant differences in relative expression levels between both control subgroups (Mann–Whitney U test: $p > 0.05$). Therefore, data from both subgroups were combined, constituting the final control group of 46 subjects.

In comparison to these controls, statistically significant different relative miRNA expression levels were observed in urine sediments from BCa patients for miR-96, -125b, -126, -145, -183, and -221. After Bonferroni's correction for multiple comparisons (Table 3 and Figure 2), the significance was retained for these miRNAs except for miR-96 ($p = 0.05$). While the miRNAs miR-96, -126, and -183 displayed higher relative expression levels in the BCa-derived urine sediments, the miRNAs miR-125b, -145, and -221 were downregulated in these specimens compared to the control group (Table 3). Receiver operating characteristic (ROC) curve analyses also revealed a diagnostic potential for these six miRNAs with area under the curve (AUC) values ranging from 0.605 ($p = 0.369$) for miR-96 to 0.772 ($p < 0.001$) for miR-221 (Table 3 and Figure 3). The remaining three miRNAs miR-21, -205, and -210 did not show significant differences between tumor and control subjects (Table 3).

Table 3. Comparison of the relative miRNA expression levels in urine sediments from the BCa and control groups (Mann–Whitney U test) and assessment of the diagnostic power by ROC curve analyses. All p-values were adjusted by Bonferroni's correction for multiple comparisons.

miRNA	Regulation in BCa	Mann–Whitney U Test (p-Value)	ROC Curve Analysis AUC	ROC Curve Analysis p-Value
miR-21	not different	=1.000	0.581	=1.000
miR-96	up	=0.050	0.605	=0.369
miR-125b	down	<0.001	0.714	<0.001
miR-126	up	<0.01	0.667	<0.01
miR-145	down	<0.01	0.687	<0.01
miR-183	up	<0.001	0.720	<0.001
miR-205	not different	=1.000	0.537	=1.000
miR-210	not different	=1.000	0.526	=1.000
miR-221	down	<0.0001	0.772	<0.0001

95% CI, 95% confidence interval; AUC, area under the curve; ROC, receiver operating characteristic.

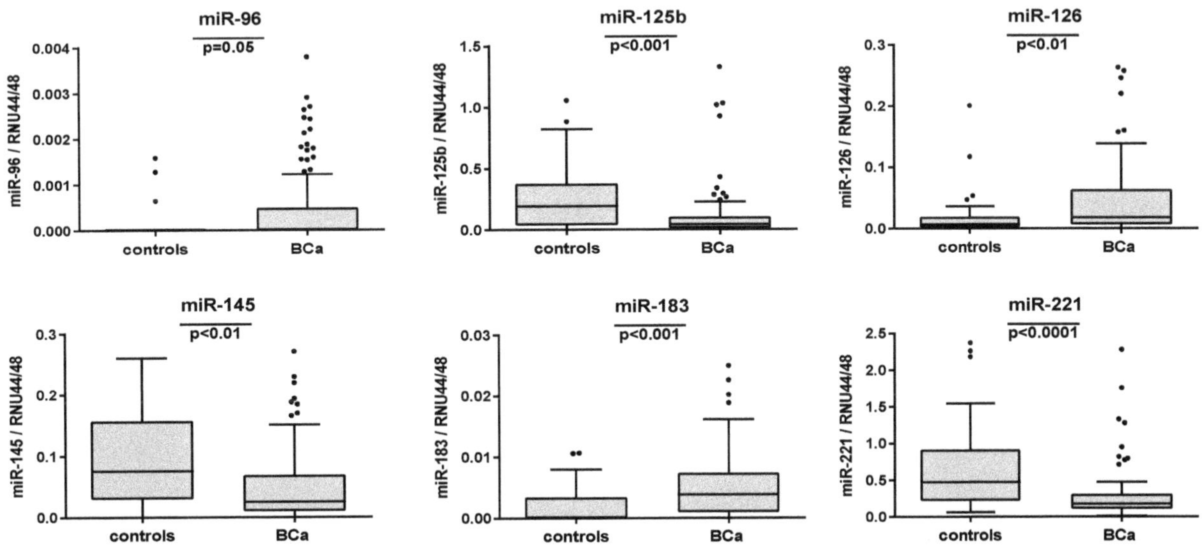

Figure 2. The distribution of the relative expression levels of the significantly altered miRNAs in urine sediments from controls and BCa patients is presented by box plots. Differences in the relative expression levels of the miRNAs (normalized to the geometric mean of the reference RNAs RNU44 and RNU48) were assessed using the Mann–Whitney U test followed by Bonferroni's correction for multiple comparisons.

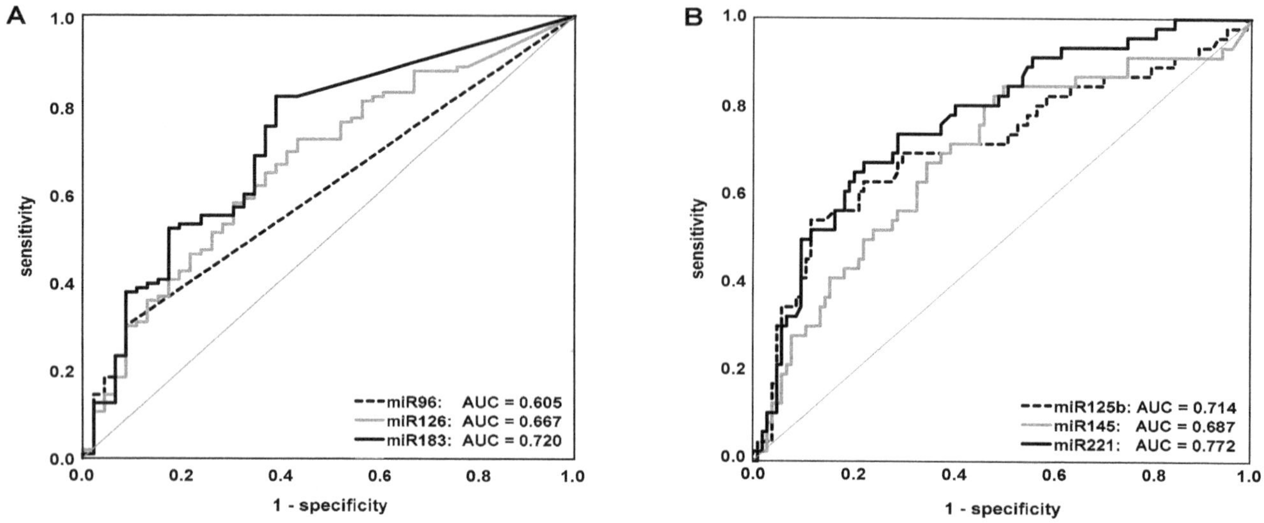

Figure 3. The diagnostic value assessed by ROC curve analysis of the six most promising miRNAs, which were significantly up- (**A**) or down-regulated (**B**) in urine sediments from BCa patients in comparison with controls. AUC, area under the curve; ROC, receiver operating characteristic.

2.5. Comparison of Diagnostic Performance of miRNA Transcript Levels and Voided Urine Cytology

To assess the diagnostic power of the single miRNAs, VUC, and combinations thereof, different statistical approaches were applied. The first approach was based on the simple classification of the measured relative miRNA expression levels and of the results of VUC assessment into positive ("1") and negative ("0") indicators of tumor detection. The diagnostic parameters calculated on this basis were assessed with regard to the best performing single BCa marker. The nine analyzed miRNAs displayed only moderate diagnostic value with accuracy rates between 48.7% for miR-96 and 78.0% for miR-125b (Table 4). None of these single miRNAs could surpass the performance of VUC, which displayed a relatively high sensitivity of 76.9% at a specificity of 100% and an accuracy of 84.0% (Table 4) in our cohort.

Table 4. Diagnostic performance of the miRNAs and VUC as single markers.

Parameter	miR-21	-96	-125b	-126	-145	-183	-205	-210	-221	VUC
SNS	0.865	0.298	0.885	0.885	0.500	0.817	0.779	0.663	0.779	0.769
SPC	0.304	0.913	0.543	0.217	0.848	0.609	0.435	0.500	0.674	1.000
PPV	0.738	0.886	0.814	0.719	0.881	0.825	0.757	0.750	0.844	1.000
NPV	0.500	0.365	0.676	0.455	0.429	0.596	0.465	0.397	0.574	0.657
pLR	1.244	3.428	1.938	1.130	3.286	2.089	1.378	1.327	2.388	n.d.
nLR	0.442	0.769	0.212	0.531	0.590	0.300	0.509	0.673	0.328	0.231
ACC	0.693	0.487	0.780	0.680	0.607	0.753	0.673	0.613	0.747	0.840

ACC, accuracy; n.d., not determinable (division by zero); nLR, negative likelihood ratio; NPV, negative predictive value; pLR, positive likelihood ratio; PPV, positive predictive value; SNS, sensitivity; SPC, specificity.

In the next step, the tumor detection values ("1" or "0") for the six miRNAs with substantially different relative expression levels between urine samples from BCa patients and controls were totaled and evaluated with regard to the best separation of these sums. In doing so, the detection of at least four of these six miRNAs as an indicator of the tumor yielded a sensitivity of 73.1%, a specificity of 93.5%, and an accuracy of 79.3% (Table 5). The combination of only the four miRNAs with the highest AUC values in ROC curve analyses (miR-125b, -145, -183, and -221) and the use of at least three positive miRNAs as a BCa indicator resulted in a slightly better diagnostic performance compared to the combination of six miRNAs and to all single miRNAs (Tables 4 and 5).

Table 5. Diagnostic performance of combinations of selected miRNAs with each other and with VUC.

Parameter	6 miRs 96/125b/126/145/183/221 0-3/4-6 pos. Markers	4 miRs 125b/145/183/221 0-2/3-4 pos. Markers	6 miRs + VUC 96/125b/126/145/183/221 0-3/4-7 pos. Markers	4 miRs + VUC 125b/145/183/221 0-2/3-5 pos. Markers
SNS	0.731	0.731	0.808	0.846
SPC	0.935	0.957	0.935	0.957
PPV	0.962	0.974	0.966	0.978
NPV	0.606	0.611	0.683	0.733
pLR	11.205	16.808	12.385	19.462
nLR	0.288	0.281	0.206	0.161
ACC	0.793	0.800	0.847	0.880

ACC, accuracy; nLR, negative likelihood ratio; NPV, negative predictive value; pos., positive; pLR, positive likelihood ratio; PPV, positive predictive value; SNS, sensitivity; SPC, specificity.

The inclusion of VUC in both miRNA combinations led to a further increase of the diagnostic power and revealed the combination of the four miRNAs with VUC as the best approach with a sensitivity of 84.6%, a specificity of 95.7%, and an accuracy of 88.0% (Table 5). This combination was able to outperform VUC as a single marker with a 4% increase in accuracy, but at the expense of specificity in the same magnitude. However, it also resulted in a gain of nearly 8% each in sensitivity and NPV.

In the second statistical approach, the diagnostic power was analyzed using penalized linear regression applied to standardized miRNA values. This regression analysis (Figure 4) indicated that miR-210, -125b, and -221 had the strongest diagnostic power, while the influence of miR-145 and -205 was much weaker and the one of miR-21, -126, and -183 the weakest. In 10,000 simulations, each performed for a sample set of 20 patients from the original dataset, the penalized regression model correctly classified the tumor status in about 75% of the cases.

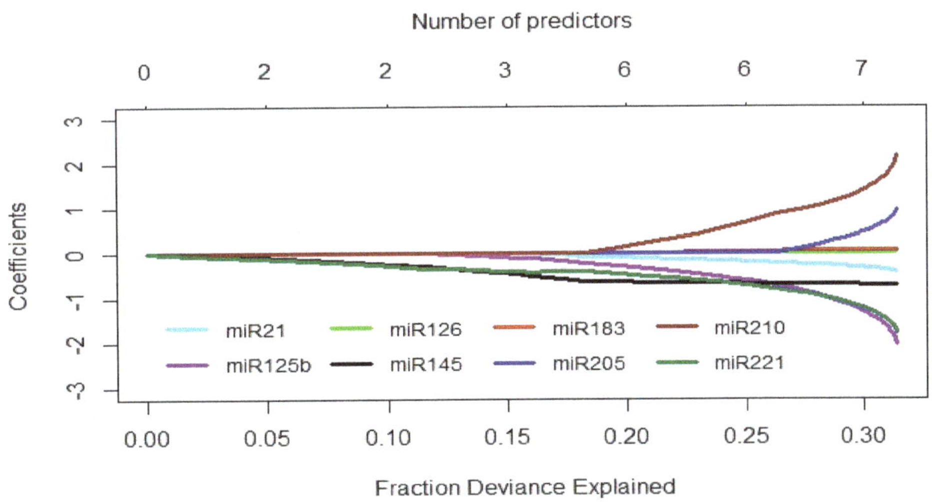

Figure 4. Diagnostic value of the miRNAs assessed by penalized linear regression. The deviance profile plot corresponding to standardized miRNAs as predictor variables in the *glmnet* model is shown. The slope of each path changes each time as another miRNA enters the model. The miRNAs, which explain a larger fraction of deviance, play a more important role in the prediction of the tumor status.

The order of importance of the miRNAs (miR-125b, -221, -145, -183, -205, -126, -210, -21) obtained using the random forest method as the third statistical approach was in concordance with the results of penalized linear regression. The percentage of cases correctly classified with this approach was 82.6%. The classification error in the random forest analysis was 20% (based on 100 simulations). Because of too many observed zero values for miR-96 in the control group, this variable was excluded from the analyses with *glmnet* and *randomForest*. In the overview of all statistical evaluation methods used herein, the miRNAs miR-125b, -145, -183, and -221 appeared to serve as well-suited biomarkers for the non-invasive detection of BCa in urine sediments independent of the chosen approach.

3. Discussion

The early and reliable detection of BCa is one of the biggest challenges to identify and treat patients at risk and to commence treatment in a timely manner. Many efforts have been made in recent years to implement new diagnostic approaches in clinical routine for the non-invasive detection of BCa using urine [6,8,9] and to replace VUC as the current gold standard. Nevertheless, none of these new biomarkers is thus far recommended for routine use in the early detection or follow-up of BCa or for replacement or reduction of the invasive procedure of cystoscopy [3]. According to current guidelines, such urinary molecular marker tests should provide a very high NPV to predict the absence of tumor reliably and eventually to avoid unnecessary cystoscopies [3]. Moreover, they should amend and strengthen the diagnostic performance of VUC and additionally overcome its main drawback: the low sensitivity, particularly for low-grade BCa [6].

For this purpose, this study focused on the diagnostic capability of miRNAs which are well known to be dysregulated in cellular pathways associated with the onset and progression of tumors including BCa [16,18,20]. Based on an extensive literature search, a number of promising miRNA candidates was selected, which were reported to be differentially expressed in bladder tissues and/or urine specimens from BCa patients and control subjects [22–32]. The diagnostic performance of the altered expression of these miRNAs in urine sediments was evaluated, revealing a certain potential of the miRNAs miR-96, -125b, -126, -145, -183, and -221 as single markers or in combination. The best diagnostic power was finally achieved by the use of four of these miRNAs in combination with VUC by simple classification of the urine samples as positive or negative for the single markers and subsequent allocation according to the total number of altered single markers (0-2 vs. 3-5 positive markers) regardless of which markers were changed. This approach resulted in a sensitivity of 84.6%, an NPV of 73.3%, and an accuracy of 88.0%, all surpassing the corresponding parameters of VUC alone (76.9%/65.7%/84.0%). In the marker combination, this was accompanied by losses of 4% in specificity and 2% in PPV compared to VUC alone where both accounted for 100%. Nevertheless, these losses appeared less severe in the face of the gain of nearly 8% each in sensitivity and NPV.

Thus, the combination of the four miRNAs miR-125b, -145, -183, and -221 with VUC seemed to have a promising potential for reliable diagnosis of BCa in urine samples prior to TUR-B. Accordingly, the diagnostic value of a reduced miR-125b expression in urine to prior tumor resection previously reported by Snowdon et al. [33], Mengual et al. [29], Zhang et al. [32], and Pospisilova et al. [34] could be confirmed in this study. This miRNA displayed a steady decrease with increasing tumor stage and grade, as also observed by Zhang et al. [32], indicating a certain prognostic power. Accordingly, Mengual et al. [29] described a prognostic panel comprising miR-125b and -92a for the identification of high-grade BCa, which was, however, not assessed in our patient cohort.

Another miRNA frequently described to be downregulated in cancer and particularly in BCa is miR-145 [27,28,35,36], which was also one of the best single miRNA markers in this study. Its diagnostic power (AUC = 0.687) herein was comparable to that (AUC = 0.729) determined by Yun et al. [36]. In contrast, Mearini et al. did not observe significant differences in urinary miR-145 levels between urine sediments from BCa patients and control subjects [37].

The miRNAs miR-96 and miR-183 are encoded by the miR-183/96/182 cluster on chromosome 7 and regulated in a concerted manner in different pathologies including BCa and other cancers [27,38–40]. Therefore, their expression behavior appears to be very similar as also reflected by their correlation observed in our measurements. Both miRNAs displayed a substantial elevation in BCa-derived urine samples compared to controls with miR-183 showing the second-best diagnostic potential of all miRNAs investigated herein (AUC = 0.720). Yamada et al. analyzed urinary levels of miR-96 and miR-183 in patients with urothelial carcinoma and revealed a high diagnostic value for both miRNAs reflected by AUC values of 0.831 and 0.817, respectively [41]. Moreover, they observed a positive dependence of miR-96/-183 levels on tumor stage and grade, whereas we could only identify a weak, but significant positive correlation with tumor stage. Considerable diagnostic power with regard to the non-invasive diagnosis of BCa by determination of urinary miR-96 levels was also described in several other studies [42–44]. This miRNA showed a differential expression only with a statistical trend ($p = 0.05$) in our study, but had to be excluded from some statistical approaches due to its low expression levels. miR-183, which was better performing in our cohort than miR-96, also emerged as a possible marker for high-grade NMIBC in the report from Pardini et al., who identified promising diagnostic miRNAs by NGS in cell-free urine supernatants from BCa patients and control subjects [45]. In summary, from these data, miR-96 and/or miR-183 seemed to provide substantial information when analyzing urine specimens for BCa diagnosis.

The diagnostic usability of elevated levels of miR-126 as a urinary marker has been reported by several studies so far [33,44,46]. In 2010, Hanke et al. reported an AUC value of 0.768 for the separation of BCa patients vs. healthy donors and of 0.747 vs. healthy donors and infections for miR-126 detection in urine [46]. Interestingly, miR-126 and -183 showed a significant, but less strong positive correlation with each other than miR-96 and -183, but they were both useful as BCa markers in contrast to miR-96.

Remarkably, miR-221 (our best performing BCa marker (AUC = 0.772)) was not found to be a promising candidate in previous studies despite its reported differential expression in BCa tissues [44,47]. In contrast, the remaining candidates (miR-21, -205, and -210), which did not show differential urinary expression levels in this study, were described as promising urinary BCa markers in selected reports [43,45,48–50]. For example, Michaildi et al. obtained a diagnostic AUC value of 0.845 when comparing miR-205 levels in cell-free urine supernatants from 177 normal donors and 32 BCa patients [50]. This miRNA also seemed promising with regard to the distinction of different BCa subsets as reported by Pardini et al. [45]. In contrast, it did not allow discrimination between patients with and without BCa, neither in the urine sediment, nor in the cell-free urine supernatant, in the study performed by Wang et al. [51]. Kim et al., who selected eight miRNAs (including miR-96, -125b, -145, and -205, like in our study) for urine analyses, observed among others increased levels of miR-205, as well as decreased levels of miR-125b and -145 in BCa-derived urine samples compared to negative controls [52]. We observed strong positive correlations between the miRNAs miR-21, -125b, -205, -210, and -221, but only miR-125b and -221 proved to be useful BCa markers in our study, for which we have no conclusive explanation. At the functional level, all of the five mentioned miRNAs were reported to regulate genes involved in cell cycle control, p53, and growth factor receptor signaling, which would fit with the observed correlations [53,54].

To explain the discrepancies observed between different studies, a variety of reasons can be given. On the one hand, there is a large diversity in the type of urinary components explored for miRNA analysis ranging from whole urine over urine sediment as used herein to cell-free urine supernatant or exosomes (Suppl. Table S1). It was assumed that exfoliated tumor cells were the main constituents of cellular urine sediments from BCa patients, and miRNA levels measured therein directly reflected those of the tumor. Both increased and decreased expression of such miRNAs would indicate the presence of BCa against the background of miRNA patterns in non-malignant cells, which are also part of the urine sediment. On the other hand, the kind of miRNA determination varied from NGS- and microarray-based profiling to different kinds of qPCR with and without miRNA-specific probes and the possible inclusion of a preamplification step. Moreover, the number of included patients and controls, the kind of controls (healthy donors or patients with benign urological diseases, infection, or hematuria), and tumor subtypes (e.g., urothelial carcinoma of the bladder or the upper urinary tract, bilharziasis-associated BCa) profoundly influenced the results obtained.

As revealed in this and many other studies, marker combinations seem to be superior to the analysis of single markers. The diagnostic gain, particularly in comparison to VUC alone, was clearly shown herein by the combination of VUC with the best four miRNAs as discussed above. In analogy, Yamada et al. and Eissa et al. reached an increase in diagnostic power by the combined analysis of

VUC and miR-96 due to a considerable number of non-overlapping cancer patients who were positive only for one of these markers. This was particularly reflected by an increase in sensitivity, NPV, and overall accuracy [41,42]. The same was true for the combination of VUC and more miRNAs, as shown by Eissa et al. for miR-10b/-29c/-210 [47], as well as in our study for miR-125b/-145/-183/-221.

However, it remains to be verified whether the achieved improvement of the diagnostic performance of VUC by combination with miRNA levels in urine sediment would really be sufficient to reduce cystoscopies for the first diagnosis or for surveillance after therapy. Alternatively, other BCa-specific biomarkers could potentially fulfill these requirements. Meanwhile, several promising tests became commercially available that detect altered biomarkers in exfoliated tumor cells such as *Xpert Bladder Cancer Monitor*, *Bladder EpiCheck test*, or *AssureMDx test* (reviewed in [55]). The *Xpert test*, which is based on differential mRNA patterns in BCa cells, delivered a sensitivity of 74% and a specificity of 80% for surveillance of NMIBC patients [56]. This was comparable to the results of the *EpiCheck test*, which reflects altered DNA methylation in BCa cells, with a sensitivity of 68% and a specificity of 88% for the detection of recurrent NMIBC [57]. Similar results were reported by Trenti et al., who directly compared the two tests with VUC in the follow-up of NMIBC patients [58]. The *AssureMDx test* (a combined DNA methylation and mutation urine assay) was reported to serve as a useful diagnostic tool to select patients with hematuria for cystoscopy with a sensitivity of 93% and a specificity of 86%, indicating the highest diagnostic potential among the new commercially available biomarker tests [59,60]. Thus, these tests seemed to provide a similar diagnostic power as our test, but only a head-to-head comparison in defined patient cohorts would deliver conclusive results with regard to first BCa diagnosis or surveillance.

Another factor that decisively determines the significance and predictive power of calculated marker combinations is the kind of statistical analysis methods. First, we compared the simple classification of urine samples as positive or negative for the single markers and subsequent allocation according to the total number of altered single markers regardless of which markers were changed with a penalized linear regression. Interestingly, penalized regression indicated the strongest diagnostic power for miR-210, -125b, and -221, although miR-210 was not identified as a suitable marker by ROC analyses. Nevertheless, the diagnostic accuracy of 79.3% and 80.0% for the combination of six or four miRNAs, respectively, accomplished by the first calculation method was higher than that of 75% yielded by penalized linear regression. The random forest method revealed a comparable accuracy of 82.6% using the same miRNAs as our first classification method. Additional principle component analyses could not further increase the diagnostic performance of different miRNA combinations in our study, but should be kept in mind as a further alternative approach, as well as the decision-tree analyses reported by Snowdon et al. and Pospisilova et al. [33,34].

Finally, the general approach for the selection of miRNAs as potential diagnostic BCa markers seems worthy of discussion, as well. The most comprehensive, but also the most cost- and labor-intensive approach is whole transcriptome profiling by NGS, microarray, or PCR array analyses followed by validation of the best candidates by independent methods such as qPCR in independent cohorts [29,32,34,44,45,48,49]. Several other authors made the choice in the same way as in the present study on the basis of publicly accessible datasets and literature reports on differential miRNA expression in malignant and non-malignant bladder tissues and/or in urine samples from BCa patients and suitable controls [33,36,51]. This approach primarily serves the independent validation of candidates that have already been investigated and shown to be promising, supporting the identification of the best markers. On the basis of our results and the presented literature review (Suppl. Table S1), the miRNAs miR-125b and -183 could represent such promising BCa-associated markers in urine. However, further miRNA candidates with a reported considerable diagnostic potential comprised of miR-99a [32,34,52], miR-146a [61], miR-155 [62], or members of the miR-200 family [30,36,51,52] should be further evaluated in comparative analyses.

Our study was associated with several limitations including the relatively low number of control subjects, since such patients are much less common in our department than BCa patients. However, the implementation of patients with benign urological diseases as done herein seemed to be more suitable than the comparison to healthy controls without any symptoms and with fewer exfoliated cells in urine sediment. Furthermore, the BCa patient cohort analyzed in the present study was comprised of a high percentage of cases with high-grade tumors, which is typical for specialized urological clinics and not comparable to those of private urological practices.

Considering this drawback, we avoided extensive calculations of possible associations with tumor grade. However, studies including more low-grade BCa would be required to assess the usefulness of this approach to identify these patients reliably. The clear advantages of our study were the direct comparison to VUC as the current gold standard for non-invasive BCa detection in urine and the combination of miRNA markers with VUC, which resulted in a superior diagnostic power. Nevertheless, this has to be confirmed in future studies on more BCa patients at different stages and suitable controls.

4. Materials and Methods

4.1. Study Population, Data, and Sample Collection

The present study was approved by the institutional review board of the Medical Faculty at the Technische Universität Dresden. Written informed consent was obtained from every participant. Patients with suspicion of having BCa and control subjects were prospectively recruited between May 2014 and September 2016. The inclusion criteria for the cases were comprised of new-onset BCa diagnosed at TUR-B and an age between 40 and 85 years. Patients diagnosed with papilloma or papillary urothelial neoplasm of low malignant potential (PUNLMP) were not eligible. In total, one-hundred four patients undergoing TUR-B with histologically-proven BCa were included (Table 1).

Eight patients suspected to have BCa, but histopathologically diagnosed as tumor-free, were allocated to the control group. Additionally, thirty-eight patients with urolithiasis were included as controls, finally resulting in a total control group size of 46 subjects (Table 2).

The histopathological examination of the resected bladder specimens, which served as the reference standard for BCa diagnosis, was performed using the UICC TNM classification from 2011 [63]. The tumors were accordingly classified as non-muscle-invasive BCa (NMIBC), comprised of the tumor stages pTa, pT1, and pTis, or as muscle-invasive BCa (MIBC), including all tumors with an expected tumor stage of ≥pT2a. The stratification of tumor grades into G1, G2, and G3 was done in accordance with the WHO classification from 1973 and into low-grade and high-grade tumors according to the WHO classification from 2004 [64]. As a reference method for the non-invasive detection of BCa, VUC specimens were prepared from urine samples from all BCa patients and control subjects. One experienced examiner (U.H.) evaluated these VUC specimens according to the ICUD/WHO classification [65].

4.2. Processing of Urine Samples, RNA Isolation, and cDNA Synthesis

Spontaneous urine samples (20–100 mL) were collected before therapeutic intervention from all BCa patients and control subjects. Urine collection was standardized in daily clinical practice (no morning urine, 2nd or 3rd urine of the day, clean catch in a sterile cup). The presence of erythrocytes, leucocytes, and bacteria was assessed by microscopic analysis of the sediment from 5–10 mL urine. Additionally, a VUC specimen was prepared from 5–10 mL urine. It was prefixed with *Esposti's fixative* overnight, centrifuged on glass slides, fixed with *Cytofix N* (Niepötter Labortechnik, Bürstadt, Germany), and stained by the Papanicolaou procedure [66].

The remaining urine was centrifuged at 1500× *g* for 10 min at 4 °C. After removal of the supernatant, the cellular pellet was washed twice with ice-cold phosphate-buffered saline (PBS) by centrifugation at 870× *g* for 5 min at 4 °C and resuspended in 700 µL *QIAzol Lysis Reagent* (Qiagen, Hilden, Germany). The lysates were frozen and stored at −80 °C until further processing. After thawing, total RNA was isolated using the *Direct-zol RNA MiniPrep kit* (Zymo Research, Freiburg, Germany) according to the manufacturer's recommendations. The RNA was eluted from the *Zymo-Spin IIC Column* with 40 μL nuclease-free water and quantified using the *NanoDrop 2000c* spectrophotometer (PEQLAB, Erlangen, Germany) and the *Agilent RNA 6000 Pico Kit* on an *Agilent 2100 Bioanalyzer* (Agilent Technologies, Ratingen, Germany).

If available, one-hundred nanograms total RNA (at least 50 ng) were employed for reverse transcription (RT) of the miRNAs using specific *TaqMan microRNA Assays* (Thermo Fisher Scientific, Darmstadt, Germany).

A multiplex RT was performed for the nine selected target miRNAs (Table 6: miR-21, -96, -125b, -126, -145, -183, -205, -210, and -221) and two reference RNAs (RNU44 andRNU48) in a final reaction volume of 30 μL comprised of 8 μL of the diluted RNA and 22 μL of the RT master mix. The latter consisted of dNTPs (each in a final concentration of 2 mM), *MultiScribe Reverse Transcriptase* (300 U), RT buffer, RNase inhibitor (7.6 U), and the respective RT primers (each 0.6×). The following temperature program was applied for the RT reaction: 30 min at 16 °C, 30 min at 42 °C, 5 min at 85 °C, followed by cooling down to 4 °C.

Table 6. The TaqMan microRNA assays used (Thermo Fisher Scientific, Darmstadt, Germany).

miRNA	Assay Name	Assay ID
miR-21-5p	hsa-miR-21	000397
miR-96-5p	mmu-miR-96 (for hsa-miR-96-5p)	000186
miR-125b-5p	hsa-miR-125b	000449
miR-126-3p	hsa-miR-126	002228
miR-145-5p	hsa-miR-145	002278
miR-183-5p	hsa-miR-183	002269
miR-205-5p	hsa-miR-205	000509
miR-210-3p	hsa-miR-210	000512
miR-221-3p	hsa-miR-221	000524
RNU44 (NR_002750) *	RNU44	001094
RNU48 (NR_002745) *	RNU48	001006

* TaqMan microRNA control assays.

4.3. Transcript Quantitation by Quantitative PCR

The individual mature miRNAs and reference RNAs were quantified separately on the *LightCycler 480 Real-Time PCR System* (Roche Diagnostics, Mannheim, Germany). Each qPCR with a final volume of 10 μL consisted of 1 μL of the undiluted cDNA product, the respective *TaqMan MicroRNA Assay* (Table 6), *GoTaq Probe qPCR Master Mix* (Promega, Mannheim, Germany), and nuclease-free water. The qPCR temperature program comprised the following steps: 10 min initial denaturation at 95 °C, 45 cycles of 15 s denaturation at 95 °C, and 1 min annealing/extension at 60 °C. The transcript quantitation was carried out in two independent reactions, and threshold cycles (C_T) determined by the second derivative method were averaged for each transcript per sample. In cases of a mean deviation >0.25 C_T-value, the measurements were repeated. Subsequently, the delta-delta-C_T method was used for the calculation of the relative miRNA levels normalized to the reference RNAs. For this, the geometric means of the C_T-values of RNU44 and RNU48 were utilized.

4.4. Statistical Analysis

For the assessment of potential differences in the relative miRNA levels between BCa patients and control subjects, the nonparametric two-tailed Mann–Whitney U test was applied. Bonferroni's correction for multiple comparisons was performed by multiplying the uncorrected *p*-values by a factor of 9 for nine miRNAs. Spearman's rank correlation coefficients (r_s) were calculated to reveal possible correlations among the relative expression levels of the different miRNAs and with tumor stage or grade. The distribution of the relative miRNA expression levels is depicted in box plots, where the bottom and top of the boxes represent the first and third quartiles, respectively. The median is shown as a solid line within the box, and the ends of the whiskers are depicted according to the Tukey method. Data outside the whiskers represent outliers and are marked as single circle symbols.

Differences in the relative miRNA levels between patients with different tumor stages and grades were assessed by the nonparametric two-tailed Mann–Whitney U test.

The diagnostic performance of the individual miRNAs was assessed by ROC curve analyses, followed by the above-mentioned Bonferroni's correction for multiple comparisons and the corresponding AUC values. The Youden index was calculated to determine optimal cutoff values, which were used to classify the relative expression levels of the different miRNAs into positive and negative indicators for tumor detection. Subsequently, the sensitivity (SNS), specificity (SPC), positive predictive value (PPV), negative predictive value (NPV), positive likelihood ratio (pLR), negative likelihood ratio (nLR), and accuracy (ACC) were calculated for each miRNA marker and for marker combinations according to standard statistical methods. The same was done for VUC alone or in combination with different miRNAs. For all analyses, two-sided p-values < 0.05 were considered statistically significant. All analyses were performed using *IBM SPSS Statistics Version 24.0.0.2* (IBM, Ehningen, Germany) and *GraphPad Prism Version 6.05 for Windows* (GraphPad Software, Inc, San Diego, CA, USA).

In addition, the diagnostic performance was assessed using penalized linear regression with miRNAs as predictor variables and tumor status as the outcome. The analysis was performed using the *R statistical environment* [67]. The predictive strength of the miRNAs for tumor status was investigated using the elastic net method [68] implemented in the R package *glmnet*. The importance of the miRNAs in predicting the tumor status and prediction accuracy were also assessed using the random forest method [69] implemented in the R package *randomForest* [70].

5. Conclusions

The literature-based selection of promising miRNAs as potential markers for the non-invasive detection of BCa in urine as alternative or adjunct markers to VUC revealed four suitable candidates (miR-125b/-145/-183/-221). In combination with VUC, an adequate performance was obtained, and the previously reported value as BCa-associated biomarkers could be confirmed for these four miRNAs. Prospective studies are required in order to reveal the real value of miRNAs in urine-based BCa diagnosis as a potential tool for the reduction of invasive and expensive diagnostic procedures like cystoscopies.

Author Contributions: Conceptualization: K.S. and S.F.; methodology: K.E., K.S., and S.F.; validation: K.E. and K.S.; formal analysis: K.E., K.S., and S.F.; investigation: U.H., A.L.-F., and R.F.; resources: M.F. and M.P.W.; data curation: K.S., A.K., I.R., and S.F.; writing, original draft preparation: S.F.; writing, review and editing: K.E., A.K., C.T., and S.F.; supervision: C.T. and M.P.W.; project administration: M.P.W. and S.F. All authors have read and agreed to the published version of the manuscript.

Acknowledgments: We thank the individuals who consented to be included in the cohorts of this project.

Abbreviations

ACC	accuracy
AUC	area under the curve
BCa	bladder cancer
G	tumor grade
MIBC	muscle-invasive bladder cancer
miRNA or miR	microRNA
NGS	next-generation sequencing

nLR	negative likelihood ratio
NMIBC	non-muscle-invasive bladder cancer
ns	not significant
NPV	negative predictive value
pLR	positive likelihood ratio
PPV	positive predictive value
pT	pathological tumor stage
PUNLMP	papillary urothelial neoplasm of low malignant potential
qPCR	quantitative polymerase chain reaction
ROC	receiver operating characteristic
RT	reverse transcription
SNS	sensitivity
SPC	specificity
TUR-B	transurethral resection of the bladder
VUC	voided urine cytology

References

1. Richters, A.; Aben, K.K.H.; Kiemeney, L. The global burden of urinary bladder cancer: An update. *World J. Urol.* **2019**. [CrossRef] [PubMed]
2. Saginala, K.; Barsouk, A.; Aluru, J.S.; Rawla, P.; Padala, S.A.; Barsouk, A. Epidemiology of Bladder Cancer. *Med. Sci. (Basel)* **2020**, *8*, 15. [CrossRef] [PubMed]
3. Babjuk, M.; Bohle, A.; Burger, M.; Capoun, O.; Cohen, D.; Comperat, E.M.; Hernandez, V.; Kaasinen, E.; Palou, J.; Roupret, M.; et al. EAU Guidelines on Non-Muscle-invasive Urothelial Carcinoma of the Bladder: Update 2016. *Eur. Urol.* **2017**, *71*, 447–461. [CrossRef]
4. Sievert, K.D.; Amend, B.; Nagele, U.; Schilling, D.; Bedke, J.; Horstmann, M.; Hennenlotter, J.; Kruck, S.; Stenzl, A. Economic aspects of bladder cancer: What are the benefits and costs? *World J. Urol.* **2009**, *27*, 295–300. [CrossRef] [PubMed]
5. Svatek, R.S.; Hollenbeck, B.K.; Holmang, S.; Lee, R.; Kim, S.P.; Stenzl, A.; Lotan, Y. The economics of bladder cancer: Costs and considerations of caring for this disease. *Eur. Urol.* **2014**, *66*, 253–262. [CrossRef]
6. Maas, M.; Bedke, J.; Stenzl, A.; Todenhofer, T. Can urinary biomarkers replace cystoscopy? *World J. Urol.* **2019**, *37*, 1741–1749. [CrossRef]
7. Woldu, S.L.; Bagrodia, A.; Lotan, Y. Guideline of guidelines: Non-muscle-invasive bladder cancer. *BJU Int.* **2017**, *119*, 371–380. [CrossRef]
8. Chou, R.; Gore, J.L.; Buckley, D.; Fu, R.; Gustafson, K.; Griffin, J.C.; Grusing, S.; Selph, S. Urinary Biomarkers for Diagnosis of Bladder Cancer: A Systematic Review and Meta-analysis. *Ann. Intern. Med.* **2015**, *163*, 922–931. [CrossRef]
9. D'Costa, J.J.; Goldsmith, J.C.; Wilson, J.S.; Bryan, R.T.; Ward, D.G. A Systematic Review of the Diagnostic and Prognostic Value of Urinary Protein Biomarkers in Urothelial Bladder Cancer. *Bladder Cancer* **2016**, *2*, 301–317. [CrossRef]
10. Mengual, L.; Ribal, M.J.; Lozano, J.J.; Ingelmo-Torres, M.; Burset, M.; Fernandez, P.L.; Alcaraz, A. Validation study of a noninvasive urine test for diagnosis and prognosis assessment of bladder cancer: Evidence for improved models. *J. Urol.* **2014**, *191*, 261–269. [CrossRef]
11. Ribal, M.J.; Mengual, L.; Lozano, J.J.; Ingelmo-Torres, M.; Palou, J.; Rodriguez-Faba, O.; Witjes, J.A.; Van der Heijden, A.G.; Medina, R.; Conde, J.M.; et al. Gene expression test for the non-invasive diagnosis of bladder cancer: A prospective, blinded, international and multicenter validation study. *Eur. J. Cancer* **2016**, *54*, 131–138. [CrossRef] [PubMed]
12. Urquidi, V.; Netherton, M.; Gomes-Giacoia, E.; Serie, D.; Eckel-Passow, J.; Rosser, C.J.; Goodison, S. Urinary mRNA biomarker panel for the detection of urothelial carcinoma. *Oncotarget* **2016**, *7*, 38731–38740. [CrossRef]
13. Esquela-Kerscher, A.; Slack, F.J. Oncomirs—microRNAs with a role in cancer. *Nat. Rev. Cancer* **2006**, *6*, 259–269. [CrossRef] [PubMed]
14. Iorio, M.V.; Croce, C.M. microRNA involvement in human cancer. *Carcinogenesis* **2012**, *33*, 1126–1133. [CrossRef] [PubMed]

15. Frixa, T.; Donzelli, S.; Blandino, G. Oncogenic MicroRNAs: Key Players in Malignant Transformation. *Cancers* **2015**, *7*, 2466–2485. [CrossRef]
16. Dong, F.; Xu, T.; Shen, Y.; Zhong, S.; Chen, S.; Ding, Q.; Shen, Z. Dysregulation of miRNAs in bladder cancer: Altered expression with aberrant biogenesis procedure. *Oncotarget* **2017**, *8*, 27547–27568. [CrossRef]
17. Liu, X.; Liu, X.; Wu, Y.; Wu, Q.; Wang, Q.; Yang, Z.; Li, L. MicroRNAs in biofluids are novel tools for bladder cancer screening. *Oncotarget* **2017**, *8*, 32370–32379. [CrossRef]
18. Matullo, G.; Naccarati, A.; Pardini, B. MicroRNA expression profiling in bladder cancer: The challenge of next-generation sequencing in tissues and biofluids. *Int. J. Cancer* **2016**, *138*, 2334–2345. [CrossRef]
19. Ouyang, H.; Zhou, Y.; Zhang, L.; Shen, G. Diagnostic Value of MicroRNAs for Urologic Cancers: A Systematic Review and Meta-Analysis. *Medicine (Baltimore)* **2015**, *94*, e1272. [CrossRef]
20. Schubert, M.; Junker, K.; Heinzelmann, J. Prognostic and predictive miRNA biomarkers in bladder, kidney and prostate cancer: Where do we stand in biomarker development? *J. Cancer Res. Clin. Oncol.* **2016**, *142*, 1673–1695. [CrossRef]
21. Enokida, H.; Yoshino, H.; Matsushita, R.; Nakagawa, M. The role of microRNAs in bladder cancer. *Investig. Clin. Urol.* **2016**, *57*, 60–76. [CrossRef] [PubMed]
22. Canturk, K.M.; Ozdemir, M.; Can, C.; Oner, S.; Emre, R.; Aslan, H.; Cilingir, O.; Ciftci, E.; Celayir, F.M.; Aldemir, O.; et al. Investigation of key miRNAs and target genes in bladder cancer using miRNA profiling and bioinformatic tools. *Mol. Biol. Rep.* **2014**, *41*, 8127–8135. [CrossRef] [PubMed]
23. Catto, J.W.; Miah, S.; Owen, H.C.; Bryant, H.; Myers, K.; Dudziec, E.; Larre, S.; Milo, M.; Rehman, I.; Rosario, D.J.; et al. Distinct microRNA alterations characterize high- and low-grade bladder cancer. *Cancer Res.* **2009**, *69*, 8472–8481. [CrossRef] [PubMed]
24. Cheng, Y.; Deng, X.; Yang, X.; Li, P.; Zhang, X.; Li, P.; Tao, J.; Lu, Q.; Wang, Z. Urine microRNAs as biomarkers for bladder cancer: A diagnostic meta-analysis. *Onco Targets Ther.* **2015**, *8*, 2089–2096. [CrossRef]
25. Ding, M.; Li, Y.; Wang, H.; Lv, Y.; Liang, J.; Wang, J.; Li, C. Diagnostic value of urinary microRNAs as non-invasive biomarkers for bladder cancer: A meta-analysis. *Int. J. Clin. Exp. Med.* **2015**, *8*, 15432–15440.
26. Dyrskjot, L.; Ostenfeld, M.S.; Bramsen, J.B.; Silahtaroglu, A.N.; Lamy, P.; Ramanathan, R.; Fristrup, N.; Jensen, J.L.; Andersen, C.L.; Zieger, K.; et al. Genomic profiling of microRNAs in bladder cancer: miR-129 is associated with poor outcome and promotes cell death in vitro. *Cancer Res.* **2009**, *69*, 4851–4860. [CrossRef]
27. Han, Y.; Chen, J.; Zhao, X.; Liang, C.; Wang, Y.; Sun, L.; Jiang, Z.; Zhang, Z.; Yang, R.; Chen, J.; et al. MicroRNA expression signatures of bladder cancer revealed by deep sequencing. *PLoS ONE* **2011**, *6*, e18286. [CrossRef]
28. Itesako, T.; Seki, N.; Yoshino, H.; Chiyomaru, T.; Yamasaki, T.; Hidaka, H.; Yonezawa, T.; Nohata, N.; Kinoshita, T.; Nakagawa, M.; et al. The microRNA expression signature of bladder cancer by deep sequencing: The functional significance of the miR-195/497 cluster. *PLoS ONE* **2014**, *9*, e84311. [CrossRef]
29. Mengual, L.; Lozano, J.J.; Ingelmo-Torres, M.; Gazquez, C.; Ribal, M.J.; Alcaraz, A. Using microRNA profiling in urine samples to develop a non-invasive test for bladder cancer. *Int. J. Cancer* **2013**, *133*, 2631–2641. [CrossRef]
30. Sapre, N.; Macintyre, G.; Clarkson, M.; Naeem, H.; Cmero, M.; Kowalczyk, A.; Anderson, P.D.; Costello, A.J.; Corcoran, N.M.; Hovens, C.M. A urinary microRNA signature can predict the presence of bladder urothelial carcinoma in patients undergoing surveillance. *Br. J. Cancer* **2016**, *114*, 454–462. [CrossRef]
31. Zaravinos, A.; Radojicic, J.; Lambrou, G.I.; Volanis, D.; Delakas, D.; Stathopoulos, E.N.; Spandidos, D.A. Expression of miRNAs involved in angiogenesis, tumor cell proliferation, tumor suppressor inhibition, epithelial-mesenchymal transition and activation of metastasis in bladder cancer. *J. Urol.* **2012**, *188*, 615–623. [CrossRef] [PubMed]
32. Zhang, D.Z.; Lau, K.M.; Chan, E.S.; Wang, G.; Szeto, C.C.; Wong, K.; Choy, R.K.; Ng, C.F. Cell-free urinary microRNA-99a and microRNA-125b are diagnostic markers for the non-invasive screening of bladder cancer. *PLoS ONE* **2014**, *9*, e100793. [CrossRef]
33. Snowdon, J.; Boag, S.; Feilotter, H.; Izard, J.; Siemens, D.R. A pilot study of urinary microRNA as a biomarker for urothelial cancer. *Can. Urol. Assoc. J.* **2013**, *7*, 28–32. [CrossRef] [PubMed]
34. Pospisilova, S.; Pazourkova, E.; Horinek, A.; Brisuda, A.; Svobodova, I.; Soukup, V.; Hrbacek, J.; Capoun, O.; Hanus, T.; Mares, J.; et al. MicroRNAs in urine supernatant as potential non-invasive markers for bladder cancer detection. *Neoplasma* **2016**, *63*, 799–808. [CrossRef] [PubMed]
35. Dip, N.; Reis, S.T.; Srougi, M.; Dall'Oglio, M.F.; Leite, K.R. Expression profile of microrna-145 in urothelial bladder cancer. *Int. Braz. J. Urol.* **2013**, *39*, 95–101. [CrossRef] [PubMed]

36. Yun, S.J.; Jeong, P.; Kim, W.T.; Kim, T.H.; Lee, Y.S.; Song, P.H.; Choi, Y.H.; Kim, I.Y.; Moon, S.K.; Kim, W.J. Cell-free microRNAs in urine as diagnostic and prognostic biomarkers of bladder cancer. *Int. J. Oncol.* **2012**, *41*, 1871–1878. [CrossRef]
37. Mearini, E.; Poli, G.; Cochetti, G.; Boni, A.; Egidi, M.G.; Brancorsini, S. Expression of urinary miRNAs targeting NLRs inflammasomes in bladder cancer. *Onco Targets Ther.* **2017**, *10*, 2665–2673. [CrossRef]
38. Dambal, S.; Shah, M.; Mihelich, B.; Nonn, L. The microRNA-183 cluster: The family that plays together stays together. *Nucleic Acids Res.* **2015**, *43*, 7173–7188. [CrossRef]
39. Ma, Y.; Liang, A.J.; Fan, Y.P.; Huang, Y.R.; Zhao, X.M.; Sun, Y.; Chen, X.F. Dysregulation and functional roles of miR-183-96-182 cluster in cancer cell proliferation, invasion and metastasis. *Oncotarget* **2016**, *7*, 42805–42825. [CrossRef]
40. Zhang, Q.H.; Sun, H.M.; Zheng, R.Z.; Li, Y.C.; Zhang, Q.; Cheng, P.; Tang, Z.H.; Huang, F. Meta-analysis of microRNA-183 family expression in human cancer studies comparing cancer tissues with noncancerous tissues. *Gene* **2013**, *527*, 26–32. [CrossRef]
41. Yamada, Y.; Enokida, H.; Kojima, S.; Kawakami, K.; Chiyomaru, T.; Tatarano, S.; Yoshino, H.; Kawahara, K.; Nishiyama, K.; Seki, N.; et al. MiR-96 and miR-183 detection in urine serve as potential tumor markers of urothelial carcinoma: Correlation with stage and grade, and comparison with urinary cytology. *Cancer Sci.* **2011**, *102*, 522–529. [CrossRef] [PubMed]
42. Eissa, S.; Habib, H.; Ali, E.; Kotb, Y. Evaluation of urinary miRNA-96 as a potential biomarker for bladder cancer diagnosis. *Med. Oncol.* **2015**, *32*, 413. [CrossRef] [PubMed]
43. Eissa, S.; Matboli, M.; Essawy, N.O.; Kotb, Y.M. Integrative functional genetic-epigenetic approach for selecting genes as urine biomarkers for bladder cancer diagnosis. *Tumour Biol.* **2015**, *36*, 9545–9552. [CrossRef]
44. Urquidi, V.; Netherton, M.; Gomes-Giacoia, E.; Serie, D.J.; Eckel-Passow, J.; Rosser, C.J.; Goodison, S. A microRNA biomarker panel for the non-invasive detection of bladder cancer. *Oncotarget* **2016**, *7*, 86290–86299. [CrossRef]
45. Pardini, B.; Cordero, F.; Naccarati, A.; Viberti, C.; Birolo, G.; Oderda, M.; Di Gaetano, C.; Arigoni, M.; Martina, F.; Calogero, R.A.; et al. microRNA profiles in urine by next-generation sequencing can stratify bladder cancer subtypes. *Oncotarget* **2018**, *9*, 20658–20669. [CrossRef] [PubMed]
46. Hanke, M.; Hoefig, K.; Merz, H.; Feller, A.C.; Kausch, I.; Jocham, D.; Warnecke, J.M.; Sczakiel, G. A robust methodology to study urine microRNA as tumor marker: microRNA-126 and microRNA-182 are related to urinary bladder cancer. *Urol. Oncol.* **2010**, *28*, 655–661. [CrossRef] [PubMed]
47. Eissa, S.; Matboli, M.; Hegazy, M.G.; Kotb, Y.M.; Essawy, N.O. Evaluation of urinary microRNA panel in bladder cancer diagnosis: Relation to bilharziasis. *Transl. Res.* **2015**, *165*, 731–739. [CrossRef] [PubMed]
48. Long, J.D.; Sullivan, T.B.; Humphrey, J.; Logvinenko, T.; Summerhayes, K.A.; Kozinn, S.; Harty, N.; Summerhayes, I.C.; Libertino, J.A.; Holway, A.H.; et al. A non-invasive miRNA based assay to detect bladder cancer in cell-free urine. *Am. J. Transl. Res.* **2015**, *7*, 2500–2509.
49. Matsuzaki, K.; Fujita, K.; Jingushi, K.; Kawashima, A.; Ujike, T.; Nagahara, A.; Ueda, Y.; Tanigawa, G.; Yoshioka, I.; Ueda, K.; et al. MiR-21-5p in urinary extracellular vesicles is a novel biomarker of urothelial carcinoma. *Oncotarget* **2017**, *8*, 24668–24678. [CrossRef]
50. Michailidi, C.; Hayashi, M.; Datta, S.; Sen, T.; Zenner, K.; Oladeru, O.; Brait, M.; Izumchenko, E.; Baras, A.; VandenBussche, C.; et al. Involvement of epigenetics and EMT-related miRNA in arsenic-induced neoplastic transformation and their potential clinical use. *Cancer Prev. Res. (Phila)* **2015**, *8*, 208–221. [CrossRef]
51. Wang, G.; Chan, E.S.; Kwan, B.C.; Li, P.K.; Yip, S.K.; Szeto, C.C.; Ng, C.F. Expression of microRNAs in the urine of patients with bladder cancer. *Clin. Genitourin. Cancer* **2012**, *10*, 106–113. [CrossRef] [PubMed]
52. Kim, S.S.; Choi, C.; Kwon, D.D. Urinary microRNAs as potential biomarkers for differentiating the "atypical urothelial cells" category of the Paris system for reporting urine cytology. *Int. J. Clin. Exp. Pathol.* **2017**, *10*, 8303–8313. [PubMed]
53. Fendler, A.; Stephan, C.; Yousef, G.M.; Jung, K. MicroRNAs as regulators of signal transduction in urological tumors. *Clin. Chem.* **2011**, *57*, 954–968. [CrossRef] [PubMed]
54. Gulia, C.; Baldassarra, S.; Signore, F.; Rigon, G.; Pizzuti, V.; Gaffi, M.; Briganti, V.; Porrello, A.; Piergentili, R. Role of Non-Coding RNAs in the Etiology of Bladder Cancer. *Genes (Basel)* **2017**, *8*, 339. [CrossRef] [PubMed]
55. Batista, R.; Vinagre, N.; Meireles, S.; Vinagre, J.; Prazeres, H.; Leao, R.; Maximo, V.; Soares, P. Biomarkers for Bladder Cancer Diagnosis and Surveillance: A Comprehensive Review. *Diagnostics (Basel)* **2020**, *10*, 39. [CrossRef] [PubMed]

56. Valenberg, F.; Hiar, A.M.; Wallace, E.; Bridge, J.A.; Mayne, D.J.; Beqaj, S.; Sexton, W.J.; Lotan, Y.; Weizer, A.Z.; Jansz, G.K.; et al. Prospective Validation of an mRNA-based Urine Test for Surveillance of Patients with Bladder Cancer. *Eur. Urol.* **2019**, *75*, 853–860. [CrossRef] [PubMed]
57. Witjes, J.A.; Morote, J.; Cornel, E.B.; Gakis, G.; van Valenberg, F.J.P.; Lozano, F.; Sternberg, I.A.; Willemsen, E.; Hegemann, M.L.; Paitan, Y.; et al. Performance of the Bladder EpiCheck Methylation Test for Patients Under Surveillance for Non-muscle-invasive Bladder Cancer: Results of a Multicenter, Prospective, Blinded Clinical Trial. *Eur. Urol. Oncol.* **2018**, *1*, 307–313. [CrossRef]
58. Trenti, E.; Pycha, S.; Mian, C.; Schwienbacher, C.; Hanspeter, E.; Kafka, M.; Spedicato, G.A.; Vjaters, E.; Degener, S.; Pycha, A.; et al. Comparison of 2 new real-time polymerase chain reaction-based urinary markers in the follow-up of patients with non muscle-invasive bladder cancer. *Cancer Cytopathol.* **2020**, *128*, 341–347. [CrossRef]
59. Sathianathen, N.J.; Butaney, M.; Weight, C.J.; Kumar, R.; Konety, B.R. Urinary Biomarkers in the Evaluation of Primary Hematuria: A Systematic Review and Meta-Analysis. *Bladder Cancer* **2018**, *4*, 353–363. [CrossRef]
60. Van Kessel, K.E.; Beukers, W.; Lurkin, I.; Ziel-van der Made, A.; van der Keur, K.A.; Boormans, J.L.; Dyrskjot, L.; Marquez, M.; Orntoft, T.F.; Real, F.X.; et al. Validation of a DNA Methylation-Mutation Urine Assay to Select Patients with Hematuria for Cystoscopy. *J. Urol.* **2017**, *197*, 590–595. [CrossRef]
61. Sasaki, H.; Yoshiike, M.; Nozawa, S.; Usuba, W.; Katsuoka, Y.; Aida, K.; Kitajima, K.; Kudo, H.; Hoshikawa, M.; Yoshioka, Y.; et al. Expression Level of Urinary MicroRNA-146a-5p Is Increased in Patients With Bladder Cancer and Decreased in Those After Transurethral Resection. *Clin. Genitourin. Cancer* **2016**, *14*, e493–e499. [CrossRef] [PubMed]
62. Zhang, X.; Zhang, Y.; Liu, X.; Fang, A.; Wang, J.; Yang, Y.; Wang, L.; Du, L.; Wang, C. Direct quantitative detection for cell-free miR-155 in urine: A potential role in diagnosis and prognosis for non-muscle invasive bladder cancer. *Oncotarget* **2016**, *7*, 3255–3266. [CrossRef] [PubMed]
63. *TNM Classification of Malignant Tumours*; Sobin, L.H.; Gospodarowicz, M.K.; Wittekind, C.E. (Eds.) Wiley-Blackwell: Hoboken, NJ, USA, 2011.
64. Humphrey, P.A.; Moch, H.; Cubilla, A.L.; Ulbright, T.M.; Reuter, V.E. The 2016 WHO Classification of Tumours of the Urinary System and Male Genital Organs-Part B: Prostate and Bladder Tumours. *Eur. Urol.* **2016**, *70*, 106–119. [CrossRef] [PubMed]
65. Amin, M.B.; Smith, S.C.; Reuter, V.E.; Epstein, J.I.; Grignon, D.J.; Hansel, D.E.; Lin, O.; McKenney, J.K.; Montironi, R.; Paner, G.P.; et al. Update for the practicing pathologist: The International Consultation On Urologic Disease-European association of urology consultation on bladder cancer. *Mod. Pathol.* **2015**, *28*, 612–630. [CrossRef]
66. Papanicolaou, G.N.; Marshall, V.F. URINE SEDIMENT SMEARS AS A DIAGNOSTIC PROCEDURE IN CANCERS OF THE URINARY TRACT. *Science* **1945**, *101*, 519–520. [CrossRef]
67. Marano, G.; Boracchi, P.; Biganzoli, E.M.; R Core Team. R: A language and environment for statistical computing. R Foundation for Statistical Computing, Vienna. *Open J. Stat.* **2016**, *6*, 3.
68. Friedman, J.; Hastie, T.; Tibshirani, R. Regularization Paths for Generalized Linear Models via Coordinate Descent. *J. Stat. Softw.* **2010**, *33*, 1–22. [CrossRef]
69. Breiman, L. Random Forests. *Mach. Learn.* **2001**, *45*, 5–32. [CrossRef]
70. Liaw, A.; Wienertitle, M. Classification and Regression by randomForest. *R News* **2002**, *2*, 18–22.

10

Impact of Sarcopenia as a Prognostic Biomarker of Bladder Cancer

Hiroshi Fukushima, Kosuke Takemura, Hiroaki Suzuki and Fumitaka Koga *

Department of Urology, Tokyo Metropolitan Cancer and Infectious Diseases Center Komagome Hospital, 3-18-22 Honkomagome, Bunkyo-ku, Tokyo 113-8677, Japan; fukuuro@tmd.ac.jp (H.F.); takemura-urol@cick.jp (K.T.); smu.udm@gmail.com (H.S.)

* Correspondence: f-koga@cick.jp

Abstract: Sarcopenia, the degenerative and systemic loss of skeletal muscle mass, indicates patient frailty and impaired physical function. Sarcopenia can be caused by multiple factors, including advanced age, lack of exercise, poor nutritional status, inflammatory diseases, endocrine diseases, and malignancies. In patients with cancer cachexia, anorexia, poor nutrition and systemic inflammation make the metabolic state more catabolic, resulting in sarcopenia. Thus, sarcopenia is considered as one of manifestations of cancer cachexia. Recently, growing evidence has indicated the importance of sarcopenia in the management of patients with various cancers. Sarcopenia is associated with not only higher rates of treatment-related complications but also worse prognosis in cancer-bearing patients. In this article, we summarized metabolic backgrounds of cancer cachexia and sarcopenia and definitions of sarcopenia based on computed tomography (CT) images. We conducted a systematic literature review regarding the significance of sarcopenia as a prognostic biomarker of bladder cancer. We also reviewed recent studies focusing on the prognostic role of changes in skeletal muscle mass during the course of treatment in bladder cancer patients. Lastly, we discussed the impact of nutritional support, medication, and exercise on sarcopenia in cancer-bearing patients.

Keywords: sarcopenia; prognosis; biomarker; bladder cancer; urothelial carcinoma

---

1. Introduction

Bladder cancer is the most common malignancy of the urinary tract in the world, with approximately 430,000 new cases and 165,000 deaths each year [1]. The major histology of bladder cancer is urothelial carcinoma. Based on the pathological depth of tumor invasion, bladder cancer is classified into two groups: non-muscle-invasive bladder cancer (NMIBC) and muscle-invasive bladder cancer (MIBC). NMIBC is treated with bladder-preserving treatments, including transurethral resection of the bladder tumor and intravesical instillation therapy [2]. Patients with MIBC generally require total cystectomy and urinary diversion as a curative treatment [3]. However, approximately half of MIBC patients undergoing total cystectomy die within five years because MIBC is potentially an aggressive disease and frequently progresses to a metastatic disease postoperatively [4]. Once MIBC patients develop distant metastasis, their prognoses are poor despite receiving systemic chemotherapy with a median overall survival (OS) of approximately 15 months [5]. Thus, bladder cancer is still a challenging disease, although the recent advent of immuno-oncology drugs is shifting the paradigm of the management of bladder cancer patients [6]. Pre-therapeutic risk assessment based on prognostic biomarkers can help clinicians to predict their outcomes and counsel patients about treatment options. Therefore, identifying prognostic biomarkers contributes to better management for bladder cancer patients.

Sarcopenia is a syndrome representing the degenerative and systemic loss of skeletal muscle mass [7]. According to recent surveys, the prevalence of sarcopenia is relatively high, ranging from 15% at 65 years to 50% at 80 years [8]. Variations in genes, such as *MSTN*, *VDR*, and *ACE*, determine the variability in skeletal muscle phenotype and the prevalence of sarcopenia in an elderly population [9]. Sarcopenia is associated with lower physical activity, morbidity, and mortality [10,11]. Sarcopenic patients tend to have higher morbidity from infectious diseases [12], metabolic syndrome [13], insulin resistance [14], and cardiovascular diseases [15]. Sarcopenia is pathophysiologically associated with various etiologies, including advanced age, lack of exercise, poor nutritional status, inflammatory diseases, and endocrine diseases [7]. Malignant diseases can also cause sarcopenia [16]. In patients with cancer cachexia, anorexia, poor nutrition, and systemic inflammation make the metabolic state more catabolic, resulting in sarcopenia [17]. Therefore, sarcopenia is considered as one of manifestations of cancer cachexia.

Recent studies have shown the prognostic impact of sarcopenia in various cancers. Sarcopenic patients show significantly worse survival than non-sarcopenic counterparts with lung or gastrointestinal cancer [18,19], hepatic cell carcinoma [20], esophageal cancer [21], lymphoma [22], melanoma [23], or renal cell carcinoma [24,25]. In bladder cancer, the role of sarcopenia in predicting survival has been clarified. In this article, we summarized metabolic backgrounds of cancer cachexia and sarcopenia and definitions of sarcopenia based on computed tomography (CT) images. Moreover, we conducted a systematic literature review on published studies to summarize comprehensively the current clinical evidence on the prognostic role of sarcopenia in bladder cancer patients. We also reviewed recent studies focusing on the prognostic importance of changes in skeletal muscle mass during the course of treatment in bladder cancer patients. Finally, we discussed the impact of nutritional support, medications, and exercise on cancer cachexia and sarcopenia in cancer-bearing patients.

2. Metabolic Background of Cancer Cachexia and Sarcopenia

Cancer cachexia is a multifactorial syndrome characterized by progressive weight loss, which is due to the depletion of adipose tissue and skeletal muscle mass. In the early phase of cancer cachexia, adipose tissue is depleted [26]. Skeletal muscle wasting is promoted after the progression of cancer cachexia [27]. Anorexia, which is caused by cancer itself or treatment for cancer, is frequently observed in patients with cancer cachexia. Moreover, resting energy expenditure increases in patients with cancer cachexia, leading to the progressive loss of body weight [28]. In the process of the progression of cancer cachexia, lipolysis and fatty acid oxidation are activated in skeletal muscle, whereas glycolysis is suppressed [29,30]. Increased oxidative stress caused by up-regulated fatty acid oxidation can contribute to skeletal muscle wasting [30]. Several mechanisms, including epinephrine stimulation and increased secretion of cytokines, are involved in these metabolic changes [31]. Moreover, skeletal muscle depletion is caused by increased protein degradation mainly by the activated ubiquitin-proteasome pathway, in which multiple receptor-mediated signaling pathways are involved [27]. In this section, we summarize the metabolic changes and the mechanisms of the depletion of adipose tissue and skeletal muscle mass during cancer cachexia.

2.1. Adipose Tissue Depletion in Cancer Cachexia

Adipose tissue volume decreases in the early process of cancer cachexia [26]. The breakdown of adipose tissue is caused by lipolysis of triglyceride, which is mediated by adipose triglyceride lipase (ATGL) and hormonal-sensitive lipase (HSL) [32]. In a previous study of ATGL- or HSL-deficient animal models, the absence of ATGL and, to lesser degree, HSL reduces fatty acid mobilization and adipose tissue loss, leading to maintained skeletal muscle mass, suggesting that excessive depletion of adipose tissue may be involved in the progression of skeletal muscle atrophy [29]. Up-regulation of lipolysis is induced by various factors, including enhanced stimulation of β-adrenergic receptor, increased secretion of cytokines such as tumor necrosis factor (TNF)-α, interleukin (IL)-1, IL-6, and IL-8, and increased expression of lipid-mobilizing factors, such as zinc-α2 glycoprotein-1 (AZGP1) [32]. White adipose tissue browning, which is associated with increased expression of uncoupling protein 1 (UCP1), increases thermogenesis and energy expenditure during cancer cachexia [28]. This process is also affected by β-adrenergic receptor stimulation and cytokines such as TNF-α and IL-6 [28].

2.2. *Skeletal Muscle Depletion in Cancer Cachexia*

Skeletal muscle depletion occurs as a consequence of reduced protein synthesis and increased degradation of proteins in the late phase of cancer cachexia [27]. Reduced protein synthesis can be caused by low nutritional status as a result of anorexia and decreased food intake [27,32]. Skeletal muscle protein degradation is promoted mainly by the ubiquitin-proteasome pathway, which is induced by myostatin, activin A, cytokines such as TNF-α and IL-6, and proteolysis-inducing factor [31,32]. Myostatin and activin A, members of the transforming-growth factor β (TGF-β) family, bind activin type 2 receptor B (ActR2B) and activate Smad2/3 and p38 mitogen-activated protein kinase (MAPK) signaling, resulting in the up-regulation of Atrogin-1 and the muscle ring finger protein 1 (MuRF-1), which are muscle-specific E3 ligases and play roles as key regulators of ubiquitin-driven protein degradation in the skeletal muscle [27,31]. Moreover, the phosphatidylinositol-3 kinase (PI3K)/Akt/mammalian target of rapamycin (mTOR) pathway and forkhead box O (FOXO), which are general regulators of skeletal muscle mass homeostasis, are affected in cancer cachexia [31–33].

TNF-α up-regulates Atrogin-1 by increasing nuclear FOXO4 protein in skeletal muscle [34]. Glucocorticoid receptor regulates the expression of Atrogin-1 and MuRF-1 [27,31]. The binding of insulin-like growth factor-1 (IGF-1) to its receptor causes the activation of PI3K/Akt/mTOR pathway, which down-regulates FOXO3 and results in decreased expression of Atrogin-1 and MuRF-1 [27,31]. Taken together, various signaling pathways are related to the regulation of skeletal muscle protein degradation. Their inhibition may contribute to the prevention of cancer cachexia and sarcopenia.

Oxidative stress promotes skeletal muscle wasting. Fukawa et al. revealed up-regulation of fatty acid oxidation and down-regulation of glycolysis in the skeletal muscle using transcriptomics of human muscle stem cell-based models and human cancer-induced cachexia models in mice [30]. Interestingly, they also showed that increased oxidative stress caused by excessive fatty acid oxidation could impair muscle growth [30]. Therefore, increased oxidative stress can cause sarcopenia through excessive fatty acid oxidation in the process of the progression of cancer cachexia. Inhibiting the process of fatty acid oxidation could be efficacious in preventing cancer cachexia and sarcopenia. In contrast, skeletal muscle mitochondrial oxidative capacities decrease without alteration of adenosine triphosphate (ATP) production efficiency in a rat model of cancer cachexia [35], which appears to be inconsistent with the results reported by Fukawa et al. [30], but this may contribute to lipid droplet accumulation in skeletal muscle mass [36].

3. Evaluation of Sarcopenia Using Computed Tomography (CT) Images

According to the European Working Group of Sarcopenia in Older People (EWGSOP), sarcopenia is determined based on three factors: lower skeletal muscle mass, lower skeletal muscle strength, and lower physical performance [7]. Skeletal muscle strength can be evaluated by upper-limb hand-grip dynamometry and lower-limb extension strength testing. The assessment of physical function is generally based on walking speed. As for skeletal muscle mass, bioimpedance analysis, anthropometry, dual energy X-ray imaging, CT, and magnetic resonance imaging (MRI) are recommended as methods to measure skeletal muscle mass by EWGSOP [7]. In cancer-bearing patients, including bladder cancer patients, CT images are generally used in the evaluation of sarcopenia, since abdominal CT scans are routinely performed for diagnosis, staging, surveillance of recurrence after treatment, and assessment of therapeutic response [37]. Therefore, most of the previous studies on sarcopenia and bladder cancer used CT images to measure skeletal muscle mass and define sarcopenia (Figure 1). In our systematic literature review below, all the articles used CT images.

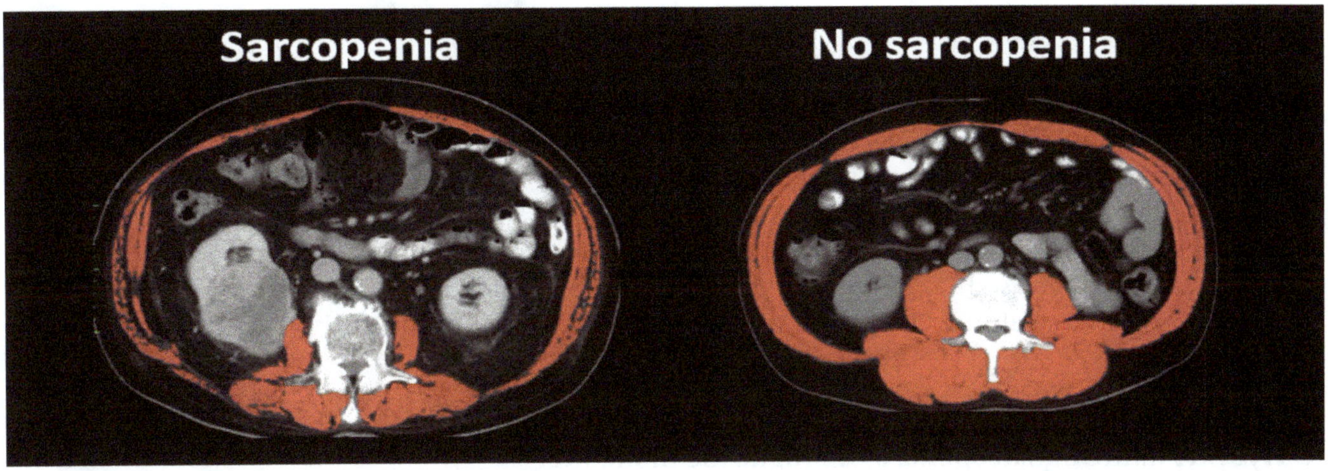

Figure 1. Computed tomography (CT) images of typical sarcopenic and non-sarcopenic cases. Skeletal muscle area is shown in red.

3.1. Measurement of Skeletal Muscle Mass Using CT Images

Axial CT images at the lumbar vertebral level are used to measure skeletal muscle areas because the total lumbar-skeletal muscle cross-sectional area is linearly correlated to the whole-body skeletal muscle mass [38]. The total skeletal muscle area at the third lumbar vertebra, including the psoas, paraspinal muscles (the erector spinae and quadratus lumborum), and abdominal wall muscles (the transversus abdominus, external and internal obliques, and rectus abdominus), is measured using software such as Slice-O-Matic (Tomovision, Montreal, QC, Canada) and OsiriX imaging software (Pixmeo, Geneva, Switzerland). The cross-sectional areas of skeletal muscle are identified using Hounsfield Unit thresholds of −29 to +150.

3.2. Skeletal Muscle Index (SMI)

Skeletal muscle index (SMI) is used widely in evaluating sarcopenia in cancer-bearing patients. SMI is calculated by normalizing skeletal muscle area for height in meters squared, as is body mass index (BMI). Two major established definitions of sarcopenia have been proposed so far. First, the International Consensus of Cancer Cachexia (ICCC) proposed cutoff values of SMI as 55 cm^2/m^2 for males and 39 cm^2/m^2 for females [16]. Second, Martin et al., defined BMI-incorporated cutoff values of SMI as <43 cm^2/m^2 for males with BMI < 25 kg/m^2, <53 cm^2/m^2 for males with BMI ≥ 25 kg/m^2, and <41 cm^2/m^2 for females [18]. Both of the two definitions were the best cutoffs to predict overall mortality using a cohort of patients with lung or gastrointestinal cancer, and either of them has been used to define sarcopenia in most previous studies on bladder cancer [37].

3.3. Psoas Muscle Index (PMI)

In some previous studies, only the psoas muscle area was measured on axial CT images at the lumbar vertebral level. The psoas muscle index (PMI) is calculated by normalizing the psoas muscle area for height in meters squared. Although a correlation between PMI and whole-body skeletal muscle mass has not yet been evaluated, the strong correlation between PMI and SMI suggests that PMI also represents whole-body skeletal muscle mass [39]. Hamaguchi et al. proposed the cutoff values of PMI to define sarcopenia as 6.36 cm^2/m^2 for males and 3.92 cm^2/m^2 for females, using a cohort of adult donors for living donor liver transplantation [39]. However, because their cohort included only Japanese patients, the use of their values may be limited to Asian populations.

3.4. *Skeletal Muscle Density*

In addition to the volume of the skeletal muscle, the quality of the skeletal muscle can be evaluated on CT scan. Skeletal muscle density is determined based on the CT density (Hounsfield unit) of the skeletal muscle [40]. Lower skeletal muscle density reflects more fat infiltration in skeletal muscle mass, which is related to lower function of the skeletal muscle and lower physical performance. Moreover, increased fat infiltration in skeletal muscle mass is involved in insulin resistance [41], which decreases glucose uptake in skeletal muscles and can eventually contribute to skeletal muscle atrophy. Because increased fat infiltration in the skeletal muscle is one of the characteristics of cancer cachexia, lower skeletal muscle density is considered as an indicator of the progression of cancer cachexia [40].

4. Hybrid Nature of Sarcopenia as a Prognostic Biomarker

Prognostic tumor biomarkers generally reflect tumor aggressiveness, including tumor stage, histological grade, lymphovascular invasion, and patient survival. Several prognostic biomarkers are related to the general condition of the host; e.g., age, sex, performance status, BMI, anemia, etc. Notably, sarcopenia reflects both tumor and host factors (Figure 2). Because sarcopenia develops as a consequence of tumor progression, tumor-induced systemic inflammation, or metabolic aberration, its presence indicates tumor aggressiveness. In addition, sarcopenic patients are characterized by poor general health and physical performance, which can contribute to worse prognosis of cancer-bearing patients. High prognostic performance of sarcopenia could be explained by its hybrid nature, which is a unique feature as a prognostic biomarker.

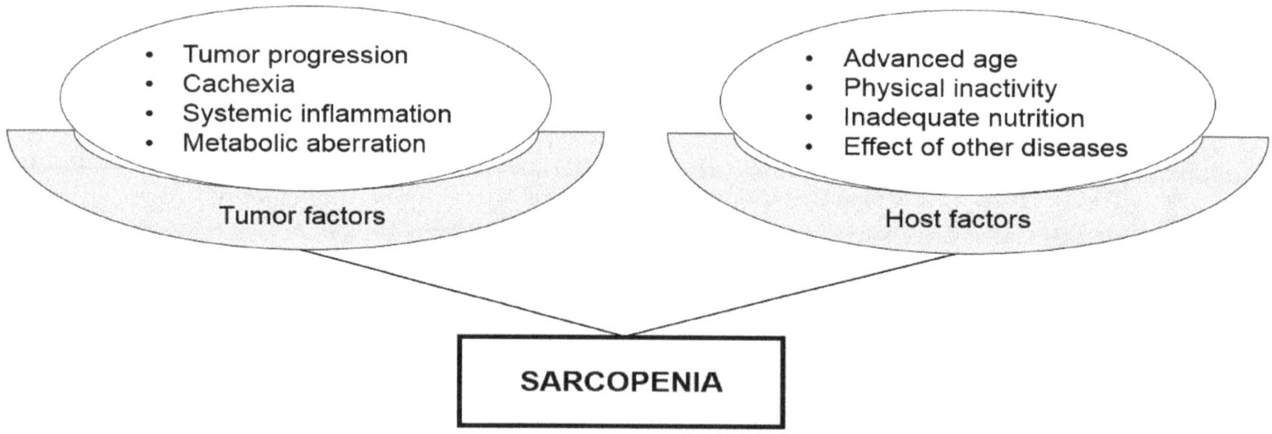

Figure 2. Hybrid nature of sarcopenia.

5. Systematic Literature Review

A systematic literature review was performed to search for studies investigating the prognostic role of sarcopenia in bladder cancer patients according to the PRISMA guidelines [42]. The search was restricted to articles written in English and performed using PubMed, Medline, and Cochrane Libraries by entering the terms "sarcopenia and urothelial carcinoma" and "sarcopenia and bladder cancer". Twenty-nine articles published from June 2014 to April 2018 were identified on 1 April 2018. There was no literature before June 2014 according to our literature search. Two independent investigators (H.F. and K.T.) conducted the literature search and selection of articles. Potential discrepancies were resolved by open discussion. Details of the search and article selection are summarized in the flow diagram (Figure 3). Studies were included if they were published as original articles investigating the prognostic role of sarcopenia in bladder cancer patients. Review articles, case reports, editorial comments, letters, meeting abstracts, and studies not meeting our inclusion criteria in their content were excluded. Our systematic literature review has several limitations. First, 12 articles were included in our systematic review, all of which were retrospective, and no study of level 1 evidence was included, indicating possible high risks of bias. Second, several different methods and definitions were used to evaluate sarcopenia using CT images in included studies.

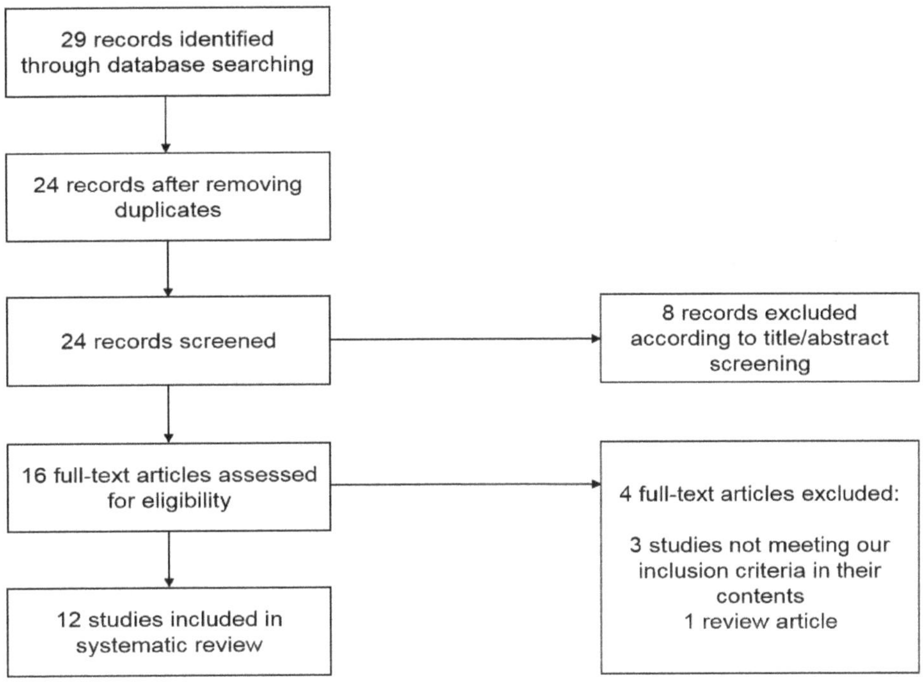

Figure 3. Flow diagram of systematic literature search.

6. Prognostic Role of Sarcopenia in Bladder Cancer

Table 1 lists published studies on the prognostic role of sarcopenia in bladder cancer patients. Most studies reported that sarcopenia was associated with worse prognosis. A systematic literature review identified six studies involving patients undergoing a radical cystectomy (due to high-risk NMIBC or MIBC) and four studies involving patients with inoperable locoregionally advanced and/or metastatic diseases. No studies investigated the association between sarcopenia and survival in low- or intermediate-risk NMIBC patients. Nine of the 10 studies used either SMI or PMI to define sarcopenia.

6.1. Survival after a Radical Cystectomy

Although a radical cystectomy with pelvic lymph node dissection is the standard of care for high-risk NMIBC and MIBC patients, its main problems include high incidences of perioperative complications [3]. In the contemporary radical cystectomy series, the incidence of major complications of Clavien–Dindo classification grade 3 or greater ranges from 5 to 26%, with a mortality rate of 0–3.9% [43]. Several studies showed that sarcopenia is significantly associated with higher rates of perioperative complications of a radical cystectomy [44,45].

Table 1. Reported series of the prognostic role of sarcopenia in bladder cancer cancers.

Study (Year)	Country	No. of Total Patients	No. of Sarcopenic Patients	Cancer Type	Therapeutic Interventions	Definition of Sarcopenia	Main Findings	Ref.
Smith et al. (2014)	United States	200	77 (39%)	Bladder cancer	Radical cystectomy	TPA † < 653 cm^2/m^2 for males and <523 cm^2/m^2 for females	The Kaplan–Meier curves showed no significant association between OS and sarcopenia ($p = 0.36$).	[45]
Psutka et al. (2014)	United States	205	141 (69%)	Bladder cancer	Radical cystectomy	SMI < 55 cm^2/m^2 for males and <39 cm^2/m^2 for females	Sarcopenia was an independent poor prognostic factor with HR 2.14 for CSS ($p = 0.007$) and 1.93 for OS ($p = 0.004$).	[46]
Hirasawa et al. (2016)	Japan	136	65 (48%)	Bladder cancer	Radical cystectomy	SMI < 43 cm^2/m^2 for males with BMI < 25 cm^2/m^2, <53 cm^2/m^2 for males with BMI ≥ 25 cm^2/m^2, and <41 cm^2/m^2 for females	Sarcopenia was an independent poor prognostic factor with HR 2.3 for CSS ($p = 0.015$).	[47]
Miyake et al. (2017)	Japan	89	22 (25%)	Bladder cancer	Radical cystectomy	SMI < 43 cm^2/m^2 for males with BMI < 25 cm^2/m^2, <53 cm^2/m^2 for males with BMI ≥ 25 cm^2/m^2, and <41 cm^2/m^2 for females	Sarcopenia was an independent poor prognostic factor with HR 2.2 for OS ($p = 0.03$).	[48]
Saitoh-Maeda et al. (2018)	Japan	63 (male only)	141 (69%)	Bladder cancer	Radical cystectomy	PMI < 400 cm^2/m^2	In male patients, non-sarcopenic patients had a significantly better OS than sarcopenic counterparts (2,889 vs. 2,009 days; $p = 0.023$).	[49]
Mayr et al. (2018)	Germany	500	189 (38%)	Bladder cancer	Radical cystectomy	SMI < 43 cm^2/m^2 for males with BMI < 25 cm^2/m^2, <53 cm^2/m^2 for males with BMI ≥ 25 cm^2/m^2, and <41 cm^2/m^2 for females	Sarcopenia was an independent poor prognostic factor with HR 1.42 for CSS ($p = 0.048$) and 1.43 for OS ($p = 0.01$).	[50]
Fukushima et al. (2015)	Japan	88	67 (76%)	Advanced urothelial carcinoma	Miscellaneous	SMI < 43 cm^2/m^2 for males with BMI < 25 cm^2/m^2, <53 cm^2/m^2 for males with BMI ≥ 25 cm^2/m^2, and <41 cm^2/m^2 for females	Sarcopenia was an independent poor prognostic factor with HR 3.36 for OS ($p < 0.001$).	[51]
Taguchi et al. (2015)	Japan	100	Not reported	Metastatic urothelial carcinoma	Systemic chemotherapy	SMI < 55 cm^2/m^2 for males and <39 cm^2/m^2 for females	Sarcopenia was an independent poor prognostic factor with HR 2.07 for CSS ($p = 0.045$).	[52]
Kasahara et al. (2017)	Japan	27	14 (52%)	Advanced bladder cancer	Systemic chemotherapy	PMI < 2.49 cm^2/m^2 for males and <2.07 cm^2/m^2 for females	The OS of the non-sarcopenic group was significantly better than that of the sarcopenic group (561 vs. 223 days; $p = 0.0150$).	[53]
Abe et al. (2018)	Japan	87	Not reported	Metastatic urothelial carcinoma	Systemic chemotherapy	SMI < 55 cm^2/m^2 for males and <39 cm^2/m^2 for females	Sarcopenia was not significantly associated with OS ($p = 0.11$). SMI stratified by BMI was an independent predictor for shorter OS ($p = 0.026$).	[54]

Abbreviations: BMI = body mass index; CSS = cancer-specific survival; HR = hazard ratio; OS = overall survival; PMI = psoas muscle index; SMI = skeletal muscle index; TPA = total psoas area. † TPA was calculated by measuring the cross-sectional area of the right and left psoas muscles on CT using 3-dimensional computerized image analysis.

As shown in Table 1, six studies reported the prognostic role of sarcopenia in bladder cancer patients undergoing a radical cystectomy [45–50]. Five of them revealed that sarcopenia is a significant predictor of cancer-specific survival (CSS) and OS [46–50]. Psutka et al., for the first time demonstrated that sarcopenia is an independent predictor for both poorer CSS and OS [46]. The 5-year CSS and OS rates were lower for sarcopenic patients than for non-sarcopenic counterparts (49% vs. 72% for CSS and 39% vs. 70% for OS, respectively). Three studies from Japan reported similar results to those of Psutka et al. [47–49]. Recently, a multi-center retrospective study from Germany demonstrated that sarcopenia is an independent predictor for both poorer CSS and OS in 500 bladder cancer patients undergoing a radical cystectomy [50]. Only one study, reported by Smith et al., showed no association between sarcopenia and OS [45]. This discrepant result may be due to the different methods for estimating skeletal muscle volume. Four studies calculated SMI, and three of them used the definition of sarcopenia proposed by Martin et al. However, Smith et al. calculated cross-sectional psoas muscle area using 3-dimensional computerized image analysis and defined sarcopenia using their own criteria.

Taken together, most previous studies demonstrated that sarcopenia is a significant poor prognostic factor in bladder cancer patients undergoing a radical cystectomy.

6.2. *Survival in Inoperable Advanced Disease*

Four studies evaluated the prognostic role of sarcopenia in patients with inoperable advanced bladder cancer (Table 1) [51–54]. Because upper tract urothelial carcinoma is histologically and biologically similar to bladder cancer, three of them included advanced upper tract urothelial carcinoma in their cohorts [51,52,54]. Fukushima et al. showed for the first time that sarcopenia is an independent predictor for shorter OS in patients with advanced urothelial carcinoma (inoperable locoregionally advanced disease and/or metastatic diseases to lymph nodes or distant organs) [51]. The median OS of sarcopenic patients was significantly shorter than that of non-sarcopenic counterparts (11 vs. 31 months). Taguchi et al. reported that sarcopenia is an independent predictor for shorter CSS in metastatic urothelial carcinoma patients receiving systemic chemotherapy as the first-line therapy [52]. Kasahara et al. showed the prognostic significance of sarcopenia in advanced bladder cancer patients receiving gemcitabine and nedaplatin therapy [53]. In addition, Abe et al. could not confirm the significance of sarcopenia in predicting OS, but they showed that SMI stratified by BMI was an independent predictor for shorter OS [54].

Thus, previous studies indicated that sarcopenia is a significant poor prognostic factor in inoperable advanced bladder cancer patients.

7. Prognostic Role of Changes in Skeletal Muscle Mass in Bladder Cancer

Because disease status and patient conditions can affect skeletal muscle mass in cancer-bearing patients, changes in skeletal muscle mass during and after treatment may represent post-therapeutic prognosis. As shown in Table 2, three studies investigated the prognostic role of changes in skeletal muscle mass during treatment in bladder cancer patients [48,55,56]. Miyake et al. reported that a 10% loss in psoas muscle volume before and after a radical cystectomy was an independent predictor for shorter OS [48]. Fukushima et al. reported that post-therapeutic skeletal muscle mass recovery was an independent predictor for both better recurrence-free survival and OS in advanced urothelial carcinoma treated with platinum-based chemotherapy as the first-line therapy [56]. Meanwhile, Zargar et al. showed that decline in psoas muscle volume during neoadjuvant chemotherapy was not predictive of OS in bladder cancer patients treated with neoadjuvant chemotherapy and a radical cystectomy [55].

Table 2. Reported series of the prognostic role of changes in skeletal muscle mass in bladder cancer cancers.

Study (Year)	Country	No. of Total Patients	Cancer Type	Therapeutic Interventions	Evaluation of Skeletal Muscle Mass	Main Findings	Ref.
Miyake et al. (2017)	Japan	89	Bladder cancer	Radical cystectomy	Postoperative changes in psoas major muscle volume were calculated after a radical cystectomy.	A 10% loss in the volume of the psoas muscle was an independent poor prognostic factor with HR 2.4 for OS ($p = 0.02$).	[48]
Zargar et al. (2017)	United States	60	Bladder cancer	NAC and a radical cystectomy	Changes in PMV were calculated from pre- and post-NAC CT images.	The proportion of PMV decline during NAC was not a predictor of OS after a radical cystectomy ($p = 0.85$).	[55]
Fukushima et al. (2018)	Japan	72	Advanced urothelial carcinoma	Systemic chemotherapy	Changes in SMI were calculated from pretherapeutic and posttherapeutic CT images.	Post-therapeutic skeletal muscle mass recovery was an independent favorable prognostic factor with HR 0.24 for RFS ($p < 0.001$) and 0.21 for OS ($p < 0.001$).	[56]

Abbreviations: CT = computed tomography; HR = hazard ratio; NAC = neoadjuvant chemotherapy; OS = overall survival; PMV = psoas muscle volume; RFS = recurrence-free survival; SMI = skeletal muscle index.

Although limited data suggest the prognostic significance of changes in skeletal muscle mass during treatments among bladder cancer patients, further studies are needed to confirm this finding. Therapeutic interventions for cancer might improve cancer cachexia and sarcopenia by eradicating cancer cells. Because adipose tissue depletion precedes skeletal muscle wasting in animal models with cancer cachexia [26], changes in fat and skeletal muscle mass and their patterns might be associated with survival of cancer-bearing patients. Indeed, patterns of fat and skeletal muscle wasting can be associated with survival of patients with pancreatic cancer [57].

8. Therapeutic Interventions for Sarcopenia

Given the prognostic significance of sarcopenia and changes in skeletal muscle mass in bladder cancer patients, prevention of or recovery from sarcopenia and cancer cachexia may contribute to improving their prognosis. There are several studies to investigate nutritional support, medication, and exercise as therapeutic interventions for cancer cachexia and sarcopenia in cancer-bearing patients. However, these current therapies, such as protein supplementation, are limited due to their inefficient efficacy for improving sarcopenia, suggesting the possibility of irreversible damage to skeletal muscles [32].

8.1. Nutritional Support

Several previous studies show the effect of nutritional support on sarcopenia in non-cancer patients. Because sarcopenia results from a decrease in protein synthesis and increase in protein degradation, protein supplementation can play a key role in nutritional support [58]. The effects of protein supplementation on skeletal muscle mass can be increased by adding anabolic agents such as growth hormones and testosterone [58]. However, accumulating evidence suggested that sarcopenia is not fully reversed by conventional nutrition in patients with cancer cachexia [32].

8.2. Medications

8.2.1. *n*-3 Fatty Acids

n-3 Fatty acids, including eicosapentaenoic acid and docosahexaenoic acid, can recover a cancer-induced hyper-catabolic state and improve sarcopenia and cachexia by its anti-inflammatory effects, involving the attenuation of NF-kB signaling, deceleration of the ubiquitin proteasome pathway, and antagonization of superoxide dismutase [59–61]. *n*-3 Fatty acids also reduce the expression of AZGP1 by interfering glucocorticoid receptor [32]. 4-Hydroxyhexenal (HHE) and 4-hydroxynonenal (HNE), lipid peroxidation products of *n*-3 fatty acids, can prevent the blocking of myosin expression and myotube formation caused by tumor cells [62]. *n*-3 Fatty acids can mediate the induction of apoptosis and the reduced proliferation of tumor cells [63]. Moreover, *n*-3 fatty acids have some effects on improving protein anabolism by activating the PI3K/Akt/mTOR pathway [64]. Recently, a randomized controlled study revealed that eicosapentaenoic acid improved postoperative survival in patients undergoing metastasectomy for liver metastases from colorectal cancer [65].

8.2.2. ActR2B Antagonist

ActR2B, a receptor for myostatin and activin A, mediate skeletal muscle protein degradation [31]. Expression of a dominant negative ActR2B in transgenic mice leads to skeletal muscle hypertrophy, which indicates that the ActR2B pathway mediates skeletal muscle growth [66]. In mice models with cancer cachexia, blockage of the ActR2B pathway suppressed skeletal muscle wasting by abolishing activated ubiquitin-proteasome system and inducing atrophy-specific ubiquitin ligases in skeletal muscles, in which tumor growth and fat loss were not inhibited [67]. Therefore, ActR2B antagonism has therapeutic potential for treating cancer cachexia and sarcopenia.

8.2.3. Medications for Insulin Resistance

Insulin resistance is basically enhanced in patients with cancer cachexia, despite the significant loss of adipose tissue [31]. Insulin resistance is related to the reduction of muscle glucose uptake and suppression of protein anabolism. Several medications for diabetes mellitus can be effective for cancer cachexia and sarcopenia. Metformin increases food intake and prolongs survival in cachectic tumor-bearing rat models [68]. Peroxisome proliferator activated receptor γ (PPAR-γ) agonists, including rosiglitazone, troglitazone, and pioglitazone, improve body weight and reduce skeletal muscle protein degradation by enhancing insulin sensitivity [69].

8.2.4. Inhibitors for Lipolysis and Fatty Acid Oxidation

ATGL and HSL regulate lipolysis of triglyceride and their inhibition reduces adipose tissue loss, contributing to maintained skeletal muscle mass [29]. Therefore, inhibitors for ATGL or HSL can be candidates for medications for cancer cachexia and sarcopenia. Moreover, increased oxidative stress caused by excessive fatty acid oxidation leads to skeletal muscle wasting [30]. Therefore, etomoxir, an inhibitor of fatty acid oxidation, can be a new approach for treating cancer cachexia and sarcopenia.

8.2.5. Hormonal Replacement Therapy

Hormonal replacement therapy is used to relieve menopausal symptoms in females. Because estrogen monotherapy can induce endometrial hyperplasia and cancer, progestogens are usually combined with estrogens. Hormonal replacement therapy is also effective for sarcopenia, which is one of the menopausal symptoms [70]. In males, testosterone is usually administered as hormonal replacement therapy. Testosterone improves sarcopenia, especially in combination with protein supplementations [58].

8.3. Exercise

Exercise, including aerobic exercise and resistance training, can contribute to the improvement of sarcopenia in cancer-bearing patients [71,72]. Exercise can overcome sarcopenia by abrogating systemic inflammation and catabolism [73]. Exercise has been reported to contribute to maintaining skeletal muscle mass and function in breast cancer patients treated with systemic chemotherapy [74]. Although the effect of exercise on metabolisms in patients with cancer cachexia is unclear, exercise may have an influence on lipolysis and insulin sensitivity. In addition, several studies demonstrated the anti-tumor effects of exercise. Exercise was shown to induce the secretion of interleukin-6 from muscles and elicit anti-tumor immunity in combination with epinephrine by redistributing natural killer cells to tumor microenvironments [75]. Because exercise enhances anti-tumor immunity, exercise might have a favorable effect on the efficacy of immune-oncology drugs for cancer [76]. Moreover, exercise was shown to inhibit tumor growth by activating the Hippo tumor suppressor pathway via β-adrenergic signaling [77].

9. Future Perspectives

Future studies are expected to clarify how cancer cachexia and sarcopenia progress in bladder cancer patients. Because the loss of adipose tissue precedes skeletal muscle wasting in animal models of cancer cachexia [26], phenotypes of cancer cachexia manifestations can be evaluated using CT images according to the level of fat and skeletal muscle depletion and may be useful in the management of bladder cancer patients [57]. Metabolic and molecular backgrounds of cancer cachexia and sarcopenia should be further elucidated to develop novel therapeutic strategies for sarcopenia. Future clinical trials are expected to assess the efficacy of novel medications and exercise in bladder cancer patients.

10. Conclusions

In this review, we summarized reported series of the prognostic role of sarcopenia in bladder cancer patients. Sarcopenia is significantly associated with unfavorable prognosis in bladder cancer patients undergoing a radical cystectomy. Moreover, sarcopenia is also a significant poor prognostic factor in patients with inoperable advanced bladder cancer. Thus, sarcopenia can be used as a prognostic biomarker in patients with bladder cancer at various stages. We reviewed reported series of the prognostic role of changes in skeletal muscle mass during treatments in bladder cancer patients. Recovery of skeletal muscle mass during treatments can be associated with the improved prognosis of bladder cancer patients, whereas decline of skeletal muscle mass can reflect poor prognosis, indicating its role not only as a prognostic biomarker but also as a surrogate marker for treatment efficacy in bladder cancer patients. In addition, nutritional support, medications, and exercise may improve sarcopenia and cancer cachexia and have a favorable influence on the management of cancer-bearing patients. Future studies may clarify the prognostic value of these interventions in cancer-bearing patients.

Author Contributions: All authors made substantial contributions to this work; acquisition and interpretation of data by online search, H.F. and K.T.; draft and supervision of the work, H.F. and F.K.; revision of the work, H.F., K.T., H.S. and F.K. All authors have approved the final version and agreed to be personally accountable for the author's own contributions.

References

1. Antoni, S.; Ferlay, J.; Soerjomataram, I.; Znaor, A.; Jemal, A.; Bray, F. Bladder Cancer Incidence and Mortality: A Global Overview and Recent Trends. *Eur. Urol.* **2017**, *71*, 96–108. [CrossRef] [PubMed]
2. Babjuk, M.; Bohle, A.; Burger, M.; Capoun, O.; Cohen, D.; Comperat, E.M.; Hernandez, V.; Kaasinen, E.; Palou, J.; Roupret, M.; et al. EAU Guidelines on Non-Muscle-invasive Urothelial Carcinoma of the Bladder: Update 2016. *Eur. Urol.* **2017**, *71*, 447–461. [CrossRef] [PubMed]
3. Witjes, J.A.; Lebret, T.; Comperat, E.M.; Cowan, N.C.; De Santis, M.; Bruins, H.M.; Hernandez, V.; Espinos, E.L.; Dunn, J.; Rouanne, M.; et al. Updated 2016 EAU Guidelines on Muscle-invasive and Metastatic Bladder Cancer. *Eur. Urol.* **2017**, *71*, 462–475. [CrossRef] [PubMed]
4. Dalbagni, G.; Genega, E.; Hashibe, M.; Zhang, Z.F.; Russo, P.; Herr, H.; Reuter, V. Cystectomy for bladder cancer: A contemporary series. *J. Urol.* **2001**, *165*, 1111–1116. [CrossRef]
5. Bellmunt, J.; von der Maase, H.; Mead, G.M.; Skoneczna, I.; De Santis, M.; Daugaard, G.; Boehle, A.; Chevreau, C.; Paz-Ares, L.; Laufman, L.R.; et al. Randomized phase III study comparing paclitaxel/cisplatin/gemcitabine and gemcitabine/cisplatin in patients with locally advanced or metastatic urothelial cancer without prior systemic therapy: EORTC Intergroup Study 30987. *J. Clin. Oncol.* **2012**, *30*, 1107–1113. [CrossRef] [PubMed]
6. Sundahl, N.; Rottey, S.; De Maeseneer, D.; Ost, P. Pembrolizumab for the treatment of bladder cancer. *Expert Rev. Anticancer Ther.* **2018**, *18*, 107–114. [CrossRef] [PubMed]
7. Cruz-Jentoft, A.J.; Baeyens, J.P.; Bauer, J.M.; Boirie, Y.; Cederholm, T.; Landi, F.; Martin, F.C.; Michel, J.P.; Rolland, Y.; Schneider, S.M.; et al. Sarcopenia: European consensus on definition and diagnosis: Report of the European Working Group on Sarcopenia in Older People. *Age Ageing* **2010**, *39*, 412–423. [CrossRef] [PubMed]
8. Kim, T.N.; Choi, K.M. Sarcopenia: Definition, epidemiology, and pathophysiology. *J. Bone Metab.* **2013**, *20*, 1–10. [CrossRef] [PubMed]
9. Garatachea, N.; Lucia, A. Genes and the ageing muscle: A review on genetic association studies. *Age* **2013**, *35*, 207–233. [CrossRef] [PubMed]
10. Brown, J.C.; Harhay, M.O.; Harhay, M.N. Sarcopenia and mortality among a population-based sample of community-dwelling older adults. *J. Cachexia Sarcopenia Muscle* **2016**, *7*, 290–298. [CrossRef] [PubMed]
11. Landi, F.; Cruz-Jentoft, A.J.; Liperoti, R.; Russo, A.; Giovannini, S.; Tosato, M.; Capoluongo, E.; Bernabei, R.; Onder, G. Sarcopenia and mortality risk in frail older persons aged 80 years and older: Results from ilSIRENTE study. *Age Ageing* **2013**, *42*, 203–209. [CrossRef] [PubMed]

12. Cosqueric, G.; Sebag, A.; Ducolombier, C.; Thomas, C.; Piette, F.; Weill-Engerer, S. Sarcopenia is predictive of nosocomial infection in care of the elderly. *Br. J. Nutr.* **2006**, *96*, 895–901. [CrossRef] [PubMed]
13. Lee, J.; Hong, Y.P.; Shin, H.J.; Lee, W. Associations of Sarcopenia and Sarcopenic Obesity With Metabolic Syndrome Considering Both Muscle Mass and Muscle Strength. *J. Prev. Med. Public Health* **2016**, *49*, 35–44. [CrossRef] [PubMed]
14. Kim, J.E.; Lee, Y.H.; Huh, J.H.; Kang, D.R.; Rhee, Y.; Lim, S.K. Early-stage chronic kidney disease, insulin resistance, and osteoporosis as risk factors of sarcopenia in aged population: The fourth Korea National Health and Nutrition Examination Survey (KNHANES IV), 2008–2009. *Osteoporos. Int.* **2014**, *25*, 2189–2198. [CrossRef] [PubMed]
15. Kim, J.H.; Cho, J.J.; Park, Y.S. Relationship between sarcopenic obesity and cardiovascular disease risk as estimated by the Framingham risk score. *J. Korean Med. Sci.* **2015**, *30*, 264–271. [CrossRef] [PubMed]
16. Fearon, K.; Strasser, F.; Anker, S.D.; Bosaeus, I.; Bruera, E.; Fainsinger, R.L.; Jatoi, A.; Loprinzi, C.; MacDonald, N.; Mantovani, G.; et al. Definition and classification of cancer cachexia: An international consensus. *Lancet Oncol.* **2011**, *12*, 489–495. [CrossRef]
17. Fearon, K.C.; Voss, A.C.; Hustead, D.S. Definition of cancer cachexia: Effect of weight loss, reduced food intake, and systemic inflammation on functional status and prognosis. *Am. J. Clin. Nutr.* **2006**, *83*, 1345–1350. [CrossRef] [PubMed]
18. Martin, L.; Birdsell, L.; Macdonald, N.; Reiman, T.; Clandinin, M.T.; McCargar, L.J.; Murphy, R.; Ghosh, S.; Sawyer, M.B.; Baracos, V.E. Cancer cachexia in the age of obesity: Skeletal muscle depletion is a powerful prognostic factor, independent of body mass index. *J. Clin. Oncol.* **2013**, *31*, 1539–1547. [CrossRef] [PubMed]
19. Prado, C.M.; Lieffers, J.R.; McCargar, L.J.; Reiman, T.; Sawyer, M.B.; Martin, L.; Baracos, V.E. Prevalence and clinical implications of sarcopenic obesity in patients with solid tumours of the respiratory and gastrointestinal tracts: A population-based study. *Lancet Oncol.* **2008**, *9*, 629–635. [CrossRef]
20. Harimoto, N.; Shirabe, K.; Yamashita, Y.I.; Ikegami, T.; Yoshizumi, T.; Soejima, Y.; Ikeda, T.; Maehara, Y.; Nishie, A.; Yamanaka, T. Sarcopenia as a predictor of prognosis in patients following hepatectomy for hepatocellular carcinoma. *Br. J. Surg.* **2013**, *100*, 1523–1530. [CrossRef] [PubMed]
21. Harada, K.; Ida, S.; Baba, Y.; Ishimoto, T.; Kosumi, K.; Tokunaga, R.; Izumi, D.; Ohuchi, M.; Nakamura, K.; Kiyozumi, Y.; et al. Prognostic and clinical impact of sarcopenia in esophageal squamous cell carcinoma. *Dis. Esophagus* **2016**, *29*, 627–633. [CrossRef] [PubMed]
22. Go, S.I.; Park, M.J.; Song, H.N.; Kim, H.G.; Kang, M.H.; Lee, H.R.; Kim, Y.; Kim, R.B.; Lee, S.I.; Lee, G.W. Prognostic impact of sarcopenia in patients with diffuse large B-cell lymphoma treated with rituximab plus cyclophosphamide, doxorubicin, vincristine, and prednisone. *J. Cachexia Sarcopenia Muscle* **2016**, *7*, 567–576. [CrossRef] [PubMed]
23. Sabel, M.S.; Lee, J.; Cai, S.; Englesbe, M.J.; Holcombe, S.; Wang, S. Sarcopenia as a prognostic factor among patients with stage III melanoma. *Ann. Surg. Oncol.* **2011**, *18*, 3579–3585. [CrossRef] [PubMed]
24. Psutka, S.P.; Boorjian, S.A.; Moynagh, M.R.; Schmit, G.D.; Costello, B.A.; Thompson, R.H.; Stewart-Merrill, S.B.; Lohse, C.M.; Cheville, J.C.; Leibovich, B.C.; et al. Decreased Skeletal Muscle Mass is Associated with an Increased Risk of Mortality after Radical Nephrectomy for Localized Renal Cell Cancer. *J. Urol.* **2016**, *195*, 270–276. [CrossRef] [PubMed]
25. Fukushima, H.; Nakanishi, Y.; Kataoka, M.; Tobisu, K.; Koga, F. Prognostic Significance of Sarcopenia in Patients with Metastatic Renal Cell Carcinoma. *J. Urol.* **2016**, *195*, 26–32. [CrossRef] [PubMed]
26. Kliewer, K.L.; Ke, J.Y.; Tian, M.; Cole, R.M.; Andridge, R.R.; Belury, M.A. Adipose tissue lipolysis and energy metabolism in early cancer cachexia in mice. *Cancer Boil. Ther.* **2015**, *16*, 886–897. [CrossRef] [PubMed]
27. Fearon, K.C.; Glass, D.J.; Guttridge, D.C. Cancer cachexia: Mediators, signaling, and metabolic pathways. *Cell Metab.* **2012**, *16*, 153–166. [CrossRef] [PubMed]
28. Petruzzelli, M.; Schweiger, M.; Schreiber, R.; Campos-Olivas, R.; Tsoli, M.; Allen, J.; Swarbrick, M.; Rose-John, S.; Rincon, M.; Robertson, G.; et al. A switch from white to brown fat increases energy expenditure in cancer-associated cachexia. *Cell Metab.* **2014**, *20*, 433–447. [CrossRef] [PubMed]
29. Das, S.K.; Eder, S.; Schauer, S.; Diwoky, C.; Temmel, H.; Guertl, B.; Gorkiewicz, G.; Tamilarasan, K.P.; Kumari, P.; Trauner, M.; et al. Adipose triglyceride lipase contributes to cancer-associated cachexia. *Science* **2011**, *333*, 233–238. [CrossRef] [PubMed]

30. Fukawa, T.; Yan-Jiang, B.C.; Min-Wen, J.C.; Jun-Hao, E.T.; Huang, D.; Qian, C.N.; Ong, P.; Li, Z.; Chen, S.; Mak, S.Y.; et al. Excessive fatty acid oxidation induces muscle atrophy in cancer cachexia. *Nat. Med.* **2016**, *22*, 666–671. [CrossRef] [PubMed]
31. Argiles, J.M.; Busquets, S.; Stemmler, B.; Lopez-Soriano, F.J. Cancer cachexia: Understanding the molecular basis. *Nat. Rev. Cancer* **2014**, *14*, 754–762. [CrossRef] [PubMed]
32. Tisdale, M.J. Mechanisms of cancer cachexia. *Physiol. Rev.* **2009**, *89*, 381–410. [CrossRef] [PubMed]
33. Schmitt, T.L.; Martignoni, M.E.; Bachmann, J.; Fechtner, K.; Friess, H.; Kinscherf, R.; Hildebrandt, W. Activity of the Akt-dependent anabolic and catabolic pathways in muscle and liver samples in cancer-related cachexia. *J. Mol. Med.* **2007**, *85*, 647–654. [CrossRef] [PubMed]
34. Moylan, J.S.; Smith, J.D.; Chambers, M.A.; McLoughlin, T.J.; Reid, M.B. TNF induction of atrogin-1/MAFbx mRNA depends on Foxo4 expression but not AKT-Foxo1/3 signaling. *Am. J. Physiol. Cell Physiol.* **2008**, *295*, C986–C993. [CrossRef] [PubMed]
35. Julienne, C.M.; Dumas, J.F.; Goupille, C.; Pinault, M.; Berri, C.; Collin, A.; Tesseraud, S.; Couet, C.; Servais, S. Cancer cachexia is associated with a decrease in skeletal muscle mitochondrial oxidative capacities without alteration of ATP production efficiency. *J. Cachexia Sarcopenia Muscle* **2012**, *3*, 265–275. [CrossRef] [PubMed]
36. Stephens, N.A.; Skipworth, R.J.; Macdonald, A.J.; Greig, C.A.; Ross, J.A.; Fearon, K.C. Intramyocellular lipid droplets increase with progression of cachexia in cancer patients. *J. Cachexia Sarcopenia Muscle* **2011**, *2*, 111–117. [CrossRef] [PubMed]
37. Fukushima, H.; Koga, F. Impact of sarcopenia in the management of urological cancer patients. *Expert Rev. Anticancer Ther.* **2017**, *17*, 455–466. [CrossRef] [PubMed]
38. Shen, W.; Punyanitya, M.; Wang, Z.; Gallagher, D.; St-Onge, M.P.; Albu, J.; Heymsfield, S.B.; Heshka, S. Total body skeletal muscle and adipose tissue volumes: Estimation from a single abdominal cross-sectional image. *J. Appl. Physiol.* **2004**, *97*, 2333–2338. [CrossRef] [PubMed]
39. Hamaguchi, Y.; Kaido, T.; Okumura, S.; Kobayashi, A.; Hammad, A.; Tamai, Y.; Inagaki, N.; Uemoto, S. Proposal for new diagnostic criteria for low skeletal muscle mass based on computed tomography imaging in Asian adults. *Nutrition* **2016**, *32*, 1200–1205. [CrossRef] [PubMed]
40. Aubrey, J.; Esfandiari, N.; Baracos, V.E.; Buteau, F.A.; Frenette, J.; Putman, C.T.; Mazurak, V.C. Measurement of skeletal muscle radiation attenuation and basis of its biological variation. *Acta Physiol.* **2014**, *210*, 489–497. [CrossRef] [PubMed]
41. Hulver, M.W.; Dohm, G.L. The molecular mechanism linking muscle fat accumulation to insulin resistance. *Proc. Nutr. Soc.* **2004**, *63*, 375–380. [CrossRef] [PubMed]
42. Moher, D.; Liberati, A.; Tetzlaff, J.; Altman, D.G. Preferred reporting items for systematic reviews and meta-analyses: The PRISMA statement. *Int. J. Surg.* **2010**, *8*, 336–341. [CrossRef] [PubMed]
43. Lawrentschuk, N.; Colombo, R.; Hakenberg, O.W.; Lerner, S.P.; Mansson, W.; Sagalowsky, A.; Wirth, M.P. Prevention and management of complications following radical cystectomy for bladder cancer. *Eur. Urol.* **2010**, *57*, 983–1001. [CrossRef] [PubMed]
44. Wan, F.; Zhu, Y.; Gu, C.; Yao, X.; Shen, Y.; Dai, B.; Zhang, S.; Zhang, H.; Cheng, J.; Ye, D. Lower skeletal muscle index and early complications in patients undergoing radical cystectomy for bladder cancer. *World J. Surg. Oncol.* **2014**, *12*, 14. [CrossRef] [PubMed]
45. Smith, A.B.; Deal, A.M.; Yu, H.; Boyd, B.; Matthews, J.; Wallen, E.M.; Pruthi, R.S.; Woods, M.E.; Muss, H.; Nielsen, M.E. Sarcopenia as a predictor of complications and survival following radical cystectomy. *J. Urol.* **2014**, *191*, 1714–1720. [CrossRef] [PubMed]
46. Psutka, S.P.; Carrasco, A.; Schmit, G.D.; Moynagh, M.R.; Boorjian, S.A.; Frank, I.; Stewart, S.B.; Thapa, P.; Tarrell, R.F.; Cheville, J.C.; et al. Sarcopenia in patients with bladder cancer undergoing radical cystectomy: Impact on cancer-specific and all-cause mortality. *Cancer* **2014**, *120*, 2910–2918. [CrossRef] [PubMed]
47. Hirasawa, Y.; Nakashima, J.; Yunaiyama, D.; Sugihara, T.; Gondo, T.; Nakagami, Y.; Horiguchi, Y.; Ohno, Y.; Namiki, K.; Ohori, M.; et al. Sarcopenia as a Novel Preoperative Prognostic Predictor for Survival in Patients with Bladder Cancer Undergoing Radical Cystectomy. *Ann. Surg. Oncol.* **2016**, *23*, 1048–1054. [CrossRef] [PubMed]
48. Miyake, M.; Morizawa, Y.; Hori, S.; Marugami, N.; Shimada, K.; Gotoh, D.; Tatsumi, Y.; Nakai, Y.; Inoue, T.; Anai, S.; et al. Clinical impact of postoperative loss in psoas major muscle and nutrition index after radical cystectomy for patients with urothelial carcinoma of the bladder. *BMC Cancer* **2017**, *17*, 237. [CrossRef] [PubMed]

49. Saitoh-Maeda, Y.; Kawahara, T.; Miyoshi, Y.; Tsutsumi, S.; Takamoto, D.; Shimokihara, K.; Hayashi, Y.; Mochizuki, T.; Ohtaka, M.; Nakamura, M.; et al. A low psoas muscle volume correlates with a longer hospitalization after radical cystectomy. *BMC Urol.* **2017**, *17*, 87. [CrossRef] [PubMed]
50. Mayr, R.; Gierth, M.; Zeman, F.; Reiffen, M.; Seeger, P.; Wezel, F.; Pycha, A.; Comploj, E.; Bonatti, M.; Ritter, M.; et al. Sarcopenia as a comorbidity-independent predictor of survival following radical cystectomy for bladder cancer. *J. Cachexia Sarcopenia Muscle* **2018**, *9*, 505–513. [CrossRef] [PubMed]
51. Fukushima, H.; Yokoyama, M.; Nakanishi, Y.; Tobisu, K.; Koga, F. Sarcopenia as a prognostic biomarker of advanced urothelial carcinoma. *PLoS ONE* **2015**, *10*, e0115895. [CrossRef] [PubMed]
52. Taguchi, S.; Akamatsu, N.; Nakagawa, T.; Gonoi, W.; Kanatani, A.; Miyazaki, H.; Fujimura, T.; Fukuhara, H.; Kume, H.; Homma, Y. Sarcopenia Evaluated Using the Skeletal Muscle Index Is a Significant Prognostic Factor for Metastatic Urothelial Carcinoma. *Clin. Genitourin. Cancer* **2016**, *14*, 237–243. [CrossRef] [PubMed]
53. Kasahara, R.; Kawahara, T.; Ohtake, S.; Saitoh, Y.; Tsutsumi, S.; Teranishi, J.I.; Miyoshi, Y.; Nakaigawa, N.; Yao, M.; Kobayashi, K.; et al. A Low Psoas Muscle Index before Treatment Can Predict a Poorer Prognosis in Advanced Bladder Cancer Patients Who Receive Gemcitabine and Nedaplatin Therapy. *BioMed Res. Int.* **2017**, *2017*, 7981549. [CrossRef] [PubMed]
54. Abe, H.; Takei, K.; Uematsu, T.; Tokura, Y.; Suzuki, I.; Sakamoto, K.; Nishihara, D.; Yamaguchi, Y.; Mizuno, T.; Nukui, A.; et al. Significance of sarcopenia as a prognostic factor for metastatic urothelial carcinoma patients treated with systemic chemotherapy. *Int. J. Clin. Oncol.* **2018**, *23*, 338–346. [CrossRef] [PubMed]
55. Zargar, H.; Almassi, N.; Kovac, E.; Ercole, C.; Remer, E.; Rini, B.; Stephenson, A.; Garcia, J.A.; Grivas, P. Change in Psoas Muscle Volume as a Predictor of Outcomes in Patients Treated with Chemotherapy and Radical Cystectomy for Muscle-Invasive Bladder Cancer. *Bladder Cancer* **2017**, *3*, 57–63. [CrossRef] [PubMed]
56. Fukushima, H.; Kataoka, M.; Nakanishi, Y.; Sakamoto, K.; Takemura, K.; Suzuki, H.; Ito, M.; Tobisu, K.I.; Fujii, Y.; Koga, F. Posttherapeutic skeletal muscle mass recovery predicts favorable prognosis in patients with advanced urothelial carcinoma receiving first-line platinum-based chemotherapy. *Urol. Oncol.* **2018**, *36*, 156.e9–156.e16. [CrossRef] [PubMed]
57. Kays, J.K.; Shahda, S.; Stanley, M.; Bell, T.M.; O'Neill, B.H.; Kohli, M.D.; Couch, M.E.; Koniaris, L.G.; Zimmers, T.A. Three cachexia phenotypes and the impact of fat-only loss on survival in FOLFIRINOX therapy for pancreatic cancer. *J. Cachexia Sarcopenia Muscle* **2018**. [CrossRef] [PubMed]
58. Ahima, R.S.; Park, H.K. Connecting Myokines and Metabolism. *Endocrinol. Metab.* **2015**, *30*, 235–245. [CrossRef] [PubMed]
59. Vaughan, V.C.; Martin, P.; Lewandowski, P.A. Cancer cachexia: Impact, mechanisms and emerging treatments. *J. Cachexia Sarcopenia Muscle* **2013**, *4*, 95–109. [CrossRef] [PubMed]
60. Whitehouse, A.S.; Smith, H.J.; Drake, J.L.; Tisdale, M.J. Mechanism of attenuation of skeletal muscle protein catabolism in cancer cachexia by eicosapentaenoic acid. *Cancer Res.* **2001**, *61*, 3604–3609. [PubMed]
61. Oh, D.Y.; Talukdar, S.; Bae, E.J.; Imamura, T.; Morinaga, H.; Fan, W.; Li, P.; Lu, W.J.; Watkins, S.M.; Olefsky, J.M. GPR120 is an omega-3 fatty acid receptor mediating potent anti-inflammatory and insulin-sensitizing effects. *Cell* **2010**, *142*, 687–698. [CrossRef] [PubMed]
62. Muzio, G.; Ricci, M.; Traverso, N.; Monacelli, F.; Oraldi, M.; Maggiora, M.; Canuto, R.A. 4-Hydroxyhexenal and 4-hydroxynonenal are mediators of the anti-cachectic effect of n-3 and n-6 polyunsaturated fatty acids on human lung cancer cells. *Free. Radic. Boil. Med.* **2016**, *99*, 63–70. [CrossRef] [PubMed]
63. Newell, M.; Baker, K.; Postovit, L.M.; Field, C.J. A Critical Review on the Effect of Docosahexaenoic Acid (DHA) on Cancer Cell Cycle Progression. *Int. J. Mol. Sci.* **2017**, *18*, 1784. [CrossRef] [PubMed]
64. Smith, G.I.; Atherton, P.; Reeds, D.N.; Mohammed, B.S.; Rankin, D.; Rennie, M.J.; Mittendorfer, B. Omega-3 polyunsaturated fatty acids augment the muscle protein anabolic response to hyperinsulinaemia-hyperaminoacidaemia in healthy young and middle-aged men and women. *Clin. Sci.* **2011**, *121*, 267–278. [CrossRef] [PubMed]
65. Cockbain, A.J.; Volpato, M.; Race, A.D.; Munarini, A.; Fazio, C.; Belluzzi, A.; Loadman, P.M.; Toogood, G.J.; Hull, M.A. Anticolorectal cancer activity of the omega-3 polyunsaturated fatty acid eicosapentaenoic acid. *Gut* **2014**, *63*, 1760–1768. [CrossRef] [PubMed]
66. Lee, S.J.; McPherron, A.C. Regulation of myostatin activity and muscle growth. *Proc. Natl. Acad. Sci. USA* **2001**, *98*, 9306–9311. [CrossRef] [PubMed]

67. Zhou, X.; Wang, J.L.; Lu, J.; Song, Y.; Kwak, K.S.; Jiao, Q.; Rosenfeld, R.; Chen, Q.; Boone, T.; Simonet, W.S.; et al. Reversal of cancer cachexia and muscle wasting by ActRIIB antagonism leads to prolonged survival. *Cell* **2010**, *142*, 531–543. [CrossRef] [PubMed]
68. Oliveira, A.G.; Gomes-Marcondes, M.C. Metformin treatment modulates the tumour-induced wasting effects in muscle protein metabolism minimising the cachexia in tumour-bearing rats. *BMC Cancer* **2016**, *16*, 418. [CrossRef] [PubMed]
69. Beluzi, M.; Peres, S.B.; Henriques, F.S.; Sertie, R.A.; Franco, F.O.; Santos, K.B.; Knobl, P.; Andreotti, S.; Shida, C.S.; Neves, R.X.; et al. Pioglitazone treatment increases survival and prevents body weight loss in tumor-bearing animals: Possible anti-cachectic effect. *PLoS ONE* **2015**, *10*, e0122660. [CrossRef] [PubMed]
70. Dionne, I.J.; Kinaman, K.A.; Poehlman, E.T. Sarcopenia and muscle function during menopause and hormone-replacement therapy. *J. Nutr. Health Aging* **2000**, *4*, 156–161. [PubMed]
71. Stene, G.B.; Helbostad, J.L.; Balstad, T.R.; Riphagen, I.I.; Kaasa, S.; Oldervoll, L.M. Effect of physical exercise on muscle mass and strength in cancer patients during treatment—A systematic review. *Crit. Rev. Oncol. Hematol.* **2013**, *88*, 573–593. [CrossRef] [PubMed]
72. Strasser, B.; Steindorf, K.; Wiskemann, J.; Ulrich, C.M. Impact of resistance training in cancer survivors: A meta-analysis. *Med. Sci. Sports Exerc.* **2013**, *45*, 2080–2090. [CrossRef] [PubMed]
73. Gould, D.W.; Lahart, I.; Carmichael, A.R.; Koutedakis, Y.; Metsios, G.S. Cancer cachexia prevention via physical exercise: Molecular mechanisms. *J. Cachexia Sarcopenia Muscle* **2013**, *4*, 111–124. [CrossRef] [PubMed]
74. Mijwel, S.; Cardinale, D.A.; Norrbom, J.; Chapman, M.; Ivarsson, N.; Wengstrom, Y.; Sundberg, C.J.; Rundqvist, H. Exercise training during chemotherapy preserves skeletal muscle fiber area, capillarization, and mitochondrial content in patients with breast cancer. *FASEB J.* **2018**. [CrossRef] [PubMed]
75. Pedersen, L.; Idorn, M.; Olofsson, G.H.; Lauenborg, B.; Nookaew, I.; Hansen, R.H.; Johannesen, H.H.; Becker, J.C.; Pedersen, K.S.; Dethlefsen, C.; et al. Voluntary Running Suppresses Tumor Growth through Epinephrine- and IL-6-Dependent NK Cell Mobilization and Redistribution. *Cell Metab.* **2016**, *23*, 554–562. [CrossRef] [PubMed]
76. Koelwyn, G.J.; Wennerberg, E.; Demaria, S.; Jones, L.W. Exercise in Regulation of Inflammation-Immune Axis Function in Cancer Initiation and Progression. *Oncology* **2015**, *29*, 908–920, 922. [PubMed]
77. Dethlefsen, C.; Hansen, L.S.; Lillelund, C.; Andersen, C.; Gehl, J.; Christensen, J.F.; Pedersen, B.K.; Hojman, P. Exercise-Induced Catecholamines Activate the Hippo Tumor Suppressor Pathway to Reduce Risks of Breast Cancer Development. *Cancer Res.* **2017**, *77*, 4894–4904. [CrossRef] [PubMed]

11

Regulatory T Cells and Tumor-Associated Macrophages in the Tumor Microenvironment in Non-Muscle Invasive Bladder Cancer Treated with Intravesical Bacille Calmette-Guérin: A Long-Term Follow-up Study of a Japanese Cohort

Makito Miyake [1,*], Yoshihiro Tatsumi [1,2], Daisuke Gotoh [1], Sayuri Ohnishi [1], Takuya Owari [1], Kota Iida [1], Kenta Ohnishi [1], Shunta Hori [1], Yosuke Morizawa [1], Yoshitaka Itami [1], Yasushi Nakai [1], Takeshi Inoue [1], Satoshi Anai [1], Kazumasa Torimoto [1], Katsuya Aoki [1], Keiji Shimada [3], Noboru Konishi [2], Nobumichi Tanaka [1] and Kiyohide Fujimoto [1]

1 Department of Urology, Nara Medical University, 840 Shijo-cho, Kashihara-shi, Nara 634-8522, Japan; takuro.birds.nest@gmail.com (Y.T.); dgotou@gmail.com (D.G.); sayuri3@naramed-u.ac.jp (S.O.); tintherye@gmail.com (T.O.); kota1006ida@yahoo.co.jp (K.I.); kenzmedico0912@yahoo.co.jp (K.O.); horimaus@gmail.com (S.H.); tigers.yosuke@gmail.com (Y.M.); y.itami.324@gmail.com (Y.I.); nakaiyasusiuro@live.jp (Y.N.); you1513tt@yahoo.co.jp (T.I.); sanai@naramed-u.ac.jp (S.A.); torimoto@nmu-gw.naramed-u.ac.jp (K.T.); aokik@naramed-u.ac.jp (K.A.); sendo@naramed-u.ac.jp (N.T.); kiyokun@naramed-u.ac.jp (K.F.)

2 Department of Pathology, Nara Medical University, 840 Shijo-cho, Kashihara-shi, Nara 634-8522, Japan; n-konishi@takai-hp.com

3 Department of Pathology, Nara City Hospital, 1501 Higashi kidera-cho, Nara-shi, Nara 630-8305, Japan; k-shimada@nara-jadecom.jp

* Correspondence: makitomiyake@naramed-u.ac.jp

Abstract: The clinical significance of regulatory T cells (Treg) and tumor-associated macrophages (TAM) in the tumor microenvironment of human bladder cancer remains unclear. The aim of this study is to explore their relevance to oncological features in non-muscle invasive bladder cancer (NMIBC). We carried out immunohistochemical analysis of forkhead box P3 (FOXP3, Treg maker), CD204 (TAM marker), and interleukin-6 (IL6) using surgical specimens obtained from 154 NMIBC patients. The Treg and TAM counts surrounding the cancer lesion and IL6-positive cancer cell counts were evaluated against clinicopathological variables. We focused on the ability of the Treg and TAM counts around the cancer lesion to predict outcomes after adjuvant intravesical Bacille Calmette–Guérin (BCG) treatment. High Treg counts were associated with female patients, older age, T1 category, and high tumor grade. TAM count was significantly correlated with Treg count and with IL6-positive cancer cell count. In our analysis of 71 patients treated with BCG, high counts of Treg and TAM were associated with shorter recurrence-free survival, and the former was an independent predictor of recurrence. Poor response to intravesical BCG was associated with Treg and TAM in the tumor microenvironment. Disrupting the immune network can be a supplementary therapeutic approach for NMIBC patients receiving intravesical BCG.

Keywords: regulatory T cell; tumor-associated macrophage; non-muscle invasive bladder cancer; intravesical recurrence; progression; Bacille Calmette–Guérin

1. Introduction

Urothelial carcinoma (UC) of the bladder is a heterogeneous disease in terms of its clinical and biological aspects [1]. Among non-muscle invasive bladder cancer (NMIBC) patients, several factors such as age, T category, tumor grade, tumor size, and multiplicity are recognized to predict the risk of intravesical recurrence and progression after transurethral resection of bladder tumor (TURBT) [2,3]. Despite advancements in detection technologies, surgical techniques, and adjuvant intravesical treatment, clinical management of high-risk diseases remains challenging [4,5].

Intravesical administration of Bacille Calmette–Guérin (BCG) is a standard treatment for carcinoma in situ (CIS) and an adjuvant option for T1 and high-risk Ta tumors following TURBT [6]. However, a delay in radical cystectomy (RC) leads to shortened cancer-specific survival as compared to immediate RC at the time of NMIBC [7]. Thus, there is an urgent need for biomarkers to identify patients who will benefit from intravesical BCG or should undergo immediate RC. Although possible mechanisms underlying BCG-induced antitumor activity and relevant molecules have been studied [8–10], they are not fully understood. Briefly, BCG is internalized into urothelial cells through the formation of a complex with fibronectin, followed by antigen presentation to BCG-specific CD4+ T-cells by antigen-presenting cells. Pro-inflammatory cytokines such as interleukin-6 (IL6) and interferon-γ are secreted to recruit a Th1-induced immunoreaction with the recognition of cancer cells through the activation of macrophages, CD8+ T-cells, and natural killer cells.

Several previous studies have demonstrated that the pre-BCG baseline status of Th1/Th2 balance, regulatory T cell (Treg) recruitment, and tumor-associated macrophage (TAM) polarization in the tumor microenvironment could influence the clinical response to BCG [10–12]. In light of the sparse data on the clinical significance of Treg/TAM and their relevance to oncological outcomes of NMIBC treated with intravesical BCG—especially in Japanese patients—this study was conducted with the goal of improving patient care.

2. Results

2.1. *Association of Treg and TAM in the Cancerous Area with Baseline Characteristics*

Treg and TAM significantly differed in their localization patterns (Figure 1A). Most of the Treg cells localized in the stroma around the cancer lesion regardless of tumor stage and grade, whereas TAM had a tendency to infiltrate into the tumor area in high-grade tumors compared to low-grade tumors. In an analysis of 154 tumors, the median counts per high power field (HPF) of Treg and TAM were eight (interquartile range [IQR], 3–15) and 23 (IQR 16–33), respectively. The appropriate cutoff points of Treg and TAM count have not been established yet, especially in bladder UC. The cutoff values for separating low counts and high counts for Treg and TAM were set as 10 and 25 respectively, based on the median values. With these thresholds, high counts of Treg and TAM were found in 68 (44%) and 62 (41%) out of 154 tumors, respectively. The clinicopathological variables and their association with Treg and TAM in 154 patients with NMIBC are outlined in Table 1. High Treg count was associated with female patients ($p = 0.001$), older age ($p = 0.024$), T1 category ($p < 0.001$), high tumor grade ($p < 0.001$), and the presence of CIS ($p = 0.011$), whereas the count of TAM was not associated with any variable (Table 1).

Table 1. Clinicopathologic variables and association with Treg and TAM in primary NMIBC.

Variables	N	Treg (FOXP3+ Cell)			TAM (CD204+ Cell)		
		Low	High	*p* Value	Low	High	*p* Value
Total	154 (100%)	86 (56%)	68 (44%)	–	92 (59%)	62 (41%)	–
Sex				0.0012			0.45
Male	137 (89%)	83 (61%)	54 (39%)		78 (57%)	59 (43%)	
Female	17 (11%)	3 (18%)	14 (82%)		8 (47%)	9 (53%)	
Age at initial TURBT categorical				0.056			0.75

Table 1. *Cont.*

Variables	N	Treg (FOXP3+ Cell)			TAM (CD204+ Cell)		
		Low	High	*p* Value	Low	High	*p* Value
<60	18 (12%)	15 (83%)	3 (17%)		11 (61%)	7 (39%)	
60 to 70	55 (36%)	34 (62%)	21 (38%)		32 (58%)	23 (42%)	
>70	81 (52%)	43 (53%)	38 (47%)		43 (53%)	38 (47%)	
Continuous median (IQR)	71 (65–76)	69 (63–76)	73 (69–79)	0.024	71 (64–76)	71 (68–77)	0.22
T category				<0.001			0.25
Ta	68 (44%)	52 (76%)	16 (24%)		41 (60%)	27 (40%)	
T1	73 (47%)	30 (41%)	43 (59%)		36 (49%)	37 (51%)	
Tis	13 (9%)	10 (77%)	3 (23%)		9 (69%)	4 (31%)	
Tumor grade				<0.001			0.16
Low	71 (46%)	53 (75%)	18 (25%)		44 (62%)	27 (38%)	
High	83 (54%)	39 (47%)	44 (53%)		42 (51%)	41 (49%)	
Tumor architecture				0.98			0.69
Papillary	134 (87%)	80 (60%)	54 (40%)		74 (55%)	60 (45%)	
Non-papillary	20 (13%)	12 (60%)	8 (40%)		12 (60%)	8 (40%)	
Multiplicity				0.64			0.71
Single	88 (57%)	54 (61%)	34 (39%)		48 (55%)	40 (45%)	
Multiple	66 (43%)	38 (58%)	28 (42%)		38 (58%)	28 (42%)	
Tumor size				0.45			0.99
Less than 3 cm	119 (77%)	73 (61%)	46 (39%)		69 (58%)	50 (42%)	
3 cm or more	35 (23%)	19 (54%)	16 (46%)		17 (49%)	18 (51%)	
CIS				0.011			0.29
No	91 (59%)	62 (68%)	29 (32%)		54 (59%)	37 (41%)	
Yes	63 (41%)	30 (48%)	33 (52%)		32 (51%)	31 (49%)	
LVI (in T1 tumor, $n = 73$)				0.66			0.93
Negative	49 (67%)	21 (43%)	28 (57%)		24 (49%)	25 (51%)	
Positive	24 (33%)	9 (38%)	15 (62%)		12 (50%)	12 (50%)	
Intravesical adjuvant therapy				0.65			0.37
No	64 (42%)	41 (64%)	23 (36%)		40 (62%)	24 (38%)	
BCG	71 (46%)	40 (56%)	31 (44%)		36 (51%)	35 (49%)	
Chemotherapy	19 (12%)	11 (58%)	8 (42%)		10 (53%)	9 (47%)	

Treg, regulatory T cell; TAM, Tumor-associated macrophage; NMIBC, non-muscle invasive bladder cancer; TURBT, transurethral resection of bladder tumor; IQR, interquartile range; CIS, Carcinoma in situ; LVI, lymphovascular invasion; BCG, Bacillus Calmette-Guerin.

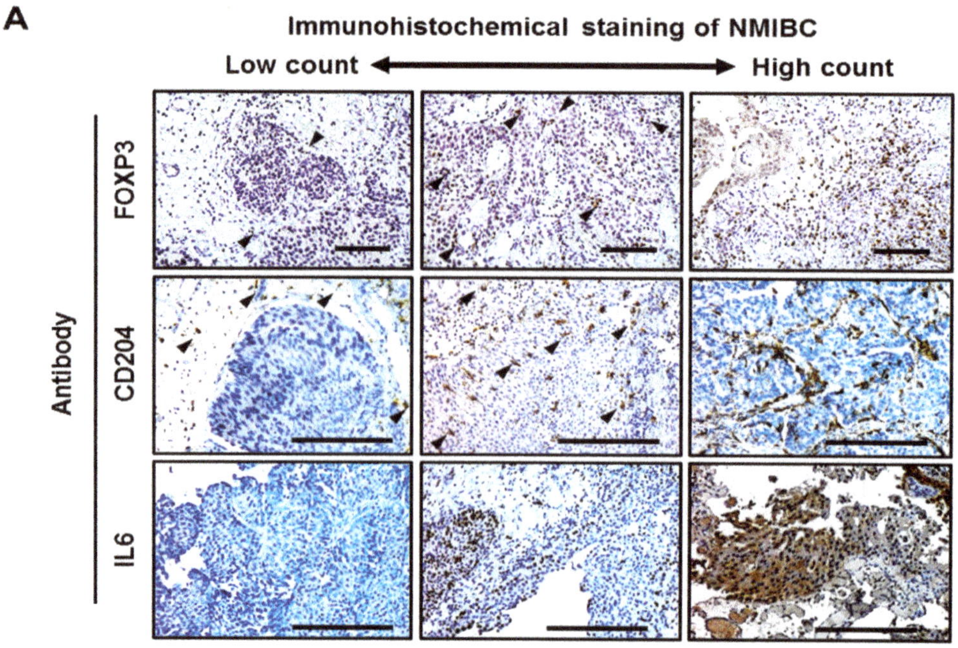

Figure 1. *Cont.*

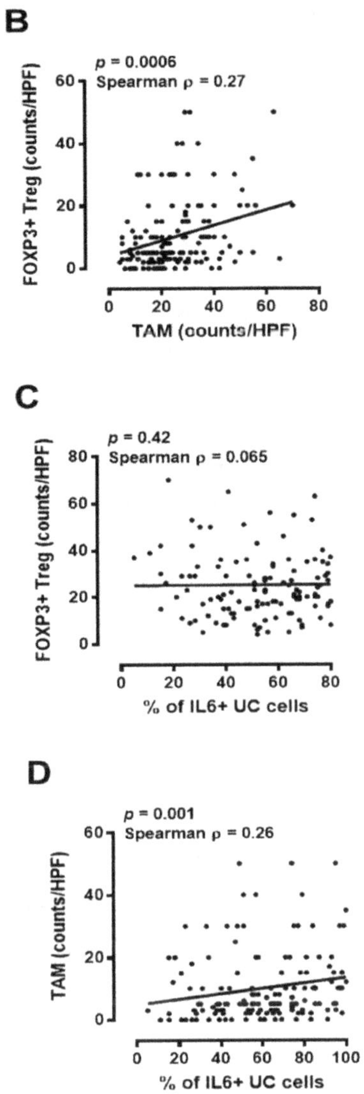

Figure 1. Immunohistochemical quantification of regulatory T cells, tumor-associated macrophages, and IL6-positive urothelial carcinoma cells. (**A**) Representative expression status of FOXP3, CD204, and IL6 in human bladder cancer tissues. Images were captured at 100× (FOXP3) or 200× (CD204 and IL6) magnification. Black arrowheads in the FOXP3 and CD204 images indicate positive-stained immune cells that exist in the stroma near the cancer cells or filtrate to the tumors. Scale bars, 200 μm. The interrelationship between (**B**) the Treg counts and TAM counts, (**C**) the Treg counts and the percentage of IL6^{+} cancer cells, and (**D**) the TAM counts and the percentage of IL6+ cancer cells were examined using Spearman's correlation. HPF, high power field; Treg, regulatory T cell; TAM, tumor-associated macrophage; UC, urothelial carcinoma.

2.2. Correlation among Treg, TAM, and IL6 in the Bladder Tumor Microenvironment

IL6 is one of the major pro-inflammatory cytokines in the tumor microenvironment, and promotes cancer progression and therapeutic resistance [13]. To investigate the correlation between Treg, TAM, and IL6+ UC cells, the Spearman correlation coefficient was analyzed among the three markers. There was a weak positive correlation between the counts of Treg and TAM ($p < 0.001$, Figure 1B). The count of TAM, but not Treg ($p = 0.42$, Figure 1C), positively correlated with counts of IL6+ cancer cells ($p = 0.001$, Figure 1D).

2.3. Prognostic Role of Baseline Treg and TAM in NMIBC Treated with Intravesical BCG

In the analysis of 71 patients treated with intravesical BCG, 40 (56%) had recurrence and 17 (24%) developed progression after a median follow-up period of 83 (IQR 61–115) months. To examine the relevance of the studied variables and prognosis, we performed univariate and multivariate analyses for recurrence-free survival (RFS) and progression-free survival (PFS) (Table 2). High counts of Treg and TAM and low tumor grade were associated with shorter recurrence-free survival in the univariate analysis (Figure 2A,B,D,E), while high count of Treg (p = 0.001, hazard ratio (HR) = 3.07, vs. low count) and low tumor grade (p = 0.01, HR = 0.27, vs. high tumor grade) were identified as independent predictors for recurrence. An additional analysis revealed that a high count of Treg was an independent predictor for progression (p = 0.021, HR = 3.43, vs. low count), whereas high counts of TAM showed marginal association with short PFS in the univariate analysis (p = 0.052, HR = 3.35, vs. low count). When patients were stratified into three groups according to the counts of Treg and TAM, 26 (37%) patients exhibited low counts of both, 24 (34%) exhibited a high count of either Treg or TAM, and the remaining 21 (29%) exhibited high counts of both. Both RFS and PFS decreased dramatically as the number of high counts of immune cells increased (Figure 2C,F).

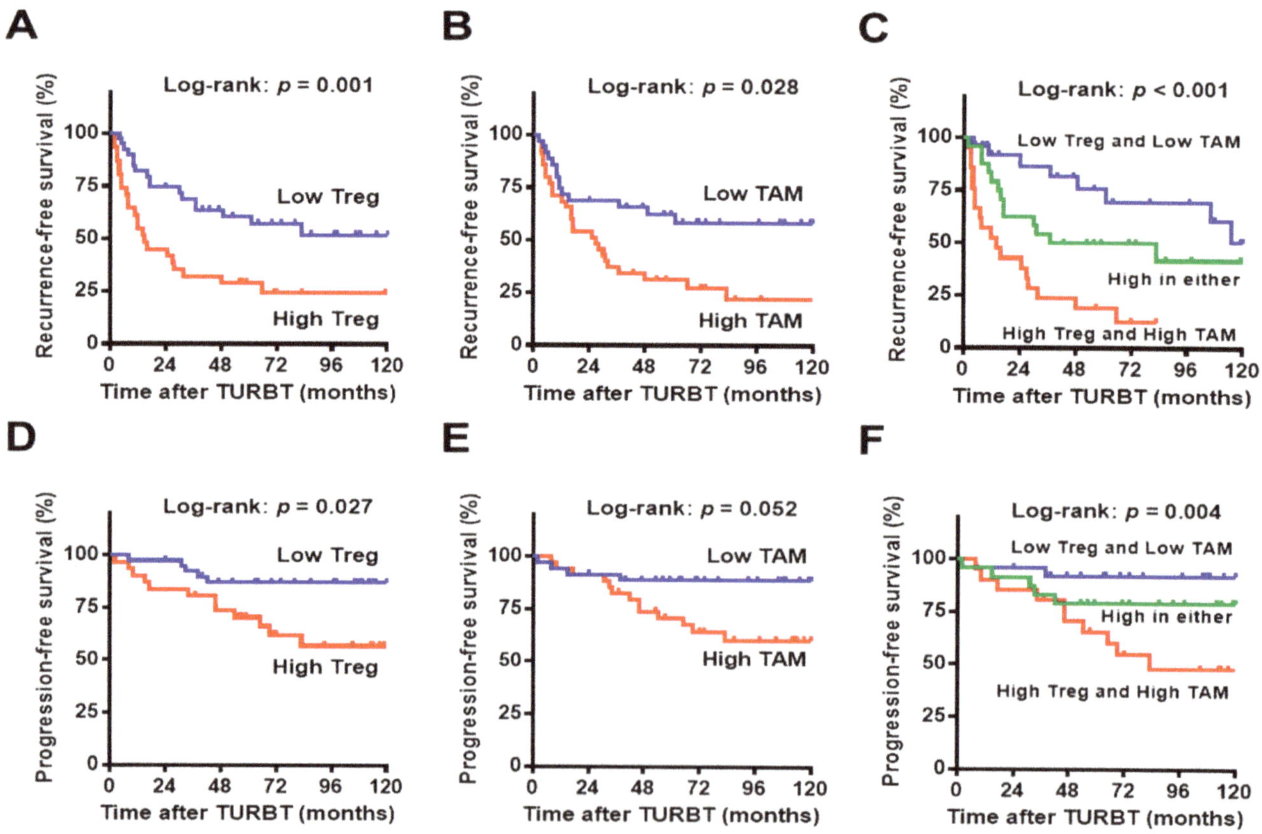

Figure 2. Kaplan–Meier plots for 71 patients treated with intravesical BCG. Intravesical recurrence-free survival (**A**–**C**) and progression-free survival (**D**–**F**) after initial TURBT are plotted. (**A**,**D**) Survival curves according to the Treg count, low (<10 cells/HPF) vs. high (≥10 cells/HPF); (**B**,**E**) survival curves according to the TAM count, low (<25 cells/HPF) vs. high (≥25 cells/HPF); (**C**,**F**) survival curves according to the number of immune cells with high counts (0, blue; 1, green; 2, red). The log-rank test was used for comparison. Treg, regulatory T cell; TAM, tumor-associated macrophage. Author 1, A.B. Title of Thesis. Level of Thesis, Degree-Granting University, Location of University, Date of Completion.

Table 2. The prognostic factors for recurrence and progression in 71 NMIBC patients treated with BCG.

Variables	N	Intravesical Recurrence-Free Survival						Progression-Free Survival					
		Univariate			Multivariate †			Univariate			Multivariate †		
		HR	95% CI	*p* Value	HR	95% CI	*p* Value	HR	95% CI	*p* Value	HR	95% CI	*p* Value
Sex													
Male	63 (89%)	1						1					
Female	8 (11%)	0.64	0.24–1.72	0.52	NA			1.24	0.25–6.21	0.98	NA		
Age													
≤70	37 (52%)	1						1					
>70	34 (48%)	1.05	0.56–1.97	0.91	NA			1.88	0.73–4.86	0.22	NA		
T stage													
Ta or isolated Tis	30 (42%)	1						1					
T1	41 (58%)	1.20	0.64–2.26	0.69	NA			1.29	0.49–3.40	0.81	NA		
Tumor grade													
Low	13 (18%)	1			1			1					
High	58 (82%)	0.68	0.26–0.96	0.04	0.81	0.24–1.16	0.10	1.85	0.56–6.09	0.48	NA		
Multiplicity													
Single	38 (54%)	1						1					
Multiple	33 (46%)	0.74	0.39–1.39	0.78	NA			1.20	0.46–3.15	0.46	NA		
Tumor size													
<3 cm	52 (73%)	1						1					
≥3 cm	19 (27%)	0.76	0.38–1.52	0.58	NA			1.05	0.39–2.87	0.89	NA		
Concomitant CIS													
No	22 (31%)	1						1					
Yes	49 (69%)	0.48	0.24–1.06	0.097	NA			2.48	0.91–6.74	0.14	NA		
Treg													
Low	31 (44%)	1			1			1			1		
High	40 (56%)	2.53	1.32–4.86	0.001	3.07	1.55–6.07	0.001	3.38	1.29–8.88	0.027	3.43	1.20–9.74	0.021
TAM													
Low	35 (49%)	1			1			1			1		
High	36 (51%)	2.31	1.27–4.30	0.029	1.39	0.68–2.84	0.37	3.35	1.29–8.66	0.052	2.50	0.79–8.02	0.12
IL6+ UC cells													
Low	32 (45%)	1						1					
High	39 (55%)	1.36	0.73–2.56	0.22	NA			1.39	0.53–3.61	0.54	NA		

NMIBC, non-muscle invasive bladder cancer; BCG, Bacillus Calmette-Guerin; HR, hazard ratio; CI, confidence interval; CIS, Carcinoma in situ; Treg, regulatory T cell; TAM, Tumor-associated macrophage; UC, urothelial carcinoma; † Multivariate Cox regression analysis; NA, not analyzed.

3. Discussion

This study demonstrates the association between poor responses to intravesical BCG and both Treg and TAM in the tumor microenvironment of human bladder UC. Although it has been decades since intravesical BCG was first introduced for bladder UC treatment in 1976 [14], no molecular biomarkers are available in clinical settings for predicting responses. There is currently little clinical evidence about associations between these tumor-supporting immune cells and resistance to intravesical BCG. A recent report by Pichler et al. investigated the baseline immune environment in NMIBC treated with intravesical BCG by IHC analysis using a total of 10 antibodies. The authors concluded that increased counts of CD4+ and GATA3+ T-cells were associated with prolonged RFS, whereas high counts of TAM and Treg were associated with shortened RFS [10]. Suriano et al. performed detailed population analyses of macrophages in the bladder tumor environment using dual immunofluorescence staining using CD68/iNOS (M1 polarization) and CD68/CD163 (M2 polarization) combinations, suggesting a prognostic value of TAM infiltration for RFS in patients with NMIBC treated with intravesical BCG [12]. One of the major drawbacks in both of these reports is the limited number of patients (only 40 each), which did not allow for multivariate analysis providing reliable prognostic values. Moreover, the topical immune environment, response pattern toward exposure of BCG, and the strains of BCG used can vary among races and countries. Therefore, we conducted the present study to explore the relevance to oncological features in a larger sample size and a Japanese cohort.

Immune cells in the tumor area or in the stroma around the tumor area can influence survival, with either poor or improved prognosis and with either sensitivity or resistance to treatment, depending on their subsets and polarization [10]. Muscle-invasive bladder cancer (MIBC) patients with FOXP3 expression in tumor cells showed shorter survival compared to those with negative cancers [15]. Another report demonstrated that an elevated FOXP3/CD8 ratio in tumor tissues was an independent predictor of poor prognosis after RC [16]. In a multivariate analysis of MIBCs, a high count of CD68+ TAM was correlated with high T category, high-grade cancer [17], and higher risk of cancer-specific death when adjusted for CD3 [18]. Although extensive studies on muscle-invasive bladder cancer have been conducted, there is little information on NMIBC, especially about its response to intravesical BCG. The present study demonstrated that high counts of Treg and TAM acted as a predictor of poor prognosis with a 2.5-fold and 2.3-fold higher risk of recurrence and a 3.38-fold and 3.35-fold higher risk of progression in univariate analysis, respectively (Table 2). These results strongly suggest a possible relationship between resistance to BCG and Treg/TAM in the tumor microenvironment.

Treg plays crucial roles in the evasion of antitumor immunity and escape from response to treatments in various malignancies, leading to poor oncological outcomes [10,19,20]. BCG treatment is known to cause Th1-polarized immunomodulation [21]. Treg can suppress effector mechanisms of the immune response in vaccination models. However, simultaneous inhibition of Th2 polarization and Tregs could promote host-protective immunity [22] and BCG-induced vaccination response using a mouse model through enhanced Th1 polarization [23]. Many studies have demonstrated that TAM cells are markedly present in various malignancies and involved in promoting neoangiogenesis and producing immunoregulatory and immunosuppressive cytokines, culminating in worsened oncological outcomes [24]. Previous studies have stated that the predominant locations of TAM are the stroma and lamina propria [10,25]. However, our analysis showed that a large number of TAM localize in the tumor area in high-grade tumors compared to low-grade tumors. Ayari et al. demonstrated that CD68+ TAM in the stroma or within tumor nests were found to have no predictive value for outcomes after intravesical BCG [26]. Further studies with larger sample sizes are needed to clarify the influence of the predominant location of Treg and TAM on prognostic significance.

IL6 is one of the major pro-inflammatory cytokines in the tumor microenvironment, and exhibits tumor-supporting activities [13,27,28]. In the present study, we examined the correlation between Treg/TAM and IL6 in the bladder tumor microenvironment. There was a positive correlation between the count of TAM and IL6+ UC cells, whereas significant correlation was not observed between the counts of Treg and IL6+ UC cells (Figure 1C,D). This finding is consistent with evidence from previous studies. Hasita et al. investigated the significance of TAM and Treg in patients with intrahepatic cholangiocarcinoma, demonstrating that IL6 production from tumor cells was correlated with the number of infiltrating TAMs, but not with the numbers of Treg cells or vessels [27]. This result supports the idea that IL6 is one of the vital molecules that differentiates macrophages. Another report by Hinz et al. revealed that specific down-regulation of FOXP3 with small interfering RNA in the pancreatic carcinoma cell line Panc89 resulted in the up-regulation of IL6 and IL8 via the activation of nuclear factor-κB (NF-κB), providing evidence for the control of inflammatory cytokine production by FOXP3 [28]. IL8 promotes angiogenesis and growth of cancer cells. However, the biological significance of FOXP3-mediated suppression of IL6 and IL8 production in malignant diseases is not fully understood.

The present study has several limitations. The first is its retrospective nature with potential selection bias; for example, some patients were excluded because of aggressive treatment (immediate radical cystectomy for T1 disease). Second, tumor tissue analysis was performed by immunohistochemistry (IHC) with possible technical biases, for example specimen fixation, antigen retrieval, antibody binding, color development, and quantification, which may affect the interpretation. Third, this study includes 71 patients, which is considered to be a relatively low sample size. Because low sample size constitutes a limitation of the work and to acknowledge this issue, further study including additional tumors and patients is needed to verify our results.

4. Materials and Methods

4.1. Data Collection of the Patients

All subjects gave their informed consent for inclusion before they participated in the study. The study was conducted in accordance with the Declaration of Helsinki, and the protocol was approved by the Ethics Committee of the Nara Medical University (Project identification code: 1630, accepted: 21 August 2017). In total, 154 patients with newly diagnosed NMIBC undergoing TURBT between 2004 and 2013 were enrolled in this study. Clinical information was retrieved from medical charts. All hematoxylin and eosin-stained specimens obtained by initial TURBT were reassessed independently by two experienced uropathologists (Keiji Shimada and Noboru Konishi) to determine T category (2010 American Joint Committee on Cancer TNM Staging system), tumor grade (2004 WHO classification), CIS, and lymphovascular invasion. Follow-up was performed according to our institutional protocol [29].

4.2. Immunohistochemical Staining and Quantification

IHC staining of paraffin-embedded, formalin-fixed tissue blocks was performed using the Histofine SAB-PO kit (Nichirei Co., Tokyo, Japan) as previously described [30,31]. Briefly, the sections were autoclaved for 10 min in 0.01 M citrate buffer (pH 6.0) for antigen retrieval. The primary antibodies were monoclonal mouse anti-FOXP3 (dilution 1/100; Ref. ab20034, Abcam, Cambridge, MA, USA), monoclonal mouse anti-MRS-A (CD204) (dilution 1/2000; Ref. KT022; Trans Genic Inc., Kobe, Japan), and polyclonal rabbit anti-IL6 (dilution 1/500; Ref. sc-1265, Santa Cruz, Dallas, TX, USA).

FOXP3-positive Treg was quantified as previously described [32]. Lymphocytes exhibiting nuclear immunostaining for FOXP3 in the cancerous area were counted in at least five independent HPFs (400×, 0.0625 μm^2). The mean count of each patient was determined by dividing the sum by the number of assessed fields. Similarly, $CD204^{-}$positive TAM in the cancerous area was counted [30]. To quantify the expression level of IL6 in the UC cells, immunoreactive tumor cells were counted in at least five independent fields, and the percentage of positive cells was calculated by dividing that number by the total counted UC cells (1–100%) [30]. The median values (IQR) of total count cells for the quantification of the FOXP3-positive Treg, CD204-positive TAM, and IL6+ cells were 185 (132–125), 185 (132–125), and 221 (158–291), respectively. Evaluation was carried out by two trained investigators (M.M. and Y.T.) in a blind manner, without knowledge of the patients' outcome or other clinicopathological characteristics.

4.3. Adjuvant Intravesical Therapy for NMIBC after TURBT

TURBT was carried out according to a standardized procedure used by all surgeons at the single institute [29]. Because of the study's retrospective nature, the criteria, dosage, and scheme for adjuvant intravesical therapy were not consistent between patients, and depended on the physician's decision. In general, patients with high-risk NMIBC, such as those positive for concomitant CIS, T1 category, and high-grade tumors, were treated with intravesical BCG. A substantial number of patients were given intravesical BCG as initial adjuvant therapy. The schedule for intravesical BCG consisted of weekly instillations for 6–8 consecutive weeks of Immunobladder (BCG Tokyo 172 strain; Japan BCG Laboratory Tokyo, Japan) or ImmuCyst (Connaught strain; Sanofi, Paris, France; currently not being supplied as of October 2017). A single immediate post-TURBT chemotherapy instillation and/or maintenance chemotherapy instillation using anthracyclines or mitomycin-C was given to a subset of the cohort.

4.4. Statistical Analysis

The clinicopathological characteristics were compared using the Mann–Whitney *U* test and Fisher's exact test as appropriate. The interrelationships among the studied parameters were examined using the Spearman correlation coefficient and linear regression analysis. RFS and progression-free survival were calculated from the date of TURBT for the initial TURBT to the date of intravesical recurrence and progression, respectively. Progression was defined as recurrent disease when there was invasion into the muscularis propria ($\geq$T2), lymph node involvement, and/or occurrence of distant metastases. Survival rates were analyzed using the Kaplan–Meier method and compared using the log-rank test for univariate analysis. Multivariate analysis was used to identify independent prognostic variables using a stepwise Cox proportional hazards regression model. IBM SPSS version 21 (SPSS, Inc., Chicago, IL, USA) and PRISM software version 7.00 (GraphPad Software, Inc., San Diego, CA, USA) were used for statistical analyses and data plotting, respectively. Statistical significance in this study was set at $p < 0.05$, and all reported p values were two-sided.

5. Conclusions

We explored the clinical significance of Treg and TAM in the bladder tumor environment, suggesting that the immunological response to intravesical BCG is a complicated mechanism involving multiple subpopulations of immune cells. Moreover, IL6 production from UC cells might play a key role in the induction of TAM and the protection of the cancer cells from BCG treatment. Therefore, disrupting the recruitment of Treg and TAM, in combination with conventional intravesical BCG could be a potential therapeutic approach. Randomized control trials are required to determine the true clinical benefit.

Acknowledgments: We would like to thank Editage (www.editage.jp) for English language editing.

Author Contributions: Makito Miyake, Daisuke Gotoh, Takuya Owari, and Kiyohide Fujimoto contributed to conception and design, and acquisition of patients' data, and analysis and interpretation of data. Yoshihiro Tatsumi, Sayuri Ohnishi, Kenta Ohnishi, Kota Iida, Shunta Hori, Yosuke Morizawa, and Yoshitaka Itami contributed to acquisition of data and interpretation of data. Yasushi Nakai, Takeshi Inoue, Satoshi Anai, Kazumasa Torimoto, and Katsuya Aoki contributed to analysis and interpretation of data. Keiji Shimada, Noboru Konishi, and Nobumichi Tanaka contributed to conception and design and review of pathologic diagnosis of surgical specimens.

Abbreviations

BCG	Bacille Calmette–Guérin
CIS	Carcinoma in situ
FR	Hazard ratio
FOXP3	Forkhead box P3
HPF	High-power microscopic fields
IHC	Immunohistochemistry
IL6	Interleukin-6
LVI	Lymphovascular invasion
MIBC	Muscle-invasive bladder cancer
NF-κB	Nuclear factor-κB
NMIBC	Non-muscle invasive bladder cancer
PFS	Progression-free survival
RC	Radical cystectomy
RFS	Recurrence-free survival
TAM	Tumor-associated macrophage
TURBT	Transurethral resection of bladder tumor
Treg	Regulatory T cell
UC	Urothelial carcinoma

References

1. Miyake, M.; Fujimoto, K.; Hirao, Y. Active surveillance for nonmuscle invasive bladder cancer. *Investig. Clin. Urol.* **2016**, *57* (Suppl. S1), S4–S13. [CrossRef] [PubMed]
2. Fernandez-Gomez, J.; Madero, R.; Solsona, E. Predicting nonmuscle invasive bladder cancer recurrence and progression in patients treated with bacillus Calmette-Guerin: The CUETO scoring model. *J. Urol.* **2009**, *182*, 2195–2203. [CrossRef] [PubMed]
3. Sylvester, R.J.; van der Meijden, A.P.; Oosterlinck, W. Predicting recurrence and progression in individual patients with stage Ta T1 bladder cancer using EORTC risk tables: A combined analysis of 2596 patients from seven EORTC trials. *Eur. Urol.* **2006**, *49*, 466–477. [CrossRef] [PubMed]
4. Witjes, J.A.; Compérat, E.; Cowan, N.C.; De Santis, M.; Gakis, G.; Lebret, T.; Ribal, M.J.; Van der Heijden, A.G.; Sherif, A.; European Association of Urology. EAU guidelines on muscle-invasive and metastatic bladder cancer: Summary of the 2013 guidelines. *Eur. Urol.* **2014**, *65*, 778–792. [CrossRef] [PubMed]
5. Reis, L.O.; Moro, J.C.; Ribeiro, L.F.; Voris, B.R.; Sadi, M.V. Are we following the guidelines on non-muscle invasive bladder cancer? *Int. Braz. J. Urol.* **2016**, *42*, 22–28. [CrossRef] [PubMed]
6. Lamm, D.L.; Blumenstein, B.A.; Crawford, E.D. A randomized trial of intravesical doxorubicin and immunotherapy with bacilli Calmette-Guerin for transitional-cell carcinoma of the bladder. *N. Engl. J. Med.* **1991**, *325*, 1205–1209. [CrossRef] [PubMed]
7. Raj, G.V.; Herr, H.; Serio, A.M.; Donat, S.M.; Bochner, B.H.; Vickers, A.J.; Dalbagni, G. Treatment paradigm shift may improve survival of patients with high risk superficial bladder cancer. *J. Urol.* **2007**, *177*, 1283–1286. [CrossRef] [PubMed]
8. Kitamura, H.; Tsukamoto, T. Immunotherapy for urothelial carcinoma: Current status and perspectives. *Cancers* **2011**, *3*, 3055–3071. [CrossRef] [PubMed]
9. Abebe, F. Is interferon-gamma the right marker for bacilli Calmette-Guérin-induced immune protection? The missing link in our understanding of tuberculosis immunology. *Clin. Exp. Immunol.* **2012**, *169*, 213–219. [CrossRef] [PubMed]
10. Pichler, R.; Fritz, J.; Zavadil, C.; Schäfer, G.; Culig, Z.; Brunner, A. Tumor-infiltrating immune cell subpopulations influence the oncologic outcome after intravesical Bacillus Calmette-Guérin therapy in bladder cancer. *Oncotarget* **2016**, *7*, 39916–39930. [CrossRef] [PubMed]
11. Nunez-Nateras, R.; Castle, E.P.; Protheroe, C.A.; Stanton, M.L.; Ocal, T.I.; Ferrigni, E.N.; Ochkur, S.I.; Jacobsen, E.A.; Hou, Y.X.; Andrews, P.E.; et al. Predicting response to bacillus Calmette-Guérin (BCG) in patients with carcinoma in situ of the bladder. *Urol. Oncol.* **2014**, *32*, e23–e30. [CrossRef] [PubMed]

12. Suriano, F.; Santini, D.; Perrone, G.; Amato, M.; Vincenzi, B.; Tonini, G.; Muda, A.; Boggia, S.; Buscarini, M.; Pantano, F. Tumor associated macrophages polarization dictates the efficacy of BCG instillation in non-muscle invasive urothelial bladder cancer. *J. Exp. Clin. Cancer Res.* **2013**, *32*, 87. [CrossRef] [PubMed]
13. Kumari, N.; Dwarakanath, B.S.; Das, A.; Bhatt, A.N. Role of interleukin-6 in cancer progression and therapeutic resistance. *Tumour Biol.* **2016**, *37*, 11553–11572. [CrossRef] [PubMed]
14. Morales, A.; Eidinger, D.; Bruce, A.W. Intracavitary Bacillus Calmette-Guerin in the treatment of superficial bladder tumors. *J. Urol.* **1976**, *116*, 180–183. [CrossRef]
15. Winerdal, M.E.; Marits, P.; Winerdal, M.; Hasan, M.; Rosenblatt, R.; Tolf, A.; Selling, K.; Sherif, A.; Winqvist, O. FOXP3 and survival in urinary bladder cancer. *BJU Int.* **2011**, *108*, 1672–1678. [CrossRef] [PubMed]
16. Horn, T.; Laus, J.; Seitz, A.K.; Maurer, T.; Schmid, S.C.; Wolf, P.; Haller, B.; Winkler, M.; Retz, M.; Nawroth, R.; et al. The prognostic effect of tumour-infiltrating lymphocytic subpopulations in bladder cancer. *World J. Urol.* **2016**, *34*, 181–187. [CrossRef] [PubMed]
17. Boström, M.M.; Irjala, H.; Mirtti, T.; Taimen, P.; Kauko, T.; Ålgars, A.; Jalkanen, S.; Boström, P.J. Tumor-Associated Macrophages Provide Significant Prognostic Information in Urothelial Bladder Cancer. *PLoS ONE* **2015**, *10*, e0133552. [CrossRef] [PubMed]
18. Sjödahl, G.; Lövgren, K.; Lauss, M.; Chebil, G.; Patschan, O.; Gudjonsson, S.; Månsson, W.; Fernö, M.; Leandersson, K.; Lindgren, D.; et al. Infiltration of CD3+ and CD68+ cells in bladder cancer is subtype specific and interacts the outcome of patients with muscle-invasive tumors. *Urol. Oncol.* **2014**, *32*, 791–797. [CrossRef] [PubMed]
19. Mahmoud, S.M.; Paish, E.C.; Powe, D.G.; Macmillan, R.D.; Lee, A.H.; Ellis, I.O.; Green, A.R. An evaluation of the clinical significance of FOXP3+ infiltrating cells in human breast cancer. *Breast Cancer Res. Treat.* **2011**, *127*, 99–108. [CrossRef] [PubMed]
20. Shimizu, K.; Nakata, M.; Hirami, Y.; Yukawa, T.; Maeda, A.; Tanemoto, K. Tumor-infiltrating FOXP3+ regulatory T cells are correlated with cyclooxygenase-2 expression and are associated with recurrence in resected non-small cell lung cancer. *J. Thorac. Oncol.* **2010**, *5*, 585–590. [CrossRef] [PubMed]
21. Ponticiello, A.; Perna, F.; Maione, S.; Stradolini, M.; Testa, G.; Terrazzano, G.; Ruggiero, G.; Malerba, M.; Sanduzzi, A. Analysis of local T lymphocyte subsets upon stimulation with intravesical BCG: A model to study tuberculosis immunity. *Respir. Med.* **2004**, *98*, 509–514. [CrossRef] [PubMed]
22. Bhattacharya, D.; Dwivedi, V.P.; Maiga, M.; Maiga, M.; Van Kaer, L.; Bishai, W.R.; Das, G. Small molecule-directed immunotherapy against recurrent infection by Mycobacterium tuberculosis. *J. Biol. Chem.* **2014**, *289*, 16508–16515. [CrossRef] [PubMed]
23. Bhattacharya, D.; Dwivedi, V.P.; Kumar, S.; Reddy, M.C.; Van Kaer, L.; Moodley, P.; Das, G. Simultaneous inhibition of T helper 2 and T regulatory cell differentiation by small molecules enhances Bacillus Calmette-Guerin vaccine efficacy against tuberculosis. *J. Biol. Chem.* **2014**, *289*, 33404–33411. [CrossRef] [PubMed]
24. Pollard, J.W. Tumour-educated macrophages promote tumour progression and metastasis. *Nat. Rev. Cancer* **2004**, *4*, 71–78. [CrossRef] [PubMed]
25. Takayama, H.; Nishimura, K.; Tsujimura, A.; Nakai, Y.; Nakayama, M.; Aozasa, K.; Okuyama, A.; Nonomura, N. Increased infiltration of tumor associated macrophages is associated with poor prognosis of bladder carcinoma in situ after intravesical bacillus Calmette-Guerin instillation. *J. Urol.* **2009**, *181*, 1894–1900. [CrossRef] [PubMed]
26. Ayari, C.; LaRue, H.; Hovington, H.; Decobert, M.; Harel, F.; Bergeron, A.; Têtu, B.; Lacombe, L.; Fradet, Y. Bladder tumor infiltrating mature dendritic cells and macrophages as predictors of response to bacillus Calmette-Guérin immunotherapy. *Eur. Urol.* **2009**, *55*, 1386–1395. [CrossRef] [PubMed]
27. Hasita, H.; Komohara, Y.; Okabe, H.; Masuda, T.; Ohnishi, K.; Lei, X.F.; Beppu, T.; Baba, H.; Takeya, M. Significance of alternatively activated macrophages in patients with intrahepatic cholangiocarcinoma. *Cancer Sci.* **2010**, *101*, 1913–1919. [CrossRef] [PubMed]
28. Hinz, S.; Pagerols-Raluy, L.; Oberg, H.H.; Ammerpohl, O.; Grüssel, S.; Sipos, B.; Grützmann, R.; Pilarsky, C.; Ungefroren, H.; Saeger, H.D.; et al. FOXP3 expression in pancreatic carcinoma cells as a novel mechanism of immune evasion in cancer. *Cancer Res.* **2007**, *67*, 8344–8350. [CrossRef] [PubMed]

29. Miyake, M.; Gotoh, D.; Shimada, K.; Tatsumi, Y.; Nakai, Y.; Anai, S.; Torimoto, K.; Aoki, K.; Tanaka, N.; Konishi, N.; et al. Exploration of risk factors predicting outcomes for primary T1 high-grade bladder cancer and validation of the Spanish Urological Club for Oncological Treatment scoring model: Long-term follow-up experience at a single institute. *Int. J. Urol.* **2015**, *22*, 541–547. [CrossRef] [PubMed]
30. Miyake, M.; Hori, S.; Morizawa, Y.; Tatsumi, Y.; Nakai, Y.; Anai, S.; Torimoto, K.; Aoki, K.; Tanaka, N.; Shimada, K.; et al. CXCL1-Mediated Interaction of Cancer Cells with Tumor-Associated Macrophages and Cancer-Associated Fibroblasts Promotes Tumor Progression in Human Bladder Cancer. *Neoplasia* **2016**, *18*, 636–646. [CrossRef] [PubMed]
31. Miyake, M.; Hori, S.; Morizawa, Y.; Tatsumi, Y.; Toritsuka, M.; Ohnishi, S.; Shimada, K.; Furuya, H.; Khadka, V.S.; Deng, Y.; et al. Collagen type IV alpha 1 (COL4A1) and collagen type XIII alpha 1 (COL13A1) produced in cancer cells promote tumor budding at the invasion front in human urothelial carcinoma of the bladder. *Oncotarget* **2017**, *8*, 36099–36114. [CrossRef] [PubMed]
32. Schwarz, S.; Butz, M.; Morsczeck, C.; Reichert, T.E.; Driemel, O. Increased number of CD25+ FOXP3+ regulatory T cells in oral squamous cell carcinomas detected by chromogenic immunohistochemical double staining. *J. Oral Pathol. Med.* **2008**, *37*, 485–489. [CrossRef] [PubMed]

12

Transgelin, a p53 and PTEN-Upregulated Gene, Inhibits the Cell Proliferation and Invasion of Human Bladder Carcinoma Cells: In Vitro and In Vivo

Ke-Hung Tsui [1,†], Yu-Hsiang Lin [1,2,†], Kang-Shuo Chang [3,4], Chen-Pang Hou [1,2], Pin-Jung Chen [3,4], Tsui-Hsia Feng [5] and Horng-Heng Juang [1,3,4,*]

1 Department of Urology, Chang Gung Memorial Hospital-Linkou, Kwei-Shan, Tao-Yuan 33302, Taiwan; t2130@cgmh.org.tw (K.-H.T.); linyh@doctorvoice.org (Y.-H.L.); glucose1979@gmail.com (C.-P.H.)
2 Graduate Institute of Clinical Medical Science, College of Medicine, Chang Gung University, Kwei-Shan, Tao-Yuan 33302, Taiwan
3 Department of Anatomy, College of Medicine, Chang Gung University, Kwei-Shan, Tao-Yuan 33302, Taiwan; D0501301@stmail.cgu.edu.tw (K.-S.C.); lulu581623@gmail.com (P.-J.C.)
4 Graduate Institute of Biomedical Sciences, College of Medicine, Chang Gung University, Kwei-Shan, Tao-Yuan 33302, Taiwan
5 School of Nursing, College of Medicine, Chang Gung University, Kwei-Shan, Tao-Yuan 33302, Taiwan; thf@mail.cgu.edu.tw
* Correspondence: hhj143@mail.cgu.edu.tw
† These authors contributed equally to this work.

Abstract: Transgelin (TAGLN/SM22-α) is a regulator of the actin cytoskeleton, affecting the survival, migration, and apoptosis of various cancer cells divergently; however, the roles of TAGLN in bladder carcinoma cells remain inconclusive. We compared expressions of TAGLN in human bladder carcinoma cells to the normal human bladder tissues to determine the potential biological functions and regulatory mechanisms of TAGLN in bladder carcinoma cells. Results of RT-qPCR and immunoblot assays indicated that TAGLN expressions were higher in bladder smooth muscle cells, fibroblast cells, and normal epithelial cells than in carcinoma cells (RT-4, HT1376, TSGH-8301, and T24) in vitro. Besides, the results of RT-qPCR revealed that TAGLN expressions were higher in normal tissues than the paired tumor tissues. In vitro, TAGLN knockdown enhanced cell proliferation and invasion, while overexpression of TAGLN had the inverse effects in bladder carcinoma cells. Meanwhile, ectopic overexpression of TAGLN attenuated tumorigenesis in vivo. Immunofluorescence and immunoblot assays showed that TAGLN was predominantly in the cytosol and colocalized with F-actin. Ectopic overexpression of either p53 or PTEN induced TAGLN expression, while p53 knockdown downregulated TAGLN expression in bladder carcinoma cells. Our results indicate that TAGLN is a p53 and PTEN-upregulated gene, expressing higher levels in normal bladder epithelial cells than carcinoma cells. Further, TAGLN inhibited cell proliferation and invasion in vitro and blocked tumorigenesis in vivo. Collectively, it can be concluded that TAGLN is an antitumor gene in the human bladder.

Keywords: bladder; TAGLN; F-actin; PTEN; p53; tumorigenesis; proliferation; invasion

---

1. Introduction

Transglin/SM22-α/WS3-10/mp27 (TAGLN), a kind of 22-kDa protein, presents primarily in smooth muscle-containing tissues of vertebrates. Cytogenetically, the human TAGLN gene is located to the chromosome 11 q23.2 [1]. When using the TAGLN-deficient mouse embryo model, TAGLN may not be required for the development of the embryo, but plays roles in the morphological transformation of the smooth muscle cell (SMC) [2]. A study has found that decreased levels of TAGLN disrupted normal actin organization leading to the changes in the motile behavior of REF52 fibroblast cells [3]. The depletion of TAGLN resulted in an increase in the capacity of cells to go initiate spontaneous podosome formation, with a concomitant increase in the ability of invasion from Matrigel assays; therefore, TAGLN seemed to be a marker of active stromal remodeling in vicinity of invasive carcinomas [4].

The reduction in the expressions of TAGLN are often found in tumor cell lines, and the TAGLN depletion increases actin dynamics and enhances tumorigenic phenotypes of the cells [3]. Early study indicated that abolition of TAGLN expression is an important early event in tumor progression and a diagnostic marker for breast and colon cancer development [5]. However, issues concerning the tumorigenesis of TAGLN in different tissues are still in controversy. Studies have reported that TAGLN is an antitumor gene in esophageal squamous cell carcinoma and regarded as an oncogene for gastric cancer [6–8]. Other studies indicated that TAGLN exerts an anti-metastasis effect in colon and colorectal cancers [9–13]. However, contrary results from different independent laboratories showed that overexpression of TAGLN causes a poor prognosis in colon cancer in vivo and contributes to colorectal cancer progression and metastasis [14,15]. Similar, contrary reports are also found in studies of lung cancer [16,17].

An early study of rabbit bladders suggested that TAGLN is an SMC-lineage marker [18]. However, previous studies indicated that *TAGLN* is one of the common differentially-expressed genes which is significantly decreased in bladder cancer compared with normal bladder tissues [19,20]. The precise functions and the regulatory mechanisms of *TAGLN* in the bladder carcinoma cells are still not illustrated and explored.

In this study, we determined the expressions of *TAGLN* in both bladder carcinoma cells and bladder tissues, and examined the regulatory mechanisms and potential functions of *TAGLN* in bladder carcinoma cells.

2. Results

2.1. *Expressions of TAGLN in Bladder Smooth Muscle Cells, Fibroblast Cells, Normal Epithelial Cells, and Carcinoma Cells*

To understand the expression of TAGLN in human bladder cells, we compared levels of TAGLN in human normal primary bladder epithelial cells (HBdEC), bladder smooth muscle cells (HBdSMC), bladder stromal fibroblasts (HBdSF), and four lines of cultured bladder carcinoma cells (RT4, HT1376, T24, and TSGH-8301). Results of RT-qPCR assays revealed that levels of *TAGLN* were higher in both HBdSMC and HBdEC cells than the bladder carcinoma cells (Figure 1A). Further immunoblot assays showed that T24 cells expressed the highest TAGLN protein levels among the four carcinoma cell lines (Figure 1B) which were similar to the results of RT-qPCR assays presented in the Figure 1A. The immunoblot assays also revealed that HBdSMC cells expressed higher protein levels of alpha-smooth muscle actin (α-SMA), and HBdEC cells exhibited higher protein levels of uroplakin-2 (UPK-2), a marker of bladder transitional cells (Figure 1C). The normal primary bladder epithelial cells (HBdEC) presented far higher TAGLN protein levels in comparison to the bladder carcinoma T24 cells (Figure 1D).

2.2. *Expressions of TAGLN in Paired Human Bladder Tissues*

The RT-qPCR analysis of paired human bladder tissues showed that means of $\Delta\Delta C_t$ between normal and cancer tissues were 3.77 ± 0.67 using *β-actin* as internal control (Figure 1E) and 4.33 ± 0.72 using *18S* as internal control (Figure 1F), respectively, suggesting significantly higher expressions of *TAGLN* mRNA levels in normal bladder tissues than that in bladder cancer tissues.

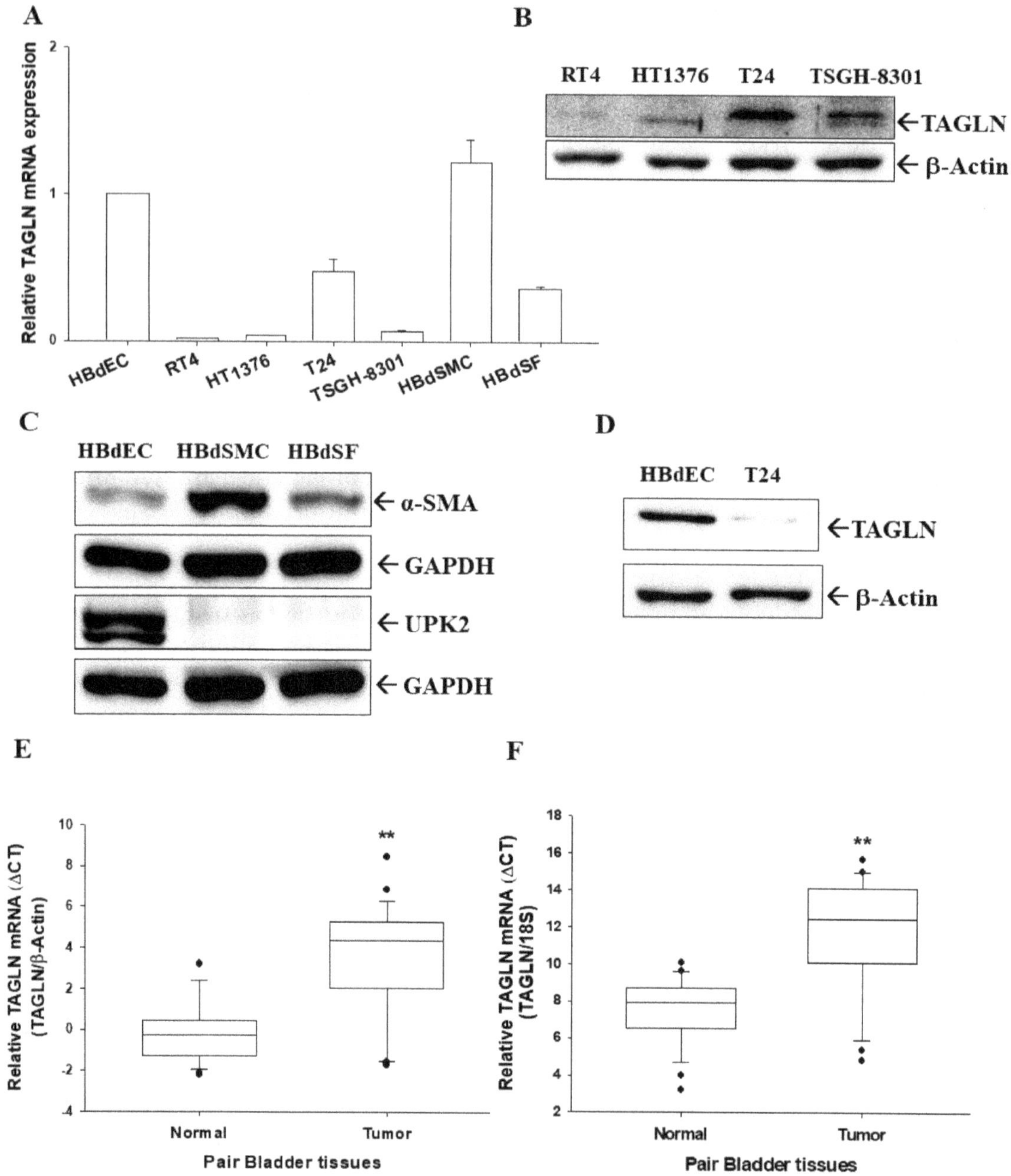

Figure 1. Gene expression of *TAGLN* in human bladder cells and tissues. (**A**) Total RNA from bladder smooth muscle cells (HBdSMC), fibroblast cells (HBdSF), normal epithelial cells (HBdEC), and carcinoma cell lines (RT4, HT1376, T24, and TSGH-8301) were extracted for RT-qPCR (± SE; $n = 3$) assays. (**B**) Bladder carcinoma cell lines (RT4, HT1376, T24, and TSGH-8301) were lysed, and TAGLN and β-actin were determined by immunoblotting. (**C**) HBdEC, HBdSMC, and HBdSF cells were lysed and α-SMA, UPK2, and GAPDH were determined by immunoblotting. (**D**) HBdEC and T24 cells were lysed and TAGLN and β-actin were determined by immunoblotting. Quantitative analysis of TAGLN expression in paired bladder cancerous and normal tissues was determined by RT-qPCR using the β-actin (**E**) or 18S (**F**) as the internal control. Box plot analysis was used to compare the TAGLN expressions in cancerous and normal bladder tissues ($n = 25$). ** represented the $p < 0.01$.

2.3. TAGLN's Localization is Predominantly Cytosolic and with F-actin

In order to understand the subcellular location of TAGLN in the bladder carcinoma cells, we transiently overexpressed TAGLN in HT1376 cells. Results of immunofluorescence staining indicated that HT-TAGLN cells expressed higher protein levels of TAGLN, located predominantly in the cytosol, in comparison to HT-DNA cells (Figure 2A,E). The cells were also stained with Texas Red X-Phalloidin to determine the F-actin (Figure 2B,F), and DAPI to highlight the nuclei of HT-DNA and HT-TAGLN cells (Figure 2C,G). Results of immunofluorescence indicated that TAGLN expression colocalized with F-actin (Figure 2D,H). Further study of immunoblot assays with subcellular extraction confirmed the ectopic-TAGLN expression in HT1376 cells (HT-TAGLN). Expression was predominantly present in the cytoplasm, with a little expression in the membrane. TAGLN did not express in the nuclei of HT-DNA and HT-TAGLN cells (Figure 2I).

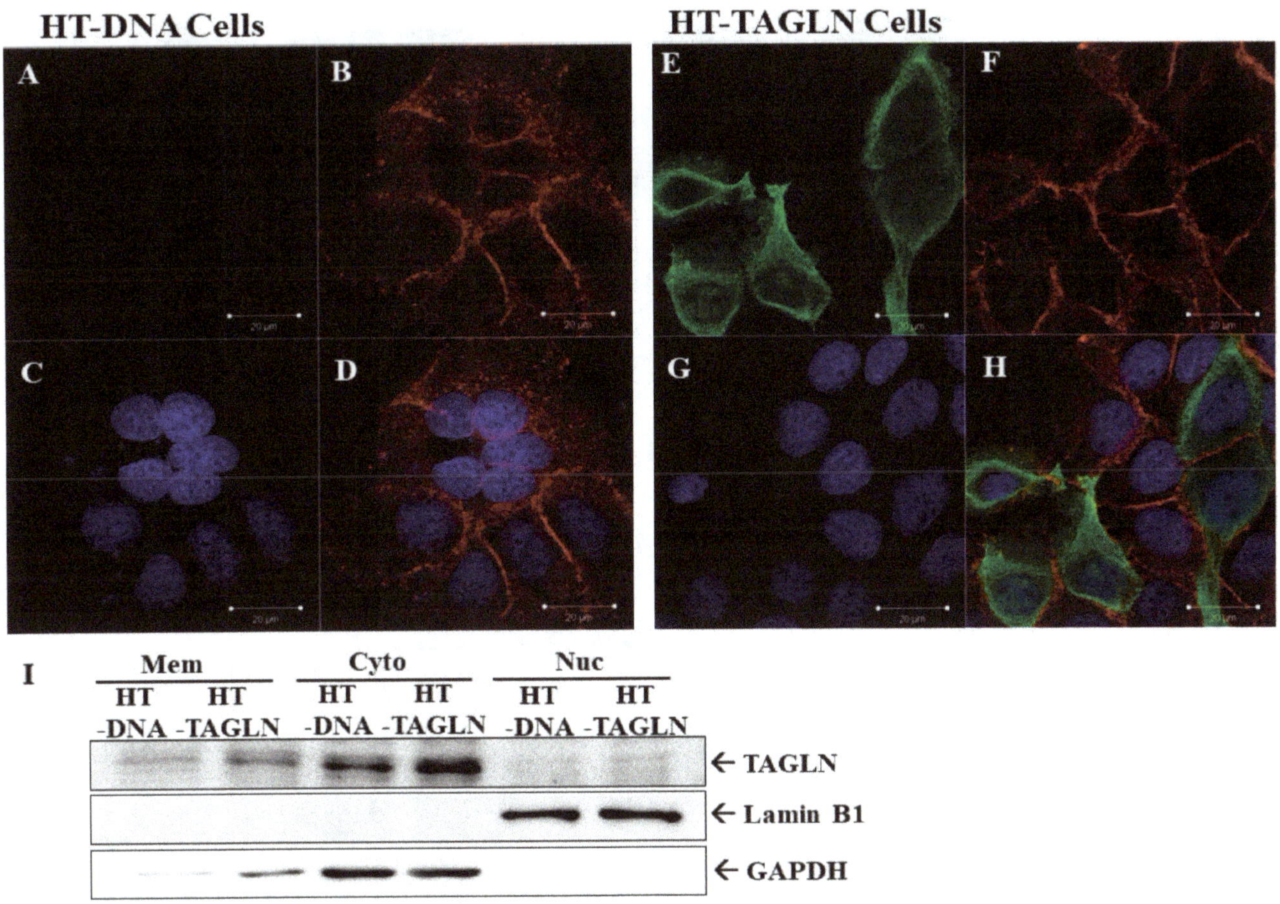

Figure 2. Immunofluorescence staining of TAGLN in TAGLN-overexpressed-HT1376 cells. Immunofluorescence detection of TAGLN in mock-transfected HT1376 (HT-DNA) (**A**) and TAGLN-overexpressed HT1376 (HT-TAGLN) (**E**) cells. The red-stained with Texas Red X-Phalloidin represents the F-actin (**B**,**F**). The blue-stained by DAPI represents nuclei of cells (**C**,**G**). All images were observed and recorded under the same settings with a confocal microscope. Immunofluorescence results indicated that TAGLN expression colocalized with F-actin (**D**,**H**). (**I**) Cells were subcellularly extracted into the membrane (Mem), cytosol (Cyto), and nuclei (Nuc). The protein levels of TAGLN, Lamin B, and GAPDH were determined using immunoblot assays.

2.4. The Effects of TAGLN on Cell Proliferation in Bladder Carcinoma Cells

Using immunoblot and RT-qPCR assays, we confirmed that expression of *TAGLN* was about 50% in the TAGLN-knockdown T24 cells compared to mock-knockdown (T24_shCOL) cells (Figure 3A). The results of EdU flow cytometry (Figure 3C) and EdU staining proliferation (Figure 3D) assays showed that knockdown of TAGLN (T24_shTAGLN) increased 10% and 9% of cells with EdU-staining compared to mock-transduced (T24_shCOL) cells, respectively. Opposite results were found for ectopic overexpression of TAGLN in HT1376 cells. Figure 3B confirmed the ectopic overexpression of TAGLN in HT1376 (HT-TAGLN) cells compared to mock-transfected HT1376 (HT-DNA) cells, as determined by immunoblot and RT-qPCR assays. When cells were overexpressed the TAGLN, the percentage of positive cells with EdU incorporation were decreased, which was determined by flow cytometry (Figure 3E) and EdU staining proliferation (Figure 3F) assays. Decreasing cell proliferation after ectopic overexpression of TAGLN was also found in the TAGLN-overexpressed HT1376 and TSGH-8301 cells, respectively, determined by Ki67 proliferation assays (Figure S1).

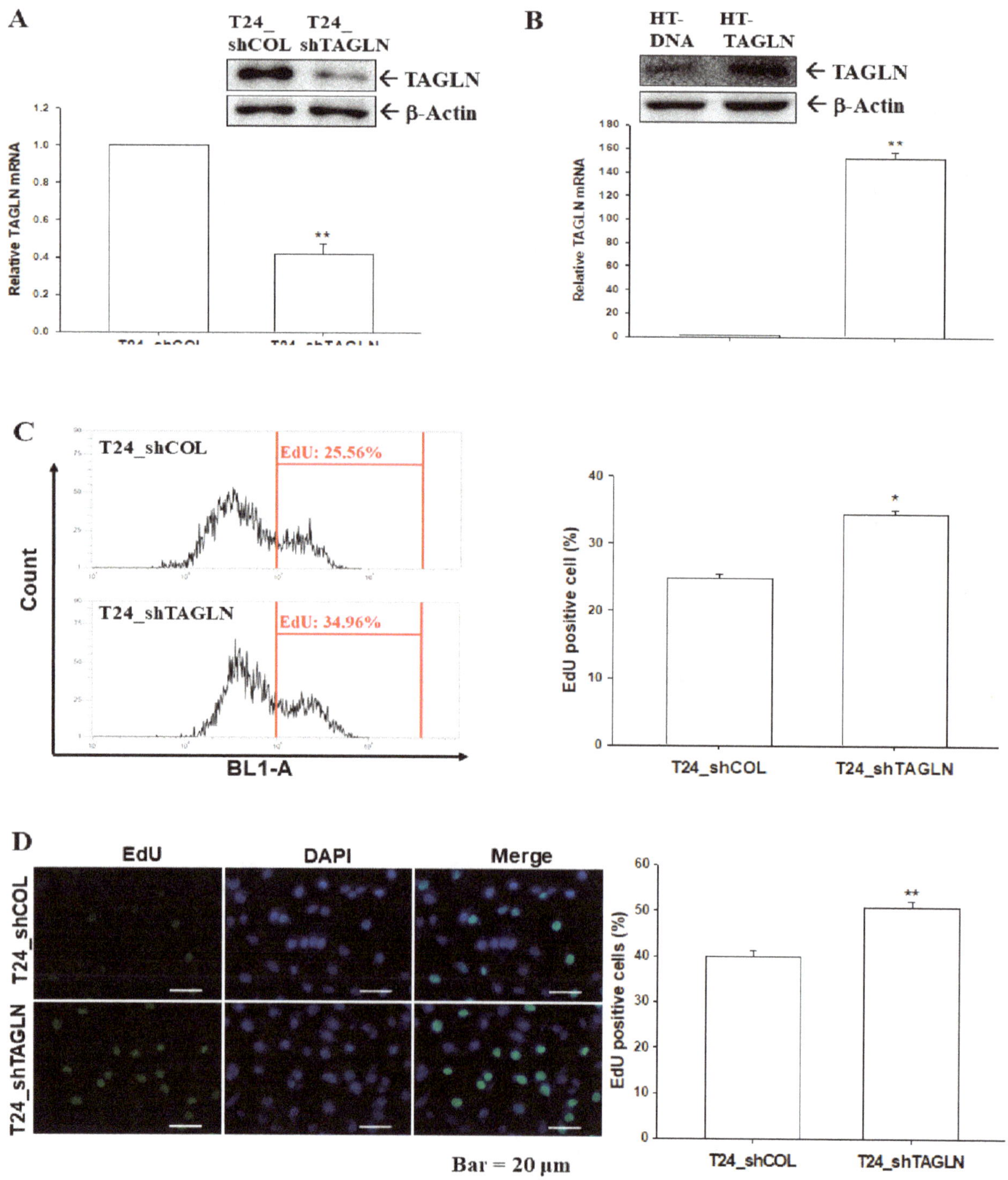

Figure 3. *Cont.*

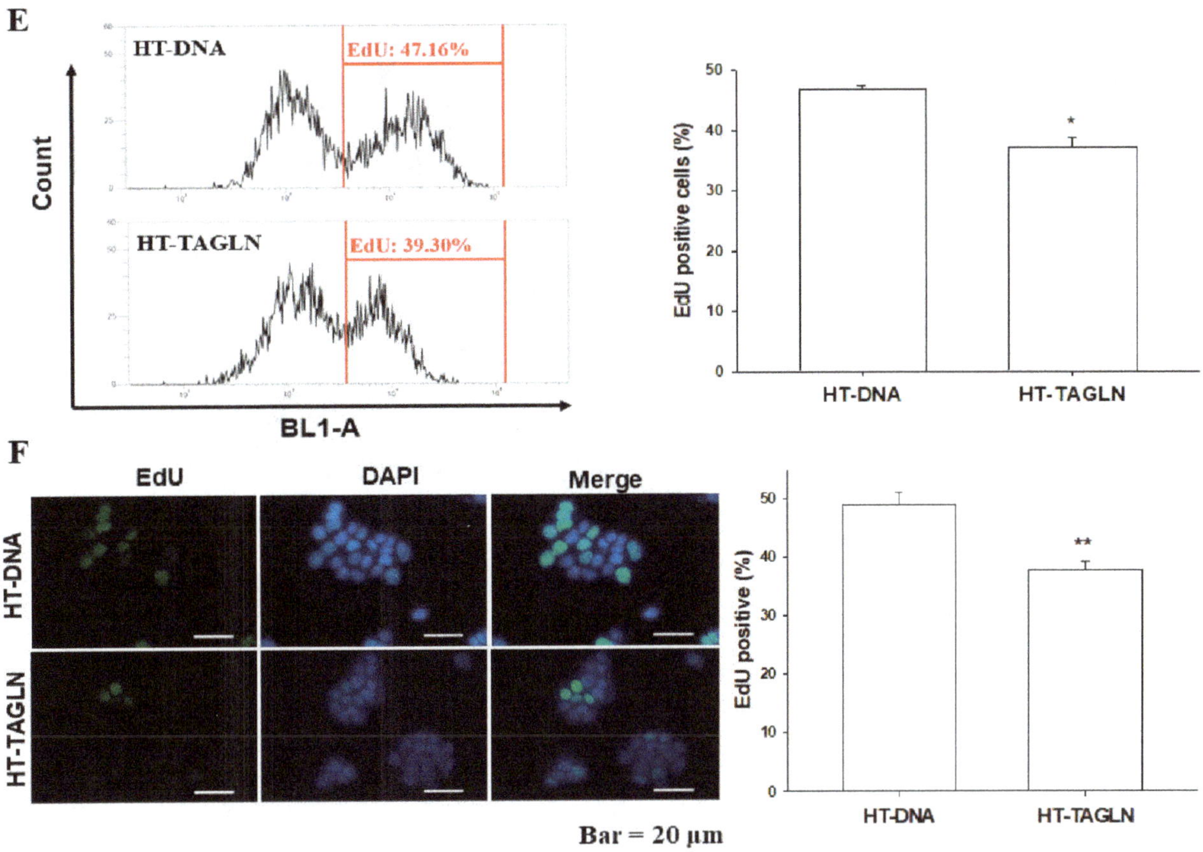

Figure 3. The effects of TAGLN on the cell proliferation of bladder carcinoma cells. The expressions of TAGLN in T24-knockdown T24 (T24_shTAGLN) cells (**A**) and ectopic TAGLN-overexpressed HT1376 (HT-TAGLN) cells (**B**) in comparison to mock-transfected control cells (T24_shCOL and HT-DNA) were determined by immunoblot (top) and RT-qPCR (bottom) assays (± SE; $n = 3$). The proliferation abilities of T24_shCOL and T24_shTAGLN cells were determined by flow cytometry with Click-iT EdU flow cytometry assays (**C**) and EdU cell immunofluorescence staining (± SE; $n = 4$) (**D**). The proliferation abilities of HT-DNA and HT-TAGLN cells were determined by flow cytometry with (**E**) Click-iT EdU flow cytometry assays and (**F**) EdU cell immunofluorescence staining (± SE; $n = 4$). * represented the $p < 0.05$ and the ** represented the $p < 0.01$.

2.5. The Effects of TAGLN on Cell Invasion in Bladder Carcinoma Cells

The results of Matrigel invasion assays indicated that the knockdown of TAGLN resulted in a two-fold increase in invasion capacity compared to T24_shCOL cells (Figure 4A). On the contrary, the invasion capacity was downregulated 45% in HT-TAGLN cell compared to HT-DNA cells (Figure 4B). We further cloned the TAGLN-overexpressed TSGH-8301 (8301-TAGLN) cells (Figure 4C) and the TAGLN-knockdown TSGH-8301 (8301_shTAGLN) cells (Figure 4D) to confirm the expression of TAGLN by immunoblot and RT-qPCR assays. The Matrigel invasion assays showed that 8301-TAGLN cells expressed markedly lower invasive capacity than 8301-DNA cells (Figure 4E), while the knockdown of TAGLN in bladder carcinoma TSGH-8301 cells enhanced cell invasion (Figure 4F). Results of wound healing assays also revealed the decreased migration ability of HT1376 cell after the ectopic overexpression of TAGLN (Figure S2).

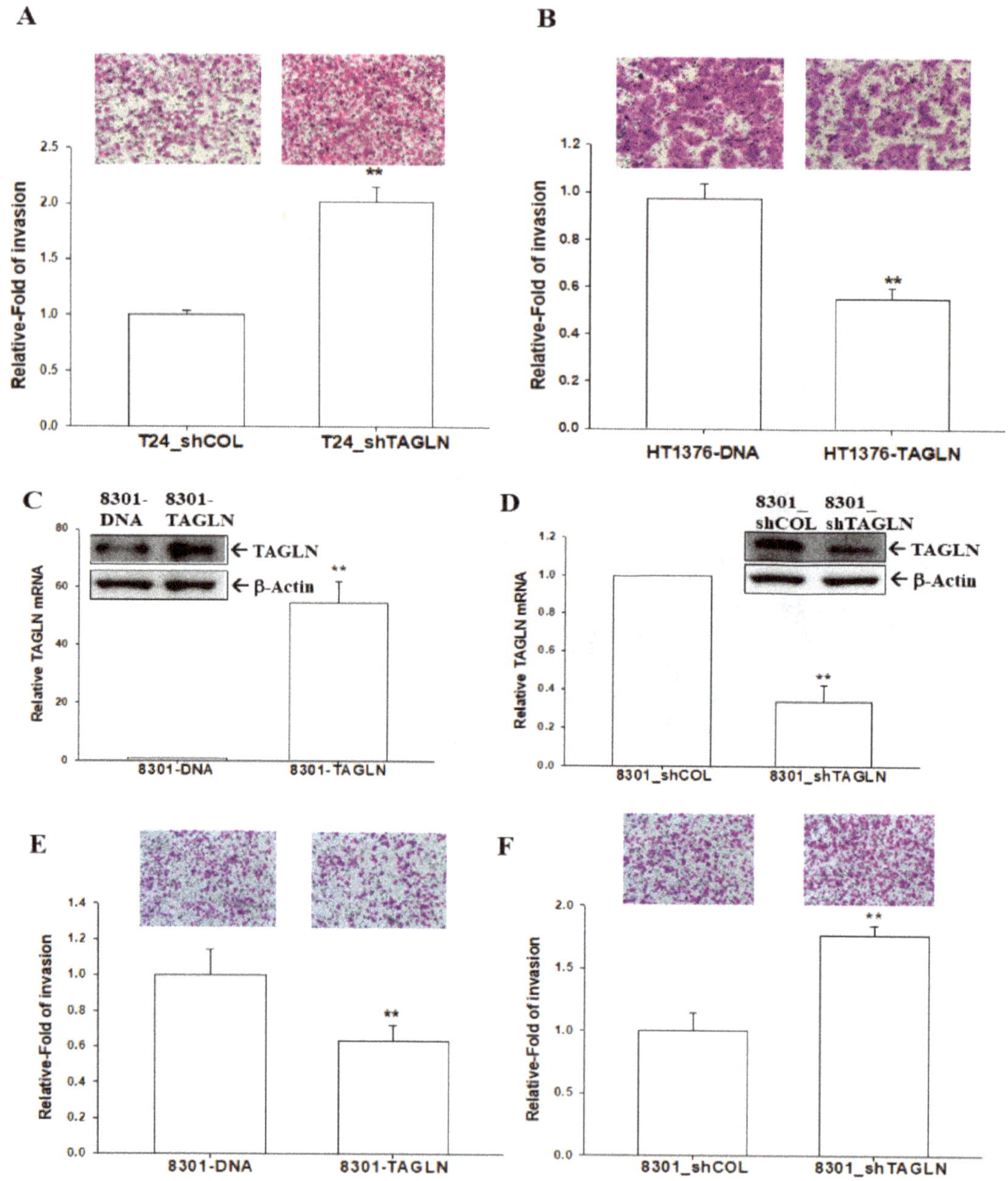

Figure 4. Modulation of TAGLN on cell invasion in bladder carcinoma cells. The invasion abilities of cells were determined by in vitro Matrigel invasion assays. Data are presented as mean percentages (± SE; $n = 3$) in relation to those of the T24_shCOL (**A**) or HT-DNA (**B**) groups. (**C**) Expressions of TAGLN in mock-transfected TSGH-8301 (8301-DNA) and ectopic TAGLN overexpression TSGH-8301 (8301-TAGLN) cells were determined by immunoblotting (top) and RT-qPCR (bottom) assays (± SE; $n = 3$). (**D**) Expressions of TAGLN in mock-knockdown TSGH-8301 (8301_shCOL) and TAGLN-knockdown TSGH-8301 (8301_shTAGLN) cells were determined using immunoblot (top) and RT-qPCR (bottom) assays (± SE; $n = 3$). The invasion abilities of cells were determined by in vitro Matrigel invasion assays. Data are presented as mean percentages (± SE; $n = 3$) in relation to those of the 8301-DNA (**E**) or (**F**) 8301_shCOL groups. ** represented the $p < 0.01$.

2.6. The Effect of the Ectopic Overexpression of TAGLN on the Tumorigenesis of Bladder Carcinoma HT1376 Cells

The effect of TAGLN on tumor growth in vivo was evaluated by using xenografts in BALB/cAnN-Foxn1^{NU} mice. Tumors generated from HT-DNA cells (Figure 5A) grew faster than those derived from HT-TAGLN cells (Figure 5B). There were no significant differences in the mean body weights of animals between the two groups (Figure 5C). Additionally, tumors generated from HT-TAGLN cells were approximately 26% smaller than the tumors generated from HT-DNA (93.11 ± 19.73 versus 364.13 ± 60.83 mm^3) after 46 days of growth (Figure 5D). The weight of tumors derived from HT-DNA cells was about four times that from the group of HT-TAGLN cells (0.40 ± 0.07 versus 0.11 ± 0.02; Figure 5E). We randomly selected five tissues from each group to perform RT-qPCR assays, and the results confirmed that TAGLN was overexpressed in the xenograft tumors derived from HT-TAGLN cells (Figure 5F).

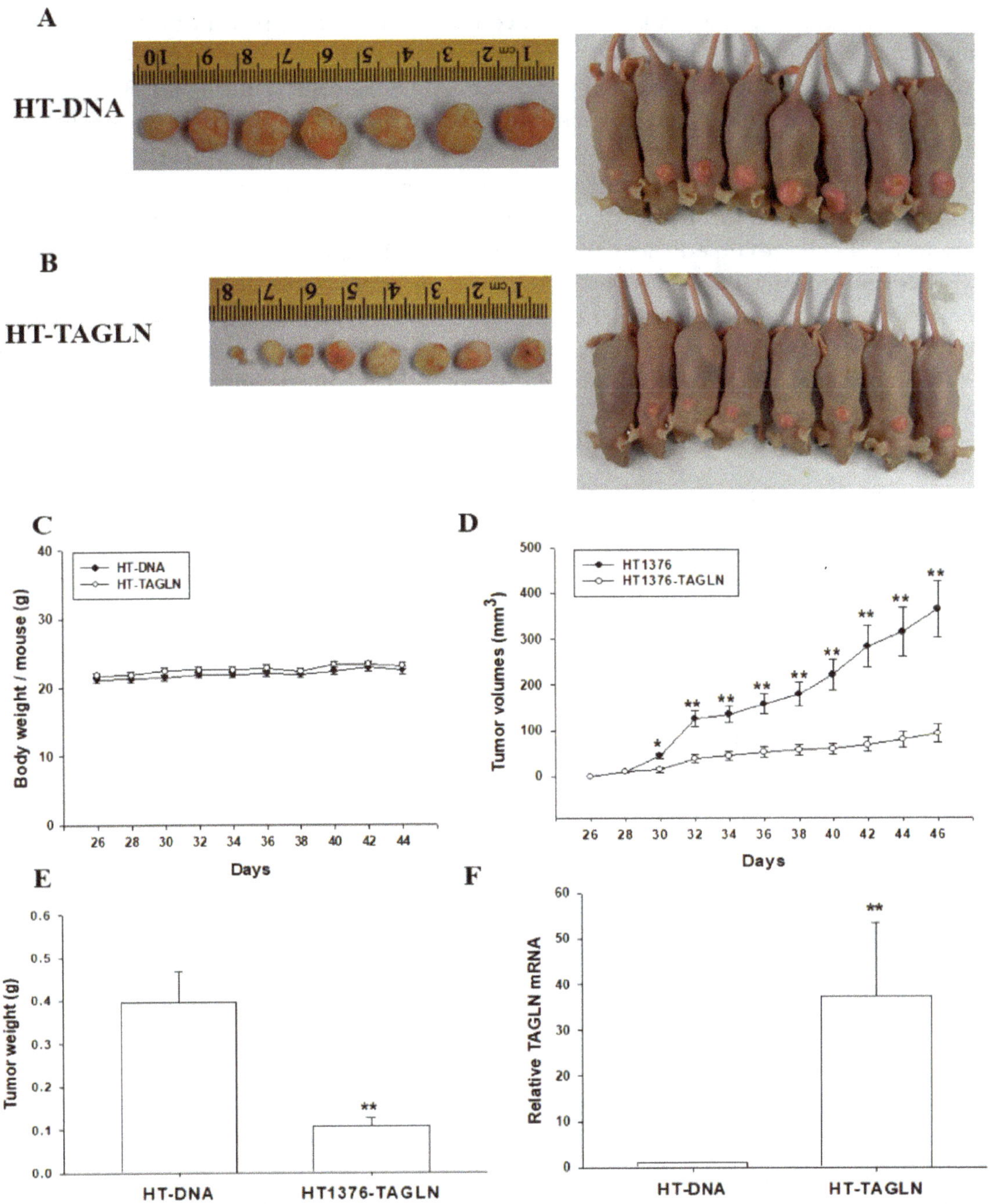

Figure 5. The ectopic overexpression of TAGLN attenuates tumorigenesis, in vivo, for bladder carcinoma HT1376 cells. Four-week-old male athymic nude (nu/nu) mice were randomized into two

groups: HT-DNA ($n = 7$; **A**) and HT-TAGLN ($n = 7$; **B**). HT-DNA cells and HT-TAGLN cells (1×10^6) were injected subcutaneously in the dorsal area of the mice, respectively. The animal body weights (**C**) and tumor growth rates (**D**) were measured every 2 days, starting at the 3-weeks-of-growth point (day 26), at which the tumors became perceptible under the skin after inoculation. The tumor weights (**E**) and levels of TAGLN mRNA (**F**) were determined after the animals were sacrificed (± SE; n =7). * represented the $p < 0.05$ and the ** represented the $p < 0.01$.

2.7. p53 and PTEN Upregulated TAGLN Expression in Bladder Carcinoma Cells

The immunoblot (Figure 6A) and RT-qPCR (Figure 6B) assays confirmed that the overexpression of p53 induced TAGLN expression in HT1376 cells. Further, the immunoblot assays showed that camptothecin, a topoisomerase inhibitor, induced not only p53 but also TAGLN expressions, while p53-knockdown attenuated these effects in p53-wild type RT-4 cells (Figure 6C). Similar results found in the reporter assays indicated that a transiently cotransfected-p53 expression vector induced the reporter activity of *TAGLN* reporter vector containing the 5′-flanking region of the human *TAGLN* gene in HT1376 cells (Figure 6D). Further immunoblot assays revealed that the ectopic overexpression of PTEN in T24 cells blocked AKT phosphorylation but enhanced TAGLN expression, whereas PTEN knockdown in RT-4 cells reversed those effects (Figure 6E). Results of RT-qPCR assays showed that ectopic overexpression of PTEN induced *TAGLN* gene expression in T24 cells (Figure 6F), while PTEN-knockdown downregulated *TAGLN* expression in RT-4 cells (Figure 6G). Further reporter assays revealed that a transiently cotransfected-PTEN expression vector upregulated the reporter activity of human *TAGLN* reporter vector in HT1376 cells (Figure 6H). Collectively, TAGLN is upregulated by p53 and PTEN in bladder carcinoma cells.

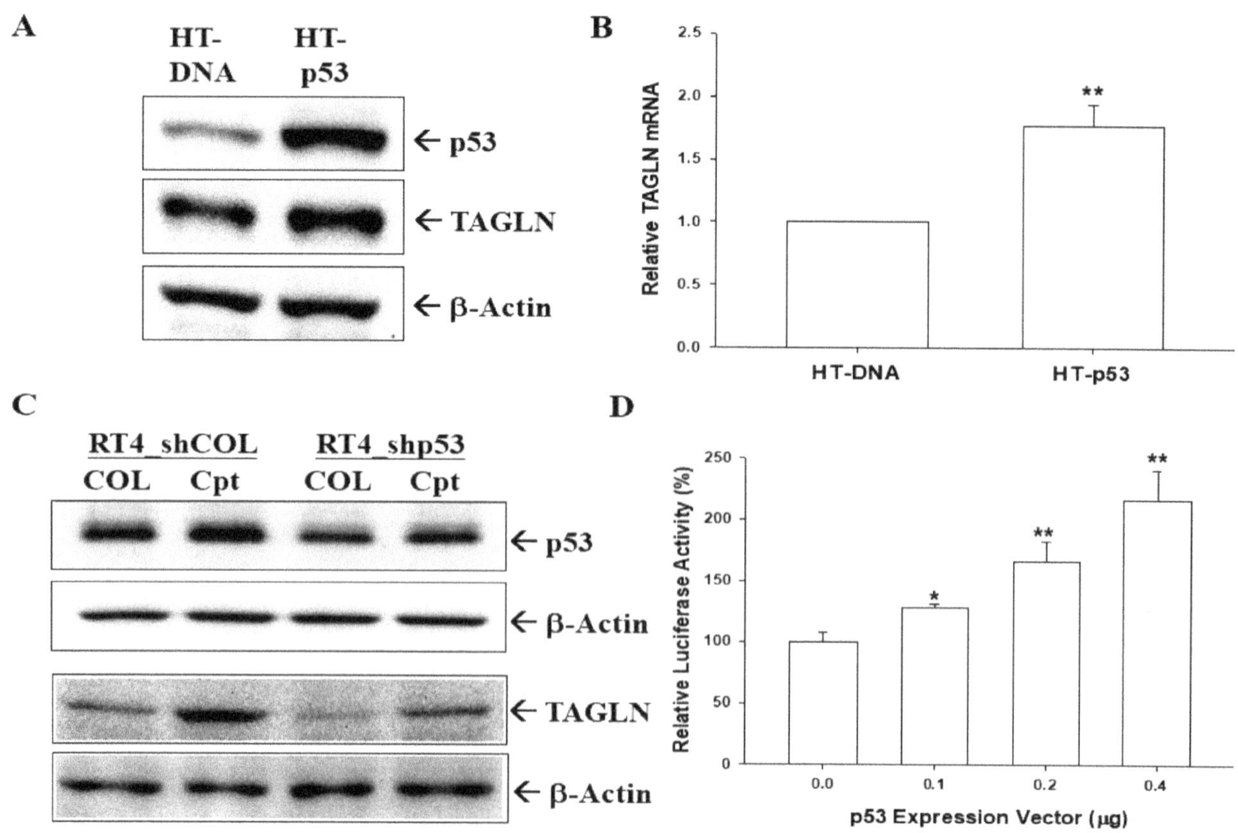

Figure 6. *Cont.*

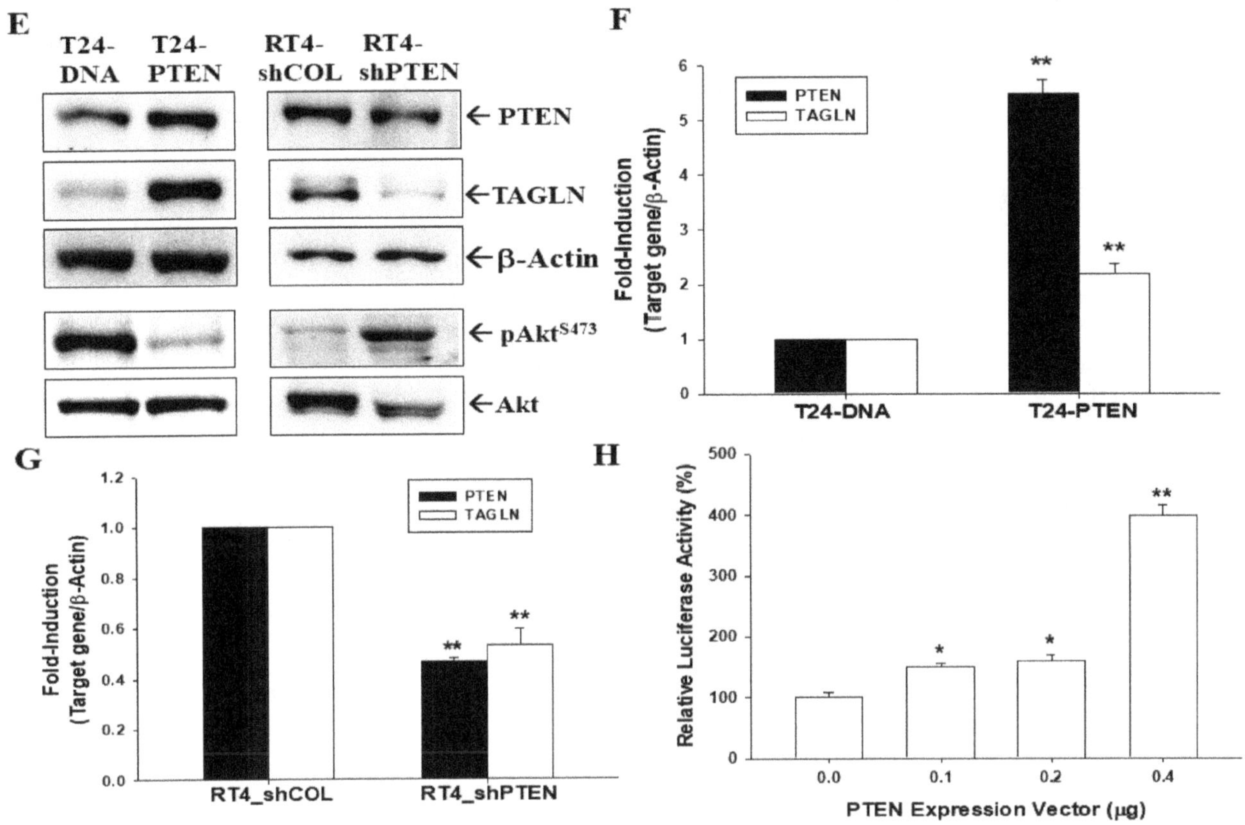

Figure 6. Modulation of p53 and PTEN on TAGLN expression in bladder carcinoma cells. The mock-transfected HT1376 (HT-DNA) and p53-overexpressed HT1376 (HT-p53) cells were lysed, and then TAGLN, p53, and β-actin were determined by immunoblotting (**A**) and RT-qPCR (**B**) assays (± SE; n = 3). The mock-knockdown RT4 (RT4_shCOL) and p53-knockdown RT4 (RT4_shp53) cells were treated with camptothecin (1 μM) for 16 h. The cells were lysed, and then TAGLN, p53, and β-actin were determined by immunoblotting (**C**). (**D**) The reporter activity of TAGLN reporter vector cotrasnfected with various dosages of p53, as indicated in HT1376 cells. Data are expressed as the mean percentages ± SEs (n = 6) of luciferase activity relative to the mock-transfected group. The mock-transfected T24 (T24-DNA), PTEN-overexpressed T24 (T24-PTEN), mock-knockdown RT4 (RT4_shCOL), and PTEN-knockdown RT4 (RT4_shpPTEN) cells were lysed, and then TAGLN, PTEN, Akt, pAkt^{S473}, and β-actin were determined by immunoblotting (**E**). Expressions of PTEN and TAGLN in T24-DNA, T24-PTEN (**F**), RT4_shCOL, and RT4_shPTEN (**G**) cells were determined by RT-qPCR assays (± SE; n = 3). (**H**) The reporter activity of TAGLN reporter vector cotrasnfected with various dosages of PTEN, as indicated in HT1376 cells. Data are expressed as the mean percentages ± SEs (n = 6) of luciferase activity relative to the mock-transfected group. * represented the $p < 0.05$ and the ** represented the $p < 0.01$.

3. Discussion

Bladder cancer is the ninth most common cancer and ranks 13th in terms of deaths worldwide, with the highest incidence rates observed in men around the world [21]. In the United States, bladder cancer is the sixth most common cancer with an estimated 79,030 new cases and 16,870 deaths in 2017 [22]. It seems critical nowadays to explore a new therapeutic molecular target for patients with bladder cancer, since multiple factors are associated with bladder cancer [23,24].

TAGLN may play roles in the morphologic transform process in smooth muscle cells, although TAGLN is not required for the normal development of mouse embryos [2]. Overexpression of TAGLN was strictly limited to the regulation of the tumor-induced, reactive, myofibroblastic stromal tissue, compartment-specific cell type's expression in tumoral stroma compared to neoplastic epithelial cells [4]. The TAGLN depletion increased the capacity of cells to form podosomes spontaneously with a concomitant increase in the ability to invade Matrigel, suggesting that TAGLN may relate to the tumorigenic properties of cells [3]. A prior study indicated that an early loss of *TAGLN* gene expression is important for tumor progression and viewed that as a diagnostic marker for breast and colon cancer development [5]. However, results from the functional assays of TAGLN in different cancers are still inconclusive. Although studies in bladder cancer suggested that *TAGLN* was one of common differentially-expressed genes, significantly decreased in cancer compared with normal tissues [19,20], the precise functions and regulatory mechanisms of *TAGLN* in bladder carcinoma cells are still unexplored.

This study illustrated that protein and mRNA levels of *TAGLN* are higher in human normal primary bladder epithelial cells (HBdEC) than in bladder carcinoma cells. Meanwhile, a recent study showed that *TAGLN* was expressed in bladder carcinoma T24 and SW780 cells at the transcription and translation levels [25]. Although our study suggested that TAGLN expressions among the bladder carcinoma cell lines could be dependent on the cell type but not relevant to the extent of neoplasia in vitro, the RT-qPCR analysis of paired human bladder tissues further demonstrated a significantly lower expression of *TAGLN* mRNA levels in bladder tumors than adjacent normal bladder tissues (Figure 1). These results are in agreement to other studies of badder cancer in vivo [19,20,26], suggesting that *TAGLN* is a tumor suppressor gene in the bladder. The family of transgelins consists of three homologs (TAGLN, transgelin-2, and transgelin-3) in human tissues. A prior study has suggested that TAGLN and trangelin-2 act as cancer biomarkers and are differentially expressed in the tumor and stroma cells [27]. Further studies implied that transgelin-2 has a potentially oncogenic function in bladder cancer, both in vitro and in vivo [28,29]. Our study presents the tumor suppressor characteristics of TAGLN in bladder cancer, both in vitro and in vivo, and agrees with the concept of that the role of transgelin-2 in tumor development might be contradictory to the role of TAGLN [27].

This study also found high levels of TAGLN expressed in the bladder's smooth muscle cells (HBdSMC) and stromal fibroblasts (HBdSF) in vitro (Figure 1). Earlier study indicated that TAGLN is an SMC-lineage marker in rabbit bladders [18]; however, TAGLN was regarded as a marker of active stromal remodeling in the vicinity of invasive carcinomas as well [4]. In the prostate study, TAGLN levels were found to be elevated in the stroma but decreased in the carcinomic epithelial cells during cancer progression [30,31]. However, further investigation into the function of TAGLN in the stroma of bladders is still necessary.

Our finding indicated that the expression of TAGLN was predominant in the cytosol and associated with F-actin during the ectopic overexpression of bladder carcinoma HT1376 cells. Further immunoblot assays with subcellular extraction confirmed that TAGLN did not express in the nuclei but in the cytoplasm, mostly with a little expression in the membrane (Figure 2). These results are in agreement with previous studies, which implied that TAGLN is localized to the cytosol where it binds to F-actin [32].

Early studies suggested that *TAGLN* was a tumor suppressor gene in various cancers, while some cancers possessed the oncogenic characteristic of *TAGLN*. The overexpression of TAGLN potentially contributed to the progression and metastasis of colorectal cancer; meanwhile, high levels of TAGLN related to a poor prognosis of colon cancer in vivo [14,15]. TAGLN was upregulated in cell lines from the human lung adenocarcinoma under hypoxic conditions that caused the migration ability of the tumor cells; moreover, a high TAGLN expression correlated with an advanced TNM stage, lymph node metastasis, and greater differentiation in lung adenocarcinoma [16]. However, other studies concluded that *TAGLN* is a tumor suppressor gene associated with a poor prognosis in colorectal carcinoma patients [9,10]. An in vitro study declared that apigenin upregulated the expression of TAGLN in mitochondria to exert its anti-tumor growth and anti-metastasis effects in colorectal cancer [11]. The restoration of the TAGLN-induced inhibition of colon carcinogenesis in vivo and in vitro suggested that TAGLN might potentially function as a novel tumor suppressor [12,13]. A previous study of prostates also identified *TAGLN* as a tumor suppressor gene in vivo and in vitro [31], and others found the same in bladder cancer, based on a gene profile analysis [19,20,26]. Our study is the first study providing direct evidence to demonstrate that *TAGLN* is an antitumor gene in the bladder carcinoma cells. Results from this study revealed that the ectopic overexpression of TAGLN decreased cell proliferation, invasion, and migration in bladder carcinoma cells in vitro, while the knockdown of *TAGLN* reversed the effects (Figure 3, Figure 4, Figures S1 and S2). The anti-tumorigenesis characteristics of *TAGLN* in bladder carcinoma cells was also demonstrated by an in vivo xenograft animal study (Figure 5).

Previous studies have indicated that *TAGLN* is a TGFβ-inducible gene of human skeletal stem cells, prostate carcinoma cells, and prostate fibroblast cells [31,33,34]. Steroid receptor coactivatior and mir-145 also modulated *TAGLN* expression in different cells [35,36]. Interestingly, *TAGLN* was regarded as an ARA54-associated AR inhibitor that suppressed AR function, and induced the apoptosis of human prostate LNCaP cells through its interaction with p53 [37]. Our study is the first to reveal that *TAGLN* is the downstream gene of *p53* and *PTEN* in bladder carcinoma cells. *p53* is a well-known tumor suppressor gene and *p53* mutations correlate with a variety of human cancers [38]. The overexpression of p53 in p53-mutant HT1376 cells, or with camptothecin (a topoisomerase I inhibitor) treatment in p53-wild type RT-4 cells, induced TAGLN expression, while p53-knockdown attenuated this effect. It was found that camptothecin induced p53 expression in RT-4 cells in a previous study that used bladder carcinoma cells [39]. Two putative p53 response elements (5′-AGGCAAGTTCTGTGTTAGTCATGCAC-3′, –2151 to –2126; and 5′-AAACTTGTTTTTATAGCTCTG CTTGAAG-3′, –1956 to –1929), which are similar to the p53 response element consensus sequence (RRRCWWGYYYN$_{0-13}$RRRCWWGYYY), as previously reported [40], were found in the promoter region of the human *TAGLN* gene—determined by in silico analysis. The precise mechanisms of the modulation *TAGLN* gene expression by p53 still need to be further investigated.

Phosphatase and tensin homolog deleted on chromosome 10 (*PTEN*) has been widely known as a tumor suppressor gene, and *PTEN* mutation or deletion is frequently noted in a lot of cancers, including bladder [39,41,42]. The most known function of PTEN is as the negative regulator of the PI3K/Akt/mTOR pathway, which is a crucial signal transduction pathway for cancer cell growth [39,43]. For bladder cancer, a loss of PTEN expression has been correlated with the cell growth and the invasion of bladder carcinoma [39,41]. In this study, we found that ectopic overexpression of PTEN in PTEN-mutant T24 cells blocked Akt phosphorylation but induced *TAGLN* expression, while knockdown of *PTEN* in PTEN-wildtype RT-4 cells reversed those effect (Figure 6). Conclusively, our study confirmed that *TAGLN* is a target gene of p53 and PTEN, and should be referred to as a tumor suppressor in bladder carcinoma cells, both in vitro and in vivo.

4. Materials and Methods

4.1. Cell Cultures and Chemicals

The four bladder-transitional carcinoma cell lines, RT-4, HT1376, TSGH-8301, and T24 cells, were purchased from the Bioresource Collection and Research Center (BCRC, Hsinchu, Taiwan) as described previously [44]. Human bladder smooth muscle cells (HBdSMC), bladder stromal fibroblasts (HBdSF), smooth muscle cell medium, and fibroblast medium were purchased from ScienCell Research Laboratories Inc. (Carlsbad, CA, USA). Human normal primary bladder epithelial cells (HBdEC; ATCC PCS-420-010) were purchased from American Type Culture Collection (ATCC; Manassas, VA, USA) and maintained in the prostate epithelial cells' basal mediums (ATCC PCS 440-030). DAPI (4,6-diamino-2-phenylindole) and camptothecin were obtained from Sigma-Aldrich Co. (St. Louis, MO, USA). Fetal calf serum (FCS) was from HyClone (Logan, UT, USA), and RPMI 1640 media was obtained from Invitrogen (Carlsbad, CA, USA).

4.2. Tissue Collection and Analysis

The specimens of the human paired bladder tissue biopsies were obtained from patients admitted to the Department of Urology, Chang Gung Memorial Hospital-Linkou (Tao-Yuan, Taiwan). Bladder tissues were classified based on the pathological examinations of the parallel preparations from respective samples by attending pathologists. The Institutional Review Board of the Chang Gung Memorial Hospital approved the protocol for tissue collection and analysis (IRB 201800981B0, 1 September 2018).

4.3. Expression Vector and Stable Transfection

The full-length human *TAGLN* cDNA (HG14991-UT) was purchased from Sino Biologic Inc. (Beijing, China). Electroporation was conducted using an ECM 830 Square Wave Electroporation System (BTX, San Diego, CA, USA), set at 180 V (for TSGH-8301 cells) or 190 V (for HT1376 cells), with a 70-msec pulse length and one pulse setting. Transfected cells (8301-TAGLN and HT-TAGLN) were selected by 100 µg/mL of hygromycin (Sigma-Aldrich Co.). For construction of the mock-transfected cells (8301-DNA and HT1376-DNA), cells were transfected with a controlled pCMV3 expression vector (Sino Biologic Inc.) and were clonally selected in the same manner as described above. The *p53* and *PTEN* expression vectors were constructed and p53-overexpressed HT1376 (HT-p53) cells and PTEN-overexpression T24 (T24-PTEN) cells were cloned as described previously [39].

4.4. Knock-Down TAGLN, p53, and PTEN

TSGH-8301 and T24 cells were transduced with control shRNA lentiviral particles-A (Sc-108080) or transgelin shRNA (h) Lentiviral Particles (sc-44163-V) that were purchased from Santa Cruz Biotechnology, Inc. (Santa Cruz, CA, USA). Two days after transduction, the cells (8301_shCOL, 8301_shTAGLN, T24_shCOL, and T24_shTAGLN) were selected by incubation with 10 µg/mL puromycin dihydrochloride for at least another 5 generations. The p53-knockdown RT-4 (RT4_shp53), PTEN-knockdown RT-4 (RT4_shPTEN), and mock-knockdown RT-4 (RT4_shCOL) cells were cloned as previously described [39].

4.5. Immunoblot Assays

Cells were cultured in RPMI-1640 medium with 10% FCS for 48 h. The nuclear and cytoplasmic fractions were separated using the subcellular protein fractionation kit (Thermo Fisher Scientific Inc., Rockford, NJ, USA) as described previously [44]. Equal amounts of whole cell, membrane, nuclear, or cytoplasmic lysates were separated on a 10%–12% SDS-polyacrylamide gel and assayed by the Western lightning plus-ECL detection system, as instructed by the manufacturer (PerkinElmer Inc, Waltham, MA, USA). The blotting membranes were probed with the antisera of p53 (DO-1, Santa Cruz Biotechnology), PTEN (#9552, Cell Signaling Technology, Danvers, MA, USA), Akt (#4691, Cell Signaling Technology), phopsho-Akt^{S473} (#9271, Cell Signaling Technology), or β-actin antiserum (MAB1501, Merck Millipore, Burlington, MA, USA). The intensities of different bands were recorded using the LuminoGraph II (Atto corporation, Tokyo, Japan).

4.6. Real-Time Reverse Transcriptase-Polymerase Chain Reaction (RT-qPCR)

Total RNA from tissues or cells was isolated using Trizol reagent (Ambion, Life Technologies, Carlsbad, CA, USA). The cDNA was synthesized using Superscript III pre-amplification system (Invitrogen), as described previously [45]. The PCR probes for human *p53* (Hs01034249_m1), *PTEN* (Hs02621230_Sl), *TAGLN* (Hs01038777_g1), *β-actin* (Hs01060665_g1), and *18S* (Hs03003631_g1) were purchased from Applied Biosystems (Foster City, CA, USA). Real-time polymerase chain reactions (qPCR) were performed using an CFX Connect Real-Time PCR system (Bio-Rad Laboratories, Foster city, CA, USA) and the mean cycle threshold (C_t) values were calculated for internal control and target genes, as described previously [44].

4.7. Cell Immunofluorescence and F-Actin Staining

Cells were seeded onto the glass bottom culture dishes (MatTek, Ashland, MD, USA) which were precoated with 50 μL fibronectin. Cells were fixed at room temperature in 4% paraformaldehyde in phosphate buffered saline (PBS) for 20 min after 24 h of attachment. After that, cells were permeabilized for 10 min in a 0.2% solution of Triton X-100 and blocked in 1% BSA for 1 h after being washed with PBS. The coverslips were incubated with 1:100 diluted anti-TAGLN antiserum overnight at 4 °C and then incubated with donkey anti-rabbit secondary antibody (A21206, Invitrogen) for 1 h. The F-actin protein expression was revealed by incubation with Texas Red X-Phalloidin (Invitrogen). The coverslips were mounted with the Prolong Gold antifade reagent with DAPI (Thermo Fisher Scientific Inc.). The immunofluorescence was examined using a confocal microscope (LSM510 Meta, Zeiss, Oberkochen, Germany) as described previously [46].

4.8. EdU Staining Proliferation Assay

Cells were seeded onto the sterile glass coverslips. After 48 h of attachment, EdU was added to the culture medium to a final concentration of 50 μM for another 2 h. Cells were washed and fixed in 3.7% paraformaldehyde in phosphate buffered saline (PBS) at room temperature for 15 min, and then washed twice with 200 μL of 3% BSA in PBS. Cells were permeabilized with saponin-based permeabilization and washing reagent for 20 min, and then incubated for 30 min with Click-iT reaction cocktail, containing fluorescent dye azide, $CuSO_4$, PBS, and reaction buffer (Thermo Fisher Scientific Inc.). Cells were washed twice with 200 μL of 3% BSA in PBS, and the coverslip was mounted with Prolong Gold antifade reagent with DAPI. The EdU fluorescence was recorded and photographed under a microscope (BX43, OLYMPUS, Tokyo, Japan).

4.9. EdU Flow Cytometry Assay

Cells (5×10^5) were serum starved for 24 h, and then incubated with RPMI1640 medium with 10% serum for another 48 h. EdU (5-ethynyl-2′-deoxyuridine; 10 μM) was added to the culture medium for further 2 h. Cells were collected, fixed, and permeabilized with saponin-based permeabilization and washing reagent for 20 min, and then incubated for 30 min with Click-iT reaction cocktail (Thermo Fisher Scientific Inc.), as described by the manufacturer. The EdU fluorescence of cells was detected using Attune NxT acoustic focusing cytometer (Thermo Fisher Scientific Inc.).

4.10. Ki67 Proliferation Assay

Cells were serum-starvated for 24 h, and then incubated with RPMI1640 medium with 10% serum for further 48 h. Cells were stained with PE Mouse Anti-Ki-67 kit (catalogue number 556027; BD Biosciences, Bedford, MA, USA) as described by the manufacturer. Briefly, cells were washed, pelleted, and fixed with cold, 70% ethanol at −20 °C overnight. The PE-conjugated anti-Ki-67 antibody and PE-conjugated mouse IgG1 were added to the cells and the mixture was incubated at room temperature for further 30 min in the dark, after the cells had been washed twice with washing buffer (PBS with 1% FBS, 0.09% NaN_3). The cells were washed with washing buffer and re-suspended in PBS, and then the Ki67 fluorescence of cells were detected using Attune NxT acoustic focusing cytometer.

4.11. Cell Migration Assay

The cell migration analysis was determined by a wound healing assay, as described previously [46]. In brief, the cell sheets were wounded with a plastic pipette tip when they attained a confluent monolayer. The wound closure (the gap width) was photographed microscopically (IX71, Olympus, Tokyo, Japan) with a digital camera during the indicated times. The quantification of cell migration was determined within a defined area using the Image J program.

4.12. Matrigel Invasion Assay

The in vitro invasion ability of cells was determined by the Matrigel invasion assay (BD Biosciences). Cells that invaded into other side of the membrane were fixed using 4% paraformaldehyde and then stained with 0.1% crystal violet solution for 10 min. The quantity of cells that invaded the Matrigel was recorded microscopically (IX71, Olympus, Tokyo, Japan) and the images were analyzed as described previously [44].

4.13. Xenograft Animal Model

The performance of animal studies was approved by the Chang Gung University Animal Research Committee (Approval No.: CGU107-092, 1 September 2018). The male nude mice (BALB/cAnN-Foxn1) were obtained from the animal center of National Science Council, Taiwan, at 4 weeks old. In all the procedures, every effort was made to minimize the suffering of the laboratory animals in accordance with the United States' National Institutes of Health Guide for the Care and Use of Laboratory Animals. The cells were detached with Gibco^{Tm} Versene solution and washed with RPMI 1640 medium with 10% FCS, and then were re-suspended in a PBS solution. The mice were anesthetized intraperitoneally and 1×10^6 cell/100 μL cells were injected subcutaneously on the right or left lateral back wall in close proximity to the shoulder of each mouse. The growth of the xenografts was measured by vernier caliper measurements on the days indicated. The tumor volume was determined by the formula volume = $\pi/6 \times W \times D^2$, as described previously [47].

4.14. TAGLN Reporter Vector and Reporter Assays

The 5′-DNA fragment (−1 to −4573) of the human *TAGLN* gene, according to the sequence from GenBank (AP005018.1), was synthesized by Invitrogen. The human *TAGLN* reporter vector was constructed by cloning the DNA fragment into the pbGL3 reporter vector (Promega Biosciences, Madison, WI, USA) with *Hind III* sites. Proper ligation was confirmed by extensive restriction mapping and sequencing. The cells were plated onto 24-well plates at 1×10^4 cells/well for 1 day prior to transfection. Cells were transiently cotransfected with reporter vectors and expression vectors as indicated, using the X-tremeGene HP DNA transfection reagent (Roche Diagnostics GmbH, Mannheim, Germany), as described previously [48]. The luciferase activity was adjusted for transfection efficiency using the normalization control plasmid pCMVSPORTβgal.

4.15. Statistical Analysis

All the results are expressed as the means ± S.Es. Statistical significance was determined by one-way ANOVA and Student's *t* tests using the SigmaPlot 10.0 (SPSS Inc., Chicago, IL, USA). The * represented the $p < 0.05$ and the ** represented the $p < 0.01$.

5. Conclusions

Our results indicated that the expression of transgelin, a regulator of the actin cytoskeleton, is higher in bladder normal epithelial cells than in carcinoma cells. Our experiments provided evidence suggesting that *TAGLN* is a p53 and PTEN-downstream gene, which attenuates cell proliferation and invasion in vitro, and tumorigenesis in vivo. *TAGLN* seems to function as a tumor suppressor gene in bladder carcinoma cells.

Supplementary Materials:
Figure S1: Effect of TAGLN on cell proliferation of bladder carcinoma HT1376 and TSGH-8301 cells determined by Ki-67 assays. Proliferation rates between (A) mock-transfected HT1376 (HT-DNA) and ectopic TAGLN overexpressed HT1376 (HT-TAGLN), and (B) between mock-transfected TSGH-8301 (8301-DNA) and ectopic TAGLN overexpressed TSGH-8301 (8301-TAGLN) cells were determined by Ki-67 assays (± SE; $n = 3$). ** is represented the $p < 0.01$. Figure S2: Effect of TAGLN on cell migration of bladder carcinoma HT1376 cells. The migration ability of HT-DNA and HT-TAGLN cells was determined by wound healing assays during the indicated times. ** is represented the $p < 0.01$.

Author Contributions: Funding acquisition, K.-H.T. and H.-H.J.; investigation, K.-H.T. and Y.-H.L.; Methodology, K.-S.C., C.-P.H. and P.-J.C.; writing–original draft, T.-H.F.; writing–review and editing, T.-H.F. and H.-H.J.

References

1. Camoretti-Mercado, B.; Forsythe, S.M.; LeBeau, M.M.; Espiosa, R.; Vieira, J.E.; Halayko, A.J.; Willadsen, S.; Kurtz, B.; Ober, C.; Evans, G.A.; et al. Expression and cytogenetic localization of the human SM22 gene (TAGLN). *Genomics* **1998**, *49*, 452–457. [CrossRef] [PubMed]
2. Yang, X.Y.; Yao, J.H.; Cheng, L.; Wei, D.W.; Xue, J.L.; Lu, D.R. Molecular cloning and expression of a smooth muscle-specific gene SM22alpha in zebrafish. *Biochem. Biophys. Res. Comm.* **2003**, *312*, 741–746. [CrossRef] [PubMed]
3. Thompson, O.; Moghraby, J.S.; Ayscough, K.R.; Winder, S.J. Depletion of the actin bundling protein SM22/transgelin increases actin dynamics and enhances the tumourigenic phenotypes of cells. *BMC Cell Biol.* **2012**, *13*, 1. [CrossRef] [PubMed]
4. Rho, J.H.; Roehrl, M.H.; Wang, J.Y. Tissue proteomics reveals differential and compartment-specific expression of the homologs transgelin and transgelin-2 in lung adenocarcinoma and its stroma. *J. Proteome Res.* **2009**, *8*, 5610–5618. [CrossRef] [PubMed]
5. Shields, J.M.; Rogers-Graham, K.; Der, C.J. Loss of transgelin in breast and colon tumors and in RIE-1 cells by Ras deregulation of gene expression through Raf-independent pathways. *J. Biol. Chem.* **2002**, *277*, 9790–9799. [CrossRef] [PubMed]
6. Zhang, J.; Wang, K.; Zhang, J.; Liu, S.S.; Dai, L.; Zhang, J.Y. Using proteomic approach to identify tumor-associated proteins as biomarkers in human esophageal squamous cell carcinoma. *J. Proteome Res.* **2011**, *10*, 2863–2872. [CrossRef]
7. Li, N.; Zhang, J.; Liang, Y.; Shao, J.; Peng, F.; Sun, M.; Xu, N.; Li, X.; Wang, R.; Liu, S.; et al. A controversial tumor marker: Is SM22 a proper biomarker for gastric cancer cells? *J. Proteome Res.* **2007**, *6*, 3304–3312. [CrossRef]
8. Yu, B.; Chen, X.; Li, J.; Qu, Y.; Su, L.; Peng, Y.; Huang, J.; Yan, J.; Yu, Y.; Gu, Q.; et al. Stromal fibroblasts in the microenvironment of gastric carcinomas promote tumor metastasis via upregulating TAGLN expression. *BMC Cell Biol.* **2013**, *14*, 17. [CrossRef]
9. Zhao, L.; Wang, H.; Deng, Y.J.; Wang, S.; Liu, C.; Jin, H.; Ding, Y.Q. Transgelin as a suppressor is associated with poor prognosis in colorectal carcinoma patients. *Modern Pathol.* **2009**, *22*, 786–796. [CrossRef]
10. Xie, X.L.; Liu, Y.B.; Liu, Y.P.; Du, B.L.; Li, Y.; Han, M.; Li, B.H. Reduced expression of SM22 is correlated with low autophagy activity in human colorectal cancer. *Pathol. Res. Prac.* **2013**, *209*, 237–243. [CrossRef]
11. Chunhua, L.; Donglan, L.; Xiuqiong, F.; Lihua, Z.; Qin, F.; Yawei, L.; Liang, Z.; Ge, W.; Linlin, J.; Ping, Z.; et al. Apigenin up-regulates transgelin and inhibits invasion and migration of colorectal cancer through decreased phosphorylation of AKT. *J. Nutr. Biochem.* **2013**, *24*, 1766–1775. [CrossRef]
12. Pang, J.; Liu, W.P.; Liu, X.P.; Li, L.Y.; Fang, Y.Q.; Sun, Q.P.; Liu, S.J.; Li, M.T.; Su, Z.L.; Gao, X. Profiling protein markers associated with lymph node metastasis in prostate cancer by DIGE-based proteomics analysis. *J. Proteome Res.* **2010**, *9*, 216–226. [CrossRef] [PubMed]
13. Yeo, M.; Park, H.J.; Kim, D.K.; Kim, Y.B.; Cheong, J.Y.; Lee, K.J.; Cho, S.W. Loss of SM22 is a characteristic signature of colon carcinogenesis and its restoration suppresses colon tumorigenicity in vivo and in vitro. *Cancer* **2010**, *116*, 2581–2589. [CrossRef] [PubMed]
14. Yokota, M.; Kojima, M.; Higuchi, Y.; Nishizawa, Y.; Kobayashi, A.; Ito, M.; Saito, N.; Ochiai, A. Gene expression profile in the activation of subperitoneal fibroblasts reflects prognosis of patients with colon cancer. *Int. J. Cancer* **2016**, *138*, 1422–1431. [CrossRef] [PubMed]
15. Zhou, H.; Zhang, Y.; Chen, Q.; Lin, Y. AKT and JNK Signaling pathways increase the metastatic potential of colorectal cancer cells by altering transgelin expression. *Dig. Dis. Sci.* **2016**, *61*, 1091–1097. [CrossRef] [PubMed]
16. Wu, X.; Dong, L.; Zhang, R.; Ying, K.; Shen, H. Transgelin overexpression in lung adenocarcinoma is associated with tumor progression. *Int. J. Mol. Med.* **2014**, *34*, 585–591. [CrossRef]

17. Li, L.S.; Kim, H.; Rhee, H.; Kim, S.H.; Shin, D.H.; Chung, K.Y.; Park, K.S.; Paik, Y.K.; Chang, J.; Kim, H. Proteomic analysis distinguishes basaloid carcinoma as a distinct subtype of nonsmall cell lung carcinoma. *Proteomics* **2004**, *4*, 3394–3400. [CrossRef]
18. Chiavegato, A.; Roelofs, M.; Franch, R.; Castellucci, E.; Sarinella, F.; Sartore, S. Differential expression of SM22 isoforms in myofibroblasts and smooth muscle cells from rabbit bladder. *J. Muscle Res. Cell Motil.* **1999**, *20*, 133–146. [CrossRef]
19. Zaravinos, A.; Lambrou, G.I.; Boulalas, I.; Delakas, D.; Spandidos, D.A. Identification of common differentially expressed genes in urinary bladder cancer. *PLoS ONE* **2011**, *6*, e18135. [CrossRef]
20. Chen, R.; Feng, C.; Xu, Y. Cyclin-dependent kinase-associated protein Cks2 is associated with bladder cancer progression. *J. Int. Med. Res.* **2011**, *39*, 533–540. [CrossRef]
21. Antomi, S.; Ferlay, J.; Soerjomataram, I.; Znaor, A.; Jemal, A.; Bray, F. Bladder cancer incidence and mortality: A global overview and recent trends. *Eur. Urol.* **2017**, *71*, 96–108. [CrossRef] [PubMed]
22. Siegel, R.L.; Miller, K.D.; Jemal, A. Cancer statistics, 2017. *CA Cancer J. Clin.* **2017**, *67*, 7–30. [CrossRef]
23. Goodison, S.; Rosser, C.J.; Urquidi, V. Bladder cancer detection and monitoring: Assessment of urine- and blood based marker tests. *Mol. Diag. Ther.* **2013**, *17*, 71–84. [CrossRef] [PubMed]
24. Narayan, V.M.; Adejoro, O.; Schwartz, I.; Ziegelmann, M.; Elliott, S.; Konety, B.R. The prevalence and impact of urinary marker testing in patients with bladder cancer. *J. Urol.* **2018**, *199*, 74–80. [CrossRef] [PubMed]
25. Chen, Z.; He, S.; Zhan, Y.; He, A.; Fang, D.; Gong, Y.; Li, X.; Zhou, L. TGF-β-induced transgelin promotes bladder cancer metastasis by upregulating epithelial-mesenchymal transition and invadopodia formation. *EBioMedicine* **2019**, *47*, 208–220. [CrossRef]
26. Ning, X.; Deng, Y. Identification of key pathways and genes influencing prognosis in bladder urothelial carcinoma. *Onco. Targets Ther.* **2017**, *10*, 1673–1686. [CrossRef] [PubMed]
27. Dvorakova, M.; Nenutil, R.; Bouchal, P. Transgelins, cytoskeletal proteins implicated in different aspects of cancer development. *Expert. Rev. Proteomics* **2014**, *11*, 149–165. [CrossRef]
28. Yoshino, H.; Chiyomaru, T.; Enokida, H.; Kawakami, K.; Tatarano, S.; Nishiyama, K.; Nohata, N.; Seki, N.; Nakagawa, M. The tumour-suppressive function of miR-1 and miR-133a targeting TAGLN2 in bladder cancer. *Br. J. Cancer* **2011**, *104*, 808–818. [CrossRef] [PubMed]
29. Zhang, H.; Jiang, M.; Liu, Q.; Han, Z.; Zhao, Y.; Ji, S. miR-145-5p inhibits the proliferation and migration of bladder cancer cells by targeting TAGLN2. *Oncol. Lett.* **2018**, *16*, 6355–6360. [CrossRef]
30. Webber, J.P.; Spary, L.K.; Mason, M.D.; Tabi, Z.; Bewis, I.A.; Clayton, A. Prostate stromal cell proteomic analysis discriminates normal from tumour reactive stroma phenotypes. *Oncotarget* **2016**, *7*, 20124–20139. [CrossRef]
31. Prasad, P.D.; Stanton, J.A.; Assinder, S.J. Expression of the actin-associated protein transgelin (SM22) is decreased in prostate cancer. *Cell Tissue Res.* **2010**, *339*, 337–347. [CrossRef] [PubMed]
32. Matsui, T.S.; Ishikawa, A.; Deguchi, S. Transgelin-1 (SM22α) interacts with actin stress fibers and podosomes in smooth muscle cells without using its actin binding site. *Biochem. Biophys. Res. Commun.* **2018**, *505*, 879–884. [CrossRef] [PubMed]
33. Elsafadi, M.; Manikandan, M.; Dawud, R.A.; Alajez, N.M.; Hamam, R.; Alfayez, M.; Kassem, M.; Aldahmash, A.; Mahmood, A. Transgelin is a TGFβ-inducible gene that regulates osteoblastic and adipogenic differentiation of human skeletal stem cells through actin cytoskeleston organization. *Cell Death Dis.* **2016**, *7*, e2321. [CrossRef] [PubMed]
34. Untergasser, G.; Gander, R.; Lilg, C.; Lepperdinger, G.; Plas, E.; Berger, P. Profiling molecular targets of TGF-beta1 in prostate fibroblast-to-myofibroblast transdifferentiation. *Mech. Ageing Dev.* **2005**, *126*, 59–69. [CrossRef] [PubMed]
35. Fenne, I.S.; Helland, T.; Flageng, M.H.; Dankel, S.N.; Mellgren, G.; Sagen, J.V. Downregulation of steroid receptor coactivator-2 modulates estrogen-responsive genes and stimulates proliferation of mcf-7 breast cancer cells. *PLoS ONE* **2013**, *8*, e70096. [CrossRef] [PubMed]
36. Pashaie, E.; Guzel, E.; Ozgurses, M.E.; Demirel, G.; Aydin, N.; Ozen, M. A meta-analysis: Identification of common mir-145 target gens that have similar behavior in different GEO datasets. *PLoS ONE* **2016**, *11*, e0161491. [CrossRef] [PubMed]

37. Zhang, Z.W.; Yang, Z.M.; Zheng, Y.C.; Chen, Z.D. Transgelin induces apoptosis of human prostate LNCaP cells through its interaction with p53. *Asian J. Androl.* **2010**, *12*, 186–195. [CrossRef] [PubMed]
38. Osman, I.; Drobnjak, M.; Fazzari, M.; Ferrara, J.; Scher, H.I.; Cordon-Cardo, C. Inactivation of the p53 pathway in prostate cancer: Impact on tumor progression. *Clin. Cancer Res.* **1999**, *5*, 2082–2088. [PubMed]
39. Tsui, K.H.; Chiang, K.C.; Feng, T.H.; Chang, K.S.; Lin, Y.H.; Juang, H.H. BTG2 is a tumor suppressor gene and upregulated by p53 and PTEN in human bladder carcinoma cells. *Cancer Med.* **2018**, *7*, 184–195. [CrossRef]
40. El-Deiry, W.S. Regulation of p53 downstream genes. *Semin. Cancer Biol.* **1998**, *8*, 345–357. [CrossRef]
41. Lee, H.; Choi, S.K.; Ro, J.Y. Overexpression of DJ-1 and HSP90alpha, and loss of PTEN associated with invasive urothelial carcinoma of urinary bladder: Possible prognostic markers. *Oncol. Lett.* **2012**, *3*, 507–512. [PubMed]
42. Boosani, C.S.; Agrawal, D.K. PTEN modulators: A patent review. *Expert. Opin. Ther. Pat.* **2013**, *23*, 569–580. [CrossRef] [PubMed]
43. Morgensztern, D.; McLeod, H.L. PI3K/Akt/mTOR pathway as a target for cancer therapy. *Anti-cancer Drugs* **2005**, *16*, 797–803. [CrossRef] [PubMed]
44. Tsui, K.H.; Hou, C.P.; Chang, K.S.; Lin, Y.H.; Feng, T.H.; Chen, C.C.; Shin, Y.S.; Juang, H.H. Metallothionein 3 is a hypoxia-upregulated oncogene enhancing cell invasion and tumorigenesis in human bladder carcinoma cells. *Int. J. Mol. Sci.* **2019**, *20*, 980. [CrossRef] [PubMed]
45. Tsui, K.H.; Hsu, S.Y.; Chung, L.C.; Lin, Y.H.; Feng, T.H.; Lee, T.Y.; Chang, P.L.; Juang, H.H. Growth differentiation factor-15: A p53- and demethylation-upregulating gene represses cell proliferation, invasion, and tumorigenesis in bladder carcinoma cells. *Sci. Rep.* **2015**, *5*, 12870. [CrossRef] [PubMed]
46. Tsui, K.H.; Chang, Y.L.; Yang, P.S.; Hou, C.P.; Lin, Y.H.; Lee, B.W.; Feng, T.H.; Juang, H.H. The inhibitory effects of capillarisin on cell proliferation and invasion of prostate carcinoma cells. *Cell Prolif.* **2018**, *51*, e12419. [CrossRef] [PubMed]
47. Chang, K.S.; Tsui, K.H.; Lin, Y.H.; Hou, C.P.; Feng, T.H.; Juang, H.H. Migration and invasion enhancer 1 is an NF-κB-inducing gene enhancing the cell proliferation and invasion ability of human prostate carcinoma cells in vitro and in vivo. *Cancers* **2019**, *11*, 1486. [CrossRef] [PubMed]
48. Tsui, K.H.; Lin, Y.H.; Chung, L.C.; Chuang, S.T.; Feng, T.H.; Chiang, K.C.; Chang, P.L.; Yen, C.L.; Juang, H.H. Prostate-derived ets factor represses tumorigenesis and modulates epithelial-to-mesenchymal transition in bladder carcinoma cells. *Cancer Lett.* **2016**, *375*, 142–151. [CrossRef]

13

Evaluation of a New Survivin ELISA and UBC® *Rapid* for the Detection of Bladder Cancer in Urine

Jan Gleichenhagen [1,*], Christian Arndt [2], Swaantje Casjens [1], Carmen Meinig [1], Holger Gerullis [3], Irina Raiko [1], Thomas Brüning [1], Thorsten Ecke [4] and Georg Johnen [1]

1 Institute for Prevention and Occupational Medicine of the German Social Accident Insurance, Institute of the Ruhr-University Bochum (IPA), 44789 Bochum, Germany; casjens@ipa-dguv.de (S.C.); meinig@ipa-dguv.de (C.M.); raiko@ipa-dguv.de (I.R.); bruening@ipa-dguv.de (T.B.); johnen@ipa-dguv.de (G.J.)

2 Department of Urology, Lukaskrankenhaus Neuss, 41464 Neuss, Germany; CArndt@lukasneuss.de

3 University Hospital for Urology, Klinikum Oldenburg, 26133 Oldenburg, Germany; holger.gerullis@gmx.net

4 Department of Urology, HELIOS Hospital, 15526 Bad Saarow, Germany; thorsten.ecke@helios-gesundheit.de

* Correspondence: Gleichenhagen@ipa-dguv.de

Abstract: Urine-based biomarkers for non-invasive diagnosis of bladder cancer are urgently needed. No single marker with sufficient sensitivity and specificity has been described so far. Thus, a combination of markers appears to be a promising approach. The aim of this case-control study was to evaluate the performance of an in-house developed enzyme-linked immunosorbent assay (ELISA) for survivin, the UBC® *Rapid* test, and the combination of both assays. A total of 290 patients were recruited. Due to prior bladder cancer, 46 patients were excluded. Urine samples were available from 111 patients with bladder cancer and 133 clinical controls without urologic diseases. Antibodies generated from recombinant survivin were utilized to develop a sandwich ELISA. The ELISA and the UBC® *Rapid* test were applied to all urine samples. Receiver operating characteristic (ROC) analysis was used to evaluate marker performance. The survivin ELISA exhibited a sensitivity of 35% with a specificity of 98%. The UBC® *Rapid* test showed a sensitivity of 56% and a specificity of 96%. Combination of both assays increased the sensitivity to 66% with a specificity of 95%. For high-grade tumors, the combination showed a sensitivity of 82% and a specificity of 95%. The new survivin ELISA and the UBC® *Rapid* test are both able to detect bladder cancer, especially high-grade tumors. However, the performance of each individual marker is moderate and efforts to improve the survivin assay should be pursued. A combination of both assays confirmed the benefit of using marker panels. The results need further testing in a prospective study and with a high-risk population.

Keywords: survivin; UBC® *Rapid*; bladder cancer; urine; biomarker combination; non-invasive

---

1. Introduction

Bladder cancer is the most common cancer of the urinary tract and ranks fifth among cancers in men in western countries [1]. It is typically diagnosed by cystoscopy followed by pathological examination of suspicious tissue. Cystoscopy is a time-consuming method that requires an experienced urologist to perform and can be painful for the patients. Thus, there is a need for an easier and non-invasive diagnostic method. Being minimally- or non-invasive is a key characteristic of biomarkers, facilitating the use of easily accessible body fluids instead of tissue, which requires invasive sampling. Because of its close proximity to the target organ, it is of general acceptance that urine might be a good source for bladder cancer-specific biomarkers [2].

Based on urine or urinary cells, only a few molecular markers have been approved by the federal Food and Drug Administration (FDA) so far. In addition, these markers are designated merely as supporting tools for monitoring bladder cancer patients instead of replacing cystoscopy [3,4]. The nuclear mitotic apparatus protein 1 (NUMA1) can be quantitated by the commercial NMP22® test or detected by the BladderChek® test [5]. The reported sensitivities of the NMP22 assays in case-control studies vary between 47% and 100%, while the specificities range from 58% to 91% [6,7]. In contrast to the results from case-control studies, in a prospective study (UroScreen), the assay reached a sensitivity of 97% and a specificity of 29% in prediagnostic samples [7]. The performance of NMP22 was limited by a relative high number of false-positive test results, which can be caused, for example, by hematuria or infections [5,7]. Using fluorescence in situ hybridization (FISH), the UroVysion test is applied to detect chromosomal copy number variations in exfoliated urothelial cells sedimented from urine samples. In a pooled analysis of FISH-based assays, the average sensitivity was 76% (65–84%) and the specificity 85% (78–92%) [8], another pooled analysis yielded 72% and 83%, respectively [9]. In the prospective study UroScreen, the UroVysion test reached a sensitivity of 45% at a specificity of 97% [10]. While UroVysion is relatively specific, it only showed a moderately increased sensitivity compared to the much cheaper classical cytology. It is also restricted by the requirement of special equipment and a time-consuming, expert-dependent procedure [11,12].

The limited performance of individual markers can be improved by combining two or more markers in a panel. For example, in the prospective study UroScreen, a combination of UroVysion and NMP22 reached a sensitivity of 67% and a specificity of 95% [11]. However, there is still a lack of easy to apply and cost-effective assays with adequate performance that would qualify as candidates for a biomarker panel.

In order to evaluate additional assays of urinary biomarkers, we focused on two candidates, UBC® *Rapid* and survivin, and tested their ability to detect bladder cancer. UBC® *Rapid* is a commercially available point-of-care test measuring cytokeratin fragments 8 and 18 in urine. Affordability and ease of use are factors that would support its implementation in routine diagnostics. Survivin is a well-known protein biomarker and detectable in almost every cancer [13,14], including bladder cancer [15,16]. Detailed information about biological function is discussed in several reviews [13,17] as well as its potential as a therapeutic target [18–20]. Most studies analyzing the expression of survivin used invasively obtained tissue samples or rely on the detection of survivin mRNA in sedimented cells from urine [21–23]. Because of our previous experience with the practical problems associated with the limited stability of mRNA, we decided to focus on the more stable survivin protein. A well-established method for the measurement of proteins in laboratory diagnostics is the enzyme-linked immunosorbent assay (ELISA). ELISAs for the detection of survivin are commercially available, but often lack sufficient performance, particularly when using urine as a sample matrix [24].

The aim of this study was to develop a new ELISA for the quantification of survivin in urine samples and to evaluate the performance of the ELISA in combination with UBC® *Rapid* for urine-based detection of bladder cancer, especially high-grade tumors.

2. Results

2.1. Survivin Production and ELISA Development

Cloning, expression, and affinity purification yielded about 2.5 mg of His_{10}-survivin fusion protein suitable for antibody generation in rabbits (Figure 1a).

Antibodies were purified and partially biotinylated for application in a sandwich ELISA. No cross-reactivity was observed for anti-survivin antibodies. The best signal-to-noise ratio was obtained with a dilution of 1:5000 for the capture antibody and a dilution of 1:10,000 for the detection antibody. The resulting sigmoidal curve could be interpolated within the range of 0.025–5 ng/mL, with a limit of detection (LoD) of about 0.033 ng/mL for the new survivin ELISA (Figure 1b). We compared our ELISA with the commercially available survivin ELISA kits of R&D and Enzo

Life Sciences by performing four-parameter logistic curve-fits for the reference curves. The standard curve of our ELISA was comparable to those of the commercial ELISA kits (Figure S1).

Reproducibility of the new survivin ELISA was investigated by measuring three defined samples of low, medium, and high survivin concentrations multiple times ($n = 24$). The resulting coefficients of variation (CVs) were 7.2% for the low, 4.6% for the medium, and 6.5% for the high concentration sample. In addition, we tested the repeatability with two different samples of medium survivin concentration at different time points. The resulting CVs were 8.8% and 19.4%. Additionally, matrix effects were investigated by spike-in experiments. Defined recombinant survivin concentrations were spiked into survivin-free urine samples. The recovery rate ranged from 74.8 to 88.9%.

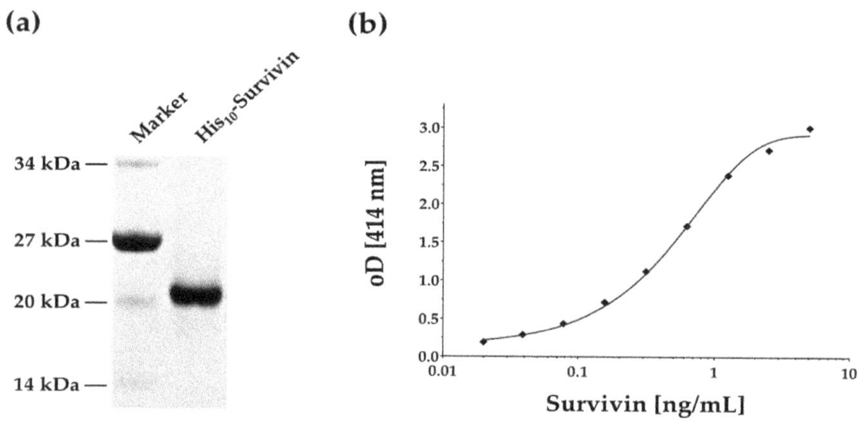

Figure 1. SDS-PAGE and ELISA reference curve. (**a**) Coomassie-blue stained SDS-PAGE of recombinant purified His_{10}-survivin; (**b**) representative four-parameter logistic curve fit for the survivin ELISA.

2.2. Study Group

Table 1 depicts the characteristics of the 244 participants, divided into tumor cases ($n = 111$), and clinical controls ($n = 133$). Most of the participants were men ($n = 175$). The median age of the tumor group and clinical controls was similar (74 vs. 71 years).

Table 1. Characteristics of the study population and patients.

Characteristics	All (n = 244)			Tumor (n = 111)			Clinical Controls (n = 133)		
Gender		Male	Female		Male	Female		Male	Female
n		175	69		83	28		92	41
	n	**Median**	**IQR**	n	**Median**	**IQR**	n	**Median**	**IQR**
Age (years)	244	73	63–80	111	74	65–80	133	71	60–79
Body mass index	244	26.5	24.0–29.8	111	26.9	24.3–30.4	133	26.3	23.6–29.6
Urine volume (mL)	244	30	16–40	111	20	14–40	133	35	20–50
Urine retention within bladder (h)	236	2.0	1.0–3.0	106	1.75	1.0–2.5	130	2.0	1.0–3.5
Specific gravity (g/L)	240	240	1015	109	1015	1015–1020	131	1020	1015–1020
pH	240	5	5.0–6.5	109	5	5–6.5	131	5	5–6.5
Survivin (ng/mL)				111	0.014 *	0–0.528	133	0	0–0.249
UBC® *Rapid* (mg/L)				111	16.3	5–300	133	5	5–28.2

IQR = interquartile range; * extrapolated value.

Among all groups, median volume of urine was 30 mL with a retention time of about 2 h within the bladder before voiding. The median pH of urinary samples was 5.0 in all groups. Additional details regarding the tumor group are listed in Table 2.

Table 2. Characteristics of the tumor group.

Characteristic	Status	(*n*)
Tumor Stage	Ta	61
	T1	14
	T2	23
	T3	9
	Carcinoma in situ	3
	Missing	1
Histological grade	Low	55
	High	55
	Missing	1
Recurrent	Yes	52
	No	58
	Missing	1
Gross hematuria	Yes	66
	No	45
Dysuria	Yes	33
	No	78
Frequent urination	Yes	51
	No	60
Bladder Stones	Yes	12
	No	99
Diabetes mellitus type II	Yes	12
	No	99
Smoking	Never	23
	Former	51
	Actual	35
	Missing	2

2.3. Survivin in Urine of Bladder Cancer Patients

Initially, we tested voided urine, supernatant, and urinary pellet for measurable amounts of survivin. Only urinary pellet exhibited detectable amounts of survivin. Therefore, all herein presented survivin-related data refer to the urinary pellet.

The distributions of survivin concentrations in tumor and control groups are shown in Figure 2a.

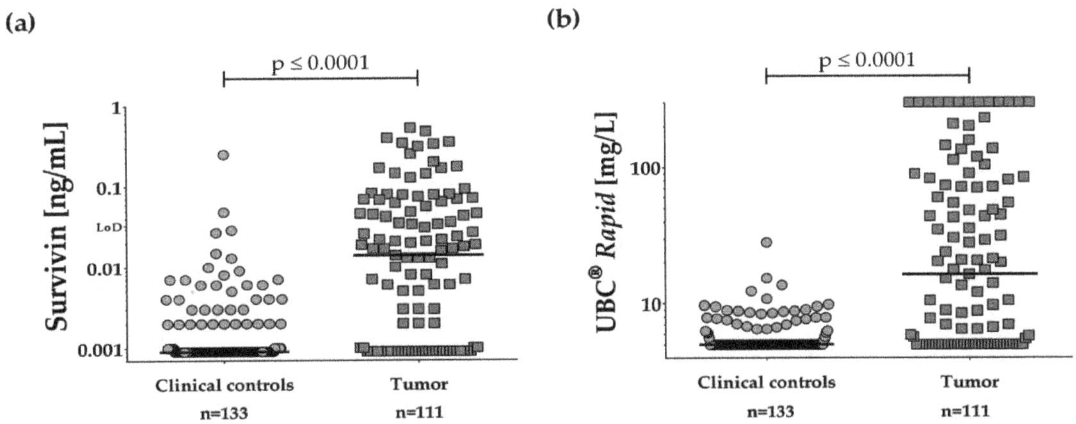

Figure 2. Dot plots of marker results in urine. Comparison of marker concentrations in urinary samples from clinical controls and bladder tumor patients. (**a**) Survivin and (**b**) UBC® *Rapid*. Lines depict the median for each group. *p*-Values were obtained from the Wilcoxon signed-rank test.

The median survivin concentration was below the LoD (<0.033 ng/mL) in both groups. Normalization by creatinine or amount of total protein was therefore not attempted. However, the median survivin concentration differed between tumor group and clinical controls ($p < 0.0001$). Survivin levels were not influenced by obtained volume of urine, retention time within the bladder, or gender. Using a cut-off of 0.033 ng/mL, our survivin ELISA showed a sensitivity of 35% (39/111 tumors true-positive) and a specificity of 98%, when comparing tumor group and clinical controls. Tumor grade had an influence on the marker performance. The survivin ELISA detected 51% (28/55) of the high-grade tumors but only 18% (10/55) of the low-grade tumors (Table 3, Figure S2a). Grading data was missing for one case. The area under the curve (AUC) was 0.77 for the ROC curve analysis of tumor versus clinical controls (Figure 3).

Table 3. Performance of survivin, UBC® *Rapid*, and combination based on single-marker cut-off for the detection of bladder cancer.

Groups	Cut-Off	Sensitivity (%)	Specificity (%)	True-Positive (*n*)	True-Negative (*n*)	False-Positive (*n*)	False-Negative (*n*)
			Survivin ELISA				
Tumor vs. Controls	0.033 ng/mL	35	98	39	131	2	72
High-grade tumor vs. Controls		51	98	28	131	2	27
Low-grade tumor vs. Controls		18	98	10	131	2	45
			UBC® *Rapid*				
Tumor vs. Controls	10.0 mg/L	56	96	62	128	5	49
High-grade tumor vs. Controls		73	96	40	128	5	15
Low-grade tumor vs. Controls		40	96	22	128	5	33
			Combination				
Tumor vs. Controls	>Survivin or >UBC® *Rapid*	66	95	73	127	6	38
High-grade tumor vs. Controls		82	95	45	127	6	10
Low-grade tumor vs. Controls		49	95	27	127	6	28

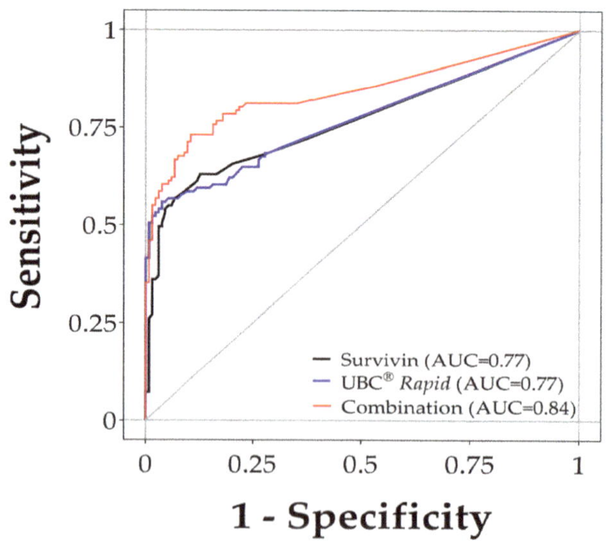

Figure 3. ROC analyses of survivin and UBC® *Rapid*. ROC curves for survivin (AUC = 0.77), UBC® *Rapid* (AUC = 0.77), and the combination of both assays (AUC = 0.84) based on comparing tumor and clinical control group.

2.4. Performance of UBC® Rapid

The distribution of the UBC® *Rapid* results for the clinical controls and the tumor group are depicted as dot plots in Figure 2b. The median UBC® *Rapid* value was <5.0 mg/L for clinical controls and 16.3 mg/L for the tumor group. The difference between the tumor group and the control group was statistically significant ($p < 0.0001$). Using the cut-off (10 mg/L) recommended by the supplier, the UBC® *Rapid* assay reached a sensitivity of 56% (62/111) at a specificity of 96%. As seen with survivin, the sensitivity of the assay increased (to 73%) in high-grade tumors in comparison to controls (Table 3, Figure S2b). ROC curves and AUC values for the UBC® *Rapid* test were similar to those of the survivin assay and are shown in Figure 3.

2.5. Combination of Survivin and UBC® Rapid

Because of the generally limited performance of individual biomarker assays, we also looked at the possible benefits of a combination of biomarkers. To our knowledge, this is the first approach exploring survivin and UBC® *Rapid* as a panel. The results of the combination of the survivin ELISA and the UBC® *Rapid* test are shown in Table 3 and depicted in Figure 3. A scatter plot of the values of the tumor samples indicates a moderate correlation between both assays (Spearman's $r_s = 0.38$; Figure S3). Further analysis by Venn-diagrams (Figure 4) revealed that, in addition to 28 tumors detected by both assays, 45 tumors were solely detected by either UBC® *Rapid* (34 tumors) or survivin (11 tumors). From the ROC analysis, an AUC of 0.84, a sensitivity of 66% and a specificity of 95% could be derived for the combination. The difference between each single marker AUC and AUC of the combination is statistically significant (combination vs. survivin: $p = 0.0025$; combination vs. UBC® *Rapid*: $p = 0.0005$). Comparing high-grade tumors with controls revealed an AUC of 0.91, a sensitivity of 82%, and a specificity of 95% (Table 3, Figures S4 and S5). Here, the difference between single marker AUC and combination AUC was not significant (combination vs. survivin: $p = 0.1826$; combination vs. UBC® *Rapid*: $p = 0.0685$).

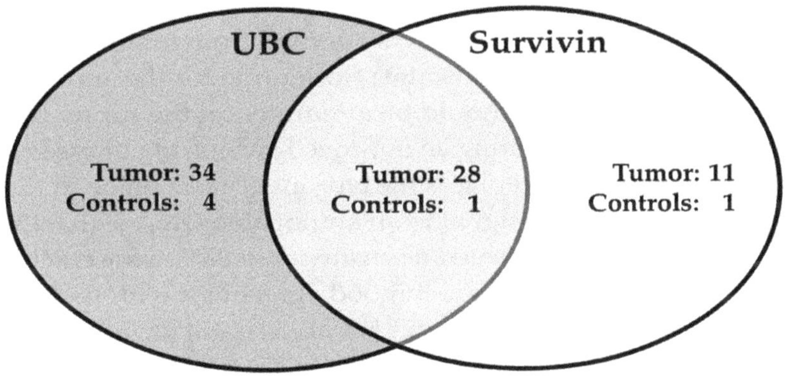

Figure 4. Venn diagrams of all positive test results. The cut-off for UBC® *Rapid* was >10 mg/L (**left**) and for survivin >0.033 ng/mL (**right**).

2.6. Possible Influence of Microhematuria

Microhematuria could be a possible influencing factor of biomarker performance. We therefore investigated the effect of microhematuria in the control group. Of the 133 controls, 28 had erythrocytes (between 5 and 250 cells [25]) in their urine. Median marker concentrations in controls with and without microhematuria did not show significant differences for both markers ($p = 0.4511$ for survivin and $p = 0.4121$ for UBC® *Rapid*).

3. Discussion

Bladder cancer is one of the most common cancers worldwide [26]. The current gold standard for bladder cancer detection is cystoscopy and cytology. Those methods are routinely applied in patients with hematuria or other symptoms suggestive of bladder cancer [8]. Clinical symptoms are more likely to occur at later stages of tumor development. Biomarkers have the potential to detect cancer at earlier stages, facilitating an earlier and therefore more curative therapy that ideally results in decreased mortality or chance of recurrence, while potentially reducing the number of invasive diagnostic procedures [27]. Urine is apparently an ideal source for non-invasive biomarkers for detection or monitoring urothelial bladder cancer [2]. Screening for bladder cancer is medically reasonable for high-risk groups, e.g., persons with a high recurrence rate or a previous exposure to bladder cancer carcinogens [4,11,15,28]. For instance, in Germany, workers with a previous occupational exposure to aromatic amines are offered free medical exams to screen for bladder cancer [11].

Examples for urine-based biomarkers that have been suggested for screening are UroVysion, uCyt+, or NMP22. However, the markers had some drawbacks, including observer bias, time-consuming procedures, confounders, and/or large variations in reported performance [5,11,29,30]. Survivin is another possible target for biomarker development that has been well published [21]. Unfortunately, most studies relied on immunohistochemistry of tissue samples or mRNA-based approaches [21–23,30]. ELISA-based techniques are an easy-to-use assay format frequently used in routine applications for protein quantification, but less commonly applied to urinary samples [24]. To overcome the limitations associated with survivin mRNA [22], we investigated a newly developed ELISA to detect survivin at the protein level. The ELISA featured a LoD (0.033 ng/mL) and detection range comparable to commercially available ELISAs. We performed a four-parameter curve fit for the calibration curve because this procedure is commonly recommended and appears to be more reliable for values close to the LoD [31].

We could not observe detectable amounts of survivin in urinary supernatant or unprocessed voided urine using the new ELISA. We did not attempt to detect survivin in concentrated urine [32]. Instead, we based our survivin determination on measurements in sedimented cells from urine to avoid matrix effects that might influence the assay. Urine is a dynamic and heterogenic fluid comprising varying salt concentrations and pH values [33–36]. Those parameters are important factors for antibody–antigen interaction [37]. A secretion of survivin from tumor cells via exosomes has been reported recently [38]. An enrichment of exosomes from urine for the subsequent determination of survivin is an interesting approach that should be attempted in the future but may require a more sensitive assay. Currently, we are investigating an improved version of our assay based on a solid-phase proximity ligation assay. This technique replaces the enzymatic reaction of an ELISA with quantitative PCR by transferring the original protein signal to an amplifiable DNA signal [39,40].

The presented case-control study revealed a sensitivity of 35%, a specificity of 98%, and an AUC of 0.77 for our survivin ELISA. The results are in good agreement with the reported sensitivity and specificity by Ohsawa et al. [41]. In comparison, Li et al., Eissa et al., and Srivastava et al. reported a somewhat higher performance with AUC values of 0.85, 0.87, and 0.88, respectively [32,42,43]. The composition of the study populations—e.g., variations in grade and stage of the tumors and variations in the control group—might have contributed to these differences. As seen before with immunohistochemistry and mRNA-based assays, the survivin ELISA was more sensitive for high-grade tumors [22,23,30]. This is also plausible in view of the mechanistic role of survivin, which is involved in suppression of apoptosis as well as regulation of mitosis [13,16,17,44,45].

Parallel to survivin, we examined the commercial point-of-care test UBC® *Rapid*. Compared to other commercially available tests like UroVysion or uCyt+, it is affordable, simple to use and not observer-biased. In our study group, the UBC® *Rapid* test reached an AUC of 0.77 and a sensitivity of 56% at a specificity of 96%, using the recommended cut-off of 10 mg/L. This is in accordance with other reports showing sensitivities in the range of 53–64% and specificities in the range of 63–91% [46–51]. Similar to survivin, UBC® *Rapid* also has a higher sensitivity for high-grade tumors [46,50–52] in comparison to low-grade tumors, indicating that the UBC® *Rapid* test may be more useful for this subgroup. The test may be influenced by urinary tract infections as has been shown before [53].

Screening, even in high-risk populations, requires a high specificity in order to avoid unnecessary invasive diagnostic procedures and psychological burden for the patients, which can be a consequence of false-positive test results [52,54]. As has been reported before, no single marker has reproducibly shown a sufficiently high sensitivity in conjunction with the required high specificity to detect bladder cancer early [2,11]. This was also true for the two biomarkers we investigated in the present study. Both survivin and UBC® *Rapid* had relatively good specificities but moderate sensitivities at the given cut-offs. However, lower sensitivities can be compensated by the use of several biomarkers in a panel. Indeed, the combination of both markers increased the sensitivity to 66% at a specificity of 95%. For the subgroup of high-grade tumors, the sensitivity even increased to 82%. Due to the fact that high-grade tumors have a higher rate of progression and/or recurrence, it is helpful to focus on markers exhibiting a higher sensitivity for this particular subgroup.

A limitation of the markers that has been reported before is the reduced performance associated with other urologic diseases, confounders that would also be expected in a typical clinical setting [45,50,55,56]. Microhematuria apparently does not affect the survivin ELISA or UBC® *Rapid*. Another possible confounder for biomarker assays can be a urinary infection. A typical example is the protein marker NMP22 [5,7]. Because expression of survivin has been reported in some cases of inflammation [56] and links between inflammation pathways and cancer development are generally known [56,57], bladder infections could also influence urinary survivin concentrations. Therefore, a combination with other markers like UroVysion, which are less affected by confounders, and different algorithms to combine the markers may be interesting options. In addition, the aforementioned efforts to refine the survivin assay could lead to a higher sensitivity. An advantage of the survivin ELISA and UBC® *Rapid* is their affordability and ease of use, factors that are important for a future application in screening or surveillance programs. The case-control design and the selection of the control group are limitations of our study, which was intended as an initial assessment of a new assay. Thus, before an application in screening is possible, the markers have to be validated in a prospective study with an independent and larger study population. The establishment of a suitable cohort is currently under way, but the process requires time and some effort.

4. Materials and Methods

4.1. Study Population

Between January 2014 and July 2015, a total of 290 patients were recruited at the Lukaskrankenhaus (Neuss, Germany). Because of a prior bladder cancer diagnosis, 46 patients were excluded. The remaining 244 participants included 111 patients suffering from bladder cancer and 133 control patients visiting for other reasons than bladder cancer or urologic disease. The initial diagnosis of bladder cancer was based on cystoscopy and confirmed by histological and immunohistochemical examination of resected tissue. Tumors have been assigned as low- or high-grade tumors according to the 2004 WHO classification [58]. Urine was collected before transurethral resection. Tumor patients and controls were matched for age and gender. The study was approved by the ethics committee of the Landesärztekammer Brandenburg No. AS 147(bB)/2013 (17 November 2013).

4.2. Urine Sample Collection

Midstream urine samples were collected at the Urology department of the Lukaskrankenhaus Neuss, Germany. Urinary samples were processed immediately or stored at +4 °C for a maximum of 4 h. Urine status was assayed by routine dipstick analysis. For the UBC® *Rapid* assay, three drops of fresh urine were used prior to further processing of a urine sample. After taking a 2-mL aliquot, remaining urine was centrifuged at 1500× g for 10 min at +10 °C in a swinging bucket rotor. Resulting supernatant was aliquoted (4 × 2 mL) and the pellet was resuspended in 1 mL of PBS. All samples were stored at −20 °C until further analyses were carried out. For further analysis, the samples were shipped on dry ice to the IPA in Bochum.

4.3. UBC® Rapid Test

The UBC® *Rapid* test (Concile GmbH, Freiburg/Breisgau, Germany) was performed according to the manufacturers' instructions as previously described [46]. The test cartridges were read out by the photometric point-of-care (POC) system Concile® Ω100 reader (Concile GmbH) according to the manufacturers' instructions, allowing a quantitative analysis of the test results.

4.4. Expression and Purification of Recombinant Survivin

Template cDNA of survivin (BIRC5) was obtained from Sino Biologicals, Beijing, China. The standard PCR protocol included the primers p1 (5′-GTATACCATATGGGTGCCCGG-3′) and p2 (5′-CGGATCCTCAATCCATGGCAGC-3′). The PCR product was cut with NdeI and BamHI (New England Biolabs, Ipswich, MA, USA) for an in-frame ligation of the survivin coding sequence into pET16b (Merck Millipore Novagen, Darmstadt, Germany), which provides the coding sequence for an N-terminal polyhistidine-tag. Cloning products were confirmed by sequencing. The resulting pET16b_His-Survivin plasmid was transformed into *E. coli* BL 21 CodonPlus RIPL (Agilent Technologies, Santa Clara, CA, USA) cells for heterologous protein expression. The cells of a 1 L culture were harvested and lysed by urea denaturation in 20 mM Hepes, 100 mM NaCl (pH 8). Purification of the His_{10}-Survivin fusion protein was performed as described elsewhere [59]. Briefly, cell lysate was centrifuged to remove cell debris. Soluble supernatant was applied to an affinity chromatography column (HisTrap HP, GE Healthcare Life Science, Freiburg, Germany). After washing, the purified protein was eluted with elution buffer (20 mM Hepes, 100 mM NaCl, 8 M Urea, 250 mM imidazole, pH 8). Eluted affinity-purified His_{10}-Survivin showed high purity and was further processed on a size-exclusion chromatography column (SuperdexTM 75, Amersham Bioscience, Little Chalfont, Buckinghamshire, UK) for protein refolding. Final proteins in PBS was stored at −20 °C and used for immunization of rabbits for the generation of polyclonal antibodies.

4.5. Immunization and Antibody Purification

Immunization with His_{10}-Survivin was performed at Charles River (Charles River Laboratories, Chatillon-sur-Chalaronne, France) following standard immunization protocols. After 70 days, 90 mL final sera were received and 20 mL of these were further processed for antibody purification. For this purpose, sera were loaded onto a Profinity Protein A column (Bio-Rad, Munich, Germany) linked to a Next Generation Chromatography System (Bio-Rad). The column was washed with PBS and the purified antibodies were eluted with 100 mM glycine (pH 2.8). Purified anti-survivin antibodies were immediately dialyzed against PBS yielding a final IgG concentration of 2.87 mg/mL (15 mL) as determined by absorption at 280 nm.

4.6. Biotinylation of Anti-Survivin Antibody

For ELISA development, the purified survivin antibody was partly biotinylated. Briefly, purified antibody was mixed with 33× molar excess of NHS-Biotin (Thermo Fisher, Waltham, MA, USA) in 10 mM $NaHCO_3$ (pH 8.4), incubated for 3 h at room temperature and finally dialyzed against PBS. The final concentration of biotinylated antibody was 2.18 mg/mL (5 mL).

4.7. Survivin ELISA

In the experiments, 250 μL urinary cell pellet was centrifuged with 1500× *g* for 5 min at +4 °C to remove the storage solution. Afterwards, the pellet was completely dissolved in 500 μL CytoBuster (Merck Millipore, Darmstadt, Germany) and concentrated by using Vivaspin 500 spin columns (Sartorius, Stonehouse, Gloucestershire, UK) to 50 μL. To this solution, 150 μL of PBST (PBS with 0.05% Tween-20) was added and used as sample for measurement. Residual CytoBuster was tested to have no influence on antibody binding. Microtiter plates (Thermo Scientific, Roskilde, Denmark) were coated with purified polyclonal antibodies (100 μL/well, diluted 1:5000 in 100 mM carbonate/bicarbonate buffer, pH 9.6) and allowed to adhere overnight at +4 °C. They were then blocked with 1.5% casein, washed, and incubated with dilutions of the standard and samples for 1 h at room temperature. A stock solution of survivin was diluted in PBST to give standard concentrations between 5 and 0.02 ng/mL. Next, plates were washed three times with PBST and incubated for 1 h with biotinylated polyclonal antibodies (100 μL/well, dilution 1:10,000). After washing, 100 μL/well of 1:20,000 diluted horseradish-peroxidase-streptavidin conjugate (Fitzgerald Industries International, Concord, MA,

USA) was added. After 1 h, plates were washed with PBST and 100 μL H_2O_2-activated ABTS substrate solution was added to each well. The enzyme reaction was stopped by addition of 100 μL 0.32% NaF and absorbance was read at 414 nm.

The dose–response curves for standards were obtained by 4-parameter curve fitting using SoftMax Pro 4.7.1 from Molecular Devices (Sunnyvale, CA, USA). The lower detection limit of the assay was defined by adding 0.05 OD units (2-fold mean of the background standard deviation of 20 plates) to the background value of each plate. Samples were considered as positive for survivin if the measured concentration was above the cut-off. The cut-off was defined as the limit of detection. Reproducibility experiments were performed with samples containing low (0.168 ng/mL), medium (0.667 ng/mL) and high (2.240 ng/mL) survivin concentrations.

4.8. Statistics

Statistical analyses were performed with SAS/STAT and SAS/IML software version 9.4 (SAS Institute Inc., Cary, NC, USA) or Prism 5 (GraphPad Software, Inc., San Diego, CA, USA). Plots were generated with Prism 5. Median and inter-quartile ranges (IQR) were used to describe the distribution of continuous variables. Groups were compared using the non-parametric Wilcoxon signed-rank test. Spearman's correlation coefficients (r_s) and 95% confidence intervals were used to describe rank correlations between variables. The performance of the individual biomarkers and their combination was evaluated by receiver operating characteristic (ROC) analysis. For the panel, an 'or' combination of both markers was used. ROC curves were compared with a non-parametric approach [60].

5. Conclusions

In summary, a new ELISA to quantitate survivin in urine samples has been developed and evaluated alongside the UBC® *Rapid* test in a case-control study. Both assays detected bladder cancer, preferably high-grade tumors, but each with relatively low sensitivity. For the first time, survivin and UBC® *Rapid* have been tested as a panel, demonstrating an increase in sensitivity. However, the results require further testing of the assays with other control groups, like patients at suspicion for bladder cancer, and finally validation in a prospective study using a high-risk cohort.

Acknowledgments: We thank Hans-Peter Rihs for kindly providing survivin coding sequence and Beate Pesch for constructive discussion on study design. We acknowledge support by the Open Access Publication Funds of the Ruhr-University Bochum.

Author Contributions: Jan Gleichenhagen designed and performed survivin experiments, participated in the immunoassay development and data collection, and drafted the manuscript. Christian Arndt carried out the UBC® *Rapid* experiments, participated in recruitment and coordination. Swaantje Casjens performed the statistical analyses and helped to draft the manuscript. Carmen Meinig carried out immunoassays and participated in data collection. Holger Gerullis participated in recruitment and coordination. Irina Raiko carried out initial immunoassay analysis and development. Thomas Brüning participated in the study design and coordination. Thorsten Ecke participated in the study design and coordination, and helped to draft the manuscript. Georg Johnen conceived the study, participated in its design and coordination, and helped to draft the manuscript.

Abbreviations

AUC	Area under the curve
CV	Coefficient of variation
LoD	Limit of detection
ELISA	Enzyme-linked immunosorbent assay
IQR	Interquartile range
ROC	Receiver operating characteristic

References

1. Knowles, M.A.; Hurst, C.D. Molecular biology of bladder cancer: New insights into pathogenesis and clinical diversity. *Nat. Rev. Cancer* **2015**, *15*, 25–41. [CrossRef] [PubMed]
2. Schmitz-Drager, B.J.; Droller, M.; Lokeshwar, V.B.; Lotan, Y.; Hudson, M.L.A.; van Rhijn, B.W.; Marberger, M.J.; Fradet, Y.; Hemstreet, G.P.; Malmstrom, P.-U.; et al. Molecular markers for bladder cancer screening, early diagnosis, and surveillance: The WHO/ICUD consensus. *Urol. Int.* **2015**, *94*, 1–24. [CrossRef] [PubMed]
3. Tilki, D.; Burger, M.; Dalbagni, G.; Grossman, H.B.; Hakenberg, O.W.; Palou, J.; Reich, O.; Roupret, M.; Shariat, S.F.; Zlotta, A.R. Urine markers for detection and surveillance of non-muscle-invasive bladder cancer. *Eur. Urol.* **2011**, *60*, 484–492. [CrossRef] [PubMed]
4. Smith, Z.L.; Guzzo, T.J. Urinary markers for bladder cancer. *F1000prime Rep.* **2013**, *5*, 21. [CrossRef] [PubMed]
5. Miyake, M.; Goodison, S.; Giacoia, E.G.; Rizwani, W.; Ross, S.; Rosser, C.J. Influencing factors on the NMP-22 urine assay: An experimental model. *BMC Urol.* **2012**, *12*, 23. [CrossRef] [PubMed]
6. Chou, R.; Gore, J.L.; Buckley, D.; Fu, R.; Gustafson, K.; Griffin, J.C.; Grusing, S.; Selph, S. Urinary Biomarkers for Diagnosis of Bladder Cancer: A Systematic Review and Meta-analysis. *Ann. Intern. Med.* **2015**, *163*, 922–931. [CrossRef] [PubMed]
7. Huber, S.; Schwentner, C.; Taeger, D.; Pesch, B.; Nasterlack, M.; Leng, G.; Mayer, T.; Gawrych, K.; Bonberg, N.; Pelster, M.; et al. Nuclear matrix protein-22: A prospective evaluation in a population at risk for bladder cancer. Results from the UroScreen study. *BJU Int.* **2012**, *110*, 699–708. [CrossRef] [PubMed]
8. Mowatt, G.; Zhu, S.; Kilonzo, M.; Boachie, C.; Fraser, C.; Griffiths, T.R.L.; N'Dow, J.; Nabi, G.; Cook, J.; Vale, L. Systematic review of the clinical effectiveness and cost-effectiveness of photodynamic diagnosis and urine biomarkers (FISH, ImmunoCyt, NMP22) and cytology for the detection and follow-up of bladder cancer. *Health Technol. Assess.* **2010**, *14*, 1–331. [CrossRef] [PubMed]
9. Hajdinjak, T. UroVysion FISH test for detecting urothelial cancers: Meta-analysis of diagnostic accuracy and comparison with urinary cytology testing. *Urol. Oncol.* **2008**, *26*, 646–651. [CrossRef] [PubMed]
10. Banek, S.; Schwentner, C.; Täger, D.; Pesch, B.; Nasterlack, M.; Leng, G.; Gawrych, K.; Bonberg, N.; Johnen, G.; Kluckert, M.; et al. Prospective evaluation of fluorescence-in situ-hybridization to detect bladder cancer: Results from the UroScreen-Study. *Urol. Oncol.* **2013**, *31*, 1656–1662. [CrossRef] [PubMed]
11. Pesch, B.; Taeger, D.; Johnen, G.; Gawrych, K.; Bonberg, N.; Schwentner, C.; Wellhausser, H.; Kluckert, M.; Leng, G.; Nasterlack, M.; et al. Screening for bladder cancer with urinary tumor markers in chemical workers with exposure to aromatic amines. *Int. Arch. Occup. Environ. Health* **2014**, *87*, 715–724. [CrossRef] [PubMed]
12. Bonberg, N.; Taeger, D.; Gawrych, K.; Johnen, G.; Banek, S.; Schwentner, C.; Sievert, K.-D.; Wellhäußer, H.; Kluckert, M.; Leng, G.; et al. Chromosomal instability and bladder cancer: The UroVysion(TM) test in the UroScreen study. *BJU Int.* **2013**, *112*, E372–E382. [CrossRef] [PubMed]
13. Unruhe, B.; Schroder, E.; Wunsch, D.; Knauer, S.K. An Old Flame Never Dies: Survivin in Cancer and Cellular Senescence. *Gerontology* **2016**, *62*, 173–181. [CrossRef] [PubMed]
14. Jaiswal, P.K.; Goel, A.; Mittal, R.D. Survivin: A molecular biomarker in cancer. *Indian J. Med. Res.* **2015**, *141*, 389–397. [PubMed]
15. Akhtar, M.; Gallagher, L.; Rohan, S. Survivin: Role in diagnosis, prognosis, and treatment of bladder cancer. *Adv. Anat. Pathol.* **2006**, *13*, 122–126. [CrossRef] [PubMed]
16. Shariat, S.F.; Casella, R.; Khoddami, S.M.; Hernandez, G.; Sulser, T.; Gasser, T.C.; Lerner, S.P. Urine detection of survivin is a sensitive marker for the noninvasive diagnosis of bladder cancer. *J. Urol.* **2004**, *171*, 626–630. [CrossRef] [PubMed]
17. Altieri, D.C. Survivin—The inconvenient IAP. *Semin. Cell Dev. Boil.* **2015**, *39*, 91–96. [CrossRef] [PubMed]
18. Groner, B.; Weiss, A. Targeting survivin in cancer: Novel drug development approaches. *BioDrugs* **2014**, *28*, 27–39. [CrossRef] [PubMed]
19. Altieri, D.C. Targeting survivin in cancer. *Cancer Lett.* **2013**, *332*, 225–228. [CrossRef] [PubMed]
20. Chen, X.; Duan, N.; Zhang, C.; Zhang, W. Survivin and Tumorigenesis: Molecular Mechanisms and Therapeutic Strategies. *J. Cancer* **2016**, *7*, 314–323. [CrossRef] [PubMed]
21. Ku, J.H.; Godoy, G.; Amiel, G.E.; Lerner, S.P. Urine survivin as a diagnostic biomarker for bladder cancer: A systematic review. *BJU Int.* **2012**, *110*, 630–636. [CrossRef] [PubMed]

22. Johnen, G.; Gawrych, K.; Bontrup, H.; Pesch, B.; Taeger, D.; Banek, S.; Kluckert, M.; Wellhausser, H.; Eberle, F.; Nasterlack, M.; et al. Performance of survivin mRNA as a biomarker for bladder cancer in the prospective study UroScreen. *PLoS ONE* **2012**, *7*, e35363. [CrossRef] [PubMed]
23. Jeon, C.; Kim, M.; Kwak, C.; Kim, H.H.; Ku, J.H. Prognostic role of survivin in bladder cancer: A systematic review and meta-analysis. *PLoS ONE* **2013**, *8*, e76719. [CrossRef] [PubMed]
24. Chatziharalambous, D.; Lygirou, V.; Latosinska, A.; Stravodimos, K.; Vlahou, A.; Jankowski, V.; Zoidakis, J. Analytical Performance of ELISA Assays in Urine: One More Bottleneck towards Biomarker Validation and Clinical Implementation. *PLoS ONE* **2016**, *11*, e0149471. [CrossRef] [PubMed]
25. Pesch, B.; Nasterlack, M.; Eberle, F.; Bonberg, N.; Taeger, D.; Leng, G.; Feil, G.; Johnen, G.; Ickstadt, K.; Kluckert, M.; et al. The role of hematuria in bladder cancer screening among men with former occupational exposure to aromatic amines. *BJU Int.* **2011**, *108*, 546–552. [CrossRef] [PubMed]
26. Li, H.-T.; Duymich, C.E.; Weisenberger, D.J.; Liang, G. Genetic and Epigenetic Alterations in Bladder Cancer. *Int. Neurourol. J.* **2016**, *20*, S84–S94. [CrossRef] [PubMed]
27. Di Meo, A.; Bartlett, J.; Cheng, Y.; Pasic, M.D.; Yousef, G.M. Liquid biopsy: A step forward towards precision medicine in urologic malignancies. *Mol. Cancer* **2017**, *16*, 80. [CrossRef] [PubMed]
28. Burger, M.; Catto, J.W.F.; Dalbagni, G.; Grossman, H.B.; Herr, H.; Karakiewicz, P.; Kassouf, W.; Kiemeney, L.A.; la Vecchia, C.; Shariat, S.; et al. Epidemiology and risk factors of urothelial bladder cancer. *Eur. Urol.* **2013**, *63*, 234–241. [CrossRef] [PubMed]
29. Öge, Ö.; Kozaci, D.; Gemalmaz, H. The BTA Stat Test is Nonspecific for Hematuria: An Experimental Hematuria Model. *J. Urol.* **2002**, *167*, 1318–1320. [CrossRef]
30. Shariat, S.F.; Karam, J.A.; Lotan, Y.; Karakiewizc, P.I. Critical evaluation of urinary markers for bladder cancer detection and monitoring. *Rev. Urol.* **2008**, *10*, 120–135. [PubMed]
31. Findlay, J.W.A.; Dillard, R.F. Appropriate calibration curve fitting in ligand binding assays. *AAPS J.* **2007**, *9*, E260–E267. [CrossRef] [PubMed]
32. Srivastava, A.K.; Singh, P.K.; Srivastava, K.; Singh, D.; Dalela, D.; Rath, S.K.; Goel, M.M.; Bhatt, M.L.B. Diagnostic Role of Survivin in Urinary Bladder Cancer. *Asian Pac. J. Cancer Prev.* **2013**, *14*, 81–85. [CrossRef] [PubMed]
33. Fichorova, R.N.; Richardson-Harman, N.; Alfano, M.; Belec, L.; Carbonneil, C.; Chen, S.; Cosentino, L.; Curtis, K.; Dezzutti, C.S.; Donoval, B.; et al. Biological and technical variables affecting immunoassay recovery of cytokines from human serum and simulated vaginal fluid: A multicenter study. *Anal. Chem.* **2008**, *80*, 4741–4751. [CrossRef] [PubMed]
34. Wu, J.; Chen, Y.-D.; Gu, W. Urinary proteomics as a novel tool for biomarker discovery in kidney diseases. *J. Zhejiang Univ. Sci. B* **2010**, *11*, 227–237. [CrossRef] [PubMed]
35. Zoidakis, J.; Makridakis, M.; Zerefos, P.G.; Bitsika, V.; Esteban, S.; Frantzi, M.; Stravodimos, K.; Anagnou, N.P.; Roubelakis, M.G.; Sanchez-Carbayo, M.; et al. Profilin 1 is a potential biomarker for bladder cancer aggressiveness. *Mol. Cell. Proteom.* **2012**, *11*. [CrossRef] [PubMed]
36. Adachi, J.; Kumar, C.; Zhang, Y.; Olsen, J.V.; Mann, M. The human urinary proteome contains more than 1500 proteins, including a large proportion of membrane proteins. *Genome Biol.* **2006**, *7*, R80. [CrossRef] [PubMed]
37. Reverberi, R.; Reverberi, L. Factors affecting the antigen-antibody reaction. *Blood Transfus.* **2007**, *5*, 227–240. [PubMed]
38. Khan, S.; Bennit, H.F.; Wall, N.R. The emerging role of exosomes in survivin secretion. *Histol. Histopathol.* **2015**, *30*, 43–50. [PubMed]
39. Nong, R.Y.; Di, W.; Yan, J.; Hammond, M.; Gu, G.J.; Kamali-Moghaddam, M.; Landegren, U.; Darmanis, S. Solid-phase proximity ligation assays for individual or parallel protein analyses with readout via real-time PCR or sequencing. *Nat. Protoc.* **2013**, *8*, 1234–1248. [CrossRef] [PubMed]
40. Darmanis, S.; Nong, R.Y.; Hammond, M.; Gu, J.; Alderborn, A.; Vanelid, J.; Siegbahn, A.; Gustafsdottir, S.; Ericsson, O.; Landegren, U.; et al. Sensitive plasma protein analysis by microparticle-based proximity ligation assays. *Mol. Cell. Proteom.* **2010**, *9*, 327–335. [CrossRef] [PubMed]
41. Ohsawa, I.; Nishimura, T.; Kondo, Y.; Kimura, G.; Satoh, M.; Matsuzawa, I.; Hamasaki, T.; Ohta, S. Detection of urine survivin in 40 patients with bladder cancer. *J. Nippon Med. Sch.* **2004**, *71*, 379–383. [CrossRef] [PubMed]
42. Li, X.; Wang, Y.; Xu, J.; Zhang, Q. Sandwich ELISA for detecting urinary Survivin in bladder cancer. *Chin. J. Cancer Res.* **2013**, *25*, 375–381. [PubMed]

43. Eissa, S.; Badr, S.; Barakat, M.; Zaghloul, A.; Mohanad, M. The Diagnostic Efficacy of Urinary Survivin and Hyaluronidase mRNA as Urine Markers in Patients with Bladder Cancer. *Clin. Lab.* **2013**, *59*, 893–900. [CrossRef] [PubMed]
44. Garg, M. Urothelial cancer stem cells and epithelial plasticity: Current concepts and therapeutic implications in bladder cancer. *Cancer Metastasis Rev.* **2015**, *34*, 691–701. [CrossRef] [PubMed]
45. Adamowicz, J.; Pokrywczynska, M.; Tworkiewicz, J.; Wolski, Z.; Drewa, T. The relationship of cancer stem cells in urological cancers. *Cent. Eur. J. Urol.* **2013**, *66*, 273–280. [CrossRef] [PubMed]
46. Ecke, T.; Arndt, C.; Stephan, C.; Hallmann, S.; Lux, O.; Otto, T.; Ruttloff, J.; Gerullis, H. Preliminary Results of a Multicentre Study of the UBC® *Rapid* Test for Detection of Urinary Bladder Cancer. *Anticancer Res.* **2015**, *2015*, 2651–2656.
47. D'Costa, J.J.; Goldsmith, J.C.; Wilson, J.S.; Bryan, R.T.; Ward, D.G. A Systematic Review of the Diagnostic and Prognostic Value of Urinary Protein Biomarkers in Urothelial Bladder Cancer. *Bladder Cancer* **2016**, *2*, 301–317. [CrossRef] [PubMed]
48. Ritter, R.; Hennenlotter, J.; Kuhs, U.; Hofmann, U.; Aufderklamm, S.; Blutbacher, P.; Deja, A.; Hohneder, A.; Gerber, V.; Gakis, G.; et al. Evaluation of a new quantitative point-of-care test platform for urine-based detection of bladder cancer. *Urol. Oncol.* **2014**, *32*, 337–344. [CrossRef] [PubMed]
49. Hakenberg, O.W.; Fuessel, S.; Richter, K.; Froehner, M.; Oehlschlaeger, S.; Rathert, P.; Meye, A.; Wirth, M.P. Qualitative and quantitative assessment of urinary cytokeratin 8 and 18 fragments compared with voided urine cytology in diagnosis of bladder carcinoma. *Urology* **2004**, *64*, 1121–1126. [CrossRef] [PubMed]
50. Styrke, J.; Henriksson, H.; Ljungberg, B.; Hasan, M.; Silfverberg, I.; Einarsson, R.; Malmström, P.-U.; Sherif, A. Evaluation of the diagnostic accuracy of UBC® *Rapid* in bladder cancer: A Swedish multicentre study. *Scand. J. Urol.* **2017**, *51*, 293–300. [CrossRef] [PubMed]
51. Ecke, T.H.; Weiß, S.; Stephan, C.; Hallmann, S.; Barski, D.; Otto, T.; Gerullis, H. UBC® *Rapid* Test for detection of carcinoma in situ for bladder cancer. *Tumour Biol.* **2017**, *39*. [CrossRef] [PubMed]
52. Pesch, B.; Bruning, T.; Johnen, G.; Casjens, S.; Bonberg, N.; Taeger, D.; Muller, A.; Weber, D.G.; Behrens, T. Biomarker research with prospective study designs for the early detection of cancer. *Biochim. Biophys. Acta* **2014**, *1844*, 874–883. [CrossRef] [PubMed]
53. Sánchez-Carbayo, M.; Herrero, E.; Megias, J.; Mira, A.; Espasa, A.; Chinchilla, V.; Soria, F. Initial evaluation of the diagnostic performance of the new urinary bladder cancer antigen test as a tumor marker for transitional cell carcinoma of the bladder. *J. Urol.* **1999**, *161*, 1110–1115. [CrossRef]
54. Larré, S.; Catto, J.W.F.; Cookson, M.S.; Messing, E.M.; Shariat, S.F.; Soloway, M.S.; Svatek, R.S.; Lotan, Y.; Zlotta, A.R.; Grossman, H.B. Screening for bladder cancer: Rationale, limitations, whom to target, and perspectives. *Eur. Urol.* **2013**, *63*, 1049–1058. [CrossRef] [PubMed]
55. Altznauer, F.; Martinelli, S.; Yousefi, S.; Thurig, C.; Schmid, I.; Conway, E.M.; Schoni, M.H.; Vogt, P.; Mueller, C.; Fey, M.F.; et al. Inflammation-associated cell cycle-independent block of apoptosis by survivin in terminally differentiated neutrophils. *J. Exp. Med.* **2004**, *199*, 1343–1354. [CrossRef] [PubMed]
56. Atsumi, T.; Singh, R.; Sabharwal, L.; Bando, H.; Meng, J.; Arima, Y.; Yamada, M.; Harada, M.; Jiang, J.-J.; Kamimura, D.; et al. Inflammation amplifier, a new paradigm in cancer biology. *Cancer Res.* **2014**, *74*, 8–14. [CrossRef] [PubMed]
57. Guven Maiorov, E.; Keskin, O.; Gursoy, A.; Nussinov, R. The structural network of inflammation and cancer: Merits and challenges. *Semin. Cancer Biol.* **2013**, *23*, 243–251. [CrossRef] [PubMed]
58. Sauter, G.; Eble, J.N.; Epstein, J.I.; Sesterhenn, I.A. (Eds.) *World Health Organization Classification of Tumours. Pathology and Genetics of Tumours of the Urinary System and Male Genital Organs*; IARC Press: Lyon, France, 2004; Volume 6.
59. Shen, C.; Liu, W.; Buck, A.K.; Reske, S.N. Pro-apoptosis and anti-proliferation effects of a recombinant dominant-negative survivin-T34A in human cancer cells. *Anticancer Res.* **2009**, *29*, 1423–1428. [PubMed]
60. DeLong, E.R.; DeLong, D.M.; Clarke-Pearson, D.L. Comparing the Areas under Two or More Correlated Receiver Operating Characteristic Curves: A Nonparametric Approach. *Biometrics* **1988**, *44*, 837–845. [CrossRef] [PubMed]

14

Inhibition of Heparanase Expression Results in Suppression of Invasion, Migration and Adhesion Abilities of Bladder Cancer Cells

Yoshihiro Tatsumi [1,2], Makito Miyake [1], Keiji Shimada [2], Tomomi Fujii [2], Shunta Hori [1], Yosuke Morizawa [1], Yasushi Nakai [1], Satoshi Anai [1], Nobumichi Tanaka [1], Noboru Konishi [2] and Kiyohide Fujimoto [1,*]

1 Department of Urology, Nara Medical University, 840 Shijo-cho, Nara 634-8522, Japan; takuro.birds.nest@gmail.com (Y.T.); makitomiyake@yahoo.co.jp (M.M.); horimaus@gmail.com (S.H.); tigers.yosuke@gmail.com (Y.M.); nakaiyasusiuro@live.jp (Y.N.); sanai@naramed-u.ac.jp (S.A.); sendo@naramed-u.ac.jp (N.T.)

2 Department of Pathology, Nara Medical University, 840 Shijo-cho, Nara 634-8522, Japan; k-shimada@nara-jadecom.jp (K.S.); fujiit@naramed-u.ac.jp (T.F.); n-konishi@takai-hp.com (N.K.)

* Correspondence: kiyokun@naramed-u.ac.jp

Abstract: Heparan sulfate proteoglycan syndecan-1, CD138, is known to be associated with cell proliferation, adhesion, and migration in malignancies. We previously reported that syndecan-1 (CD138) may contribute to urothelial carcinoma cell survival and progression. We investigated the role of heparanase, an enzyme activated by syndecan-1 in human urothelial carcinoma. Using human urothelial cancer cell lines, MGH-U3 and T24, heparanase expression was reduced with siRNA and RK-682, a heparanase inhibitor, to examine changes in cell proliferation activity, induction of apoptosis, invasion ability of cells, and its relationship to autophagy. A bladder cancer development mouse model was treated with RK-682 and the bladder tissues were examined using immunohistochemical analysis for Ki-67, E-cadherin, LC3, and CD31 expressions. Heparanase inhibition suppressed cellular growth by approximately 40% and induced apoptosis. The heparanase inhibitor decreased cell activity in a concentration-dependent manner and suppressed invasion ability by 40%. Inhibition of heparanase was found to suppress autophagy. In N-butyl-N-(4-hydroxybutyl) nitrosamine (BBN)-induced bladder cancer mice, treatment with heparanase inhibitor suppressed the progression of cancer by 40%, compared to controls. Immunohistochemistry analysis showed that heparanase inhibitor suppressed cell growth, and autophagy. In conclusion, heparanase suppresses apoptosis and promotes invasion and autophagy in urothelial cancer.

Keywords: heparanase; syndecan-1; heparan sulfate proteoglycans (HSPGs); urothelial carcinoma

---

1. Introduction

Heparan sulfate proteoglycans (HSPGs) are glycoproteins containing heparan sulfate (HS) groups that are covalently attached [1]. They are widely expressed and play critical roles in numerous cellular processes, including endocytosis, migration, and adhesion. Their actions are mediated through interactions with ligands such as growth factors, cytokines, extracellular matrix proteins, and enzymes. HSPGs are also involved in the malignant transformation of cells. Growth factors are released through cellular degradation, which promote the invasion and proliferation of cancer cells [2,3]. Syndecan-1 (SDC1) is an HSPG that is overexpressed in both normal and malignant cells, contributing to the development of hematopoietic and carcinoma development [4–9]. Syndecan-1 regulates substance permeation and constitutes a reservoir for various growth factors and cytokines in the basement membrane of cells. It plays a critical role in the progression and invasion of urothelial cancer through enhanced angiogenesis.

We have previously reported that syndecan-1 (CD138) suppresses apoptosis and increases the capacity for cell proliferation via junB-FLIP long signal in urothelial cancer [10]. Urothelial cancers can be broadly classified into low-grade, non-invasive, and high-grade invasive cancers [11]. Invasive urothelial cancers exhibit significantly higher syndecan-1 expression. In vitro experiments showed that knocking down syndecan-1 using siRNA induces cellular apoptosis and decreases the capacity for cellular proliferation. The enzyme heparanase controls the activation of syndecan-1.

Heparanase is an endoglycosidase enzyme that targets HSPG proteins expressed in the extracellular matrix (ECM) and basement membrane (BM) for degradation [12]. Heparanase activation expedites the movement of tumor cells through the ECM and BM, facilitating metastasis. Heparanase is also known to be expressed in many types of malignant tumors, and is associated with metastasis and angiogenesis [13,14]. Heparinase cleavage of HSPGs produces soluble proteins that infiltrate into the tumor microenvironment, where they interact with ligands such as growth factors, modifying signaling pathways [15]. SDC1 in the stroma promotes breast carcinoma growth by enhancing FGF2 signaling [16]. Heparanase-neutralizing antibodies have been suggested for the treatment of diffuse non-Hodgkin's B-cell and follicular lymphomas [17] through the inhibition of cell invasion and tumor metastasis processes [17–19]. Recently, a small molecule inhibitor of heparanase was shown to reduce metastatic characteristics in a hepatocellular carcinoma model [20]. In vivo studies using heparanase inhibitors in animal tumor models have also demonstrated reductions in tumor metastasis [21–23]. As heparinase is absent or expressed at low levels in normal tissue [24,25], it may be a potential target candidate for therapeutic interventions. Various studies have investigated the underlying mechanism for heparanase activity in cancer, including enhancement of angiogenesis and promotion of apoptosis and autophagy [14,26–30]. Reports indicate that autophagy contributes to chemotherapy resistance development, making this an important research focus area.

In this study, we analyzed the function of heparanase, an activator of syndecan-1, in angiogenesis, apoptosis, and autophagy. The aim was to establish heparanase as a target for molecular therapy in urothelial carcinoma.

2. Results

2.1. *Heparanase Is Overexpressed in Human Urothelial Carcinoma of the Urinary Bladder, and Heparanase Expression Levels Are Associated with Intravesical Recurrence*

The patterns of heparanase expression in resected bladder cancer tissue samples were analyzed using immunohistochemical (IHC) staining. The relationship between heparanase expression and recurrence, metastasis, and prognosis of urothelial cancer was examined. Tissue specimens ($n = 57$) were resected from the renal pelvis, ureter, and bladder of patients with multifocal onset, relapse, metastasis, and prognosis cases of urothelial cancer. Table 1 summarizes patient clinicopathological data using the 2009 World Health Organization (WHO) grading and staging of tumors classification [31]. The total number of Ta cases was 20 and the grade was low grade:high grade, 13:7. Among the 17 cases of T1, low grade:high grade, 3:14, and all 10 cases of Tis were high grade.

Table 1. Characterization of urothelial carcinomas.

	*p*Ta ($n = 20$)	*p*T1 ($n = 17$)	*p*Tis ($n = 10$)
Age	71.3 (61–82)	72.9 (5–80)	72.4 (62–86)
Gender (M:F)	16:4	14:3	8:2
Grade			
Low grade	13	3	0
High grade	7	14	10

*p*Ta = low-grade non-muscle invasive bladder cancer; *p*T1 = intermediate risk non-muscle invasive bladder cancer; *p*Tis = in situ neoplasia.

The expression of heparanase is diffusely expressed in both the cell membrane and cytoplasm. The expression of heparanase protein was approximately 10% in normal urothelium but increased to approximately 30% in urothelial carcinoma samples ($p < 0.05$). Heparanase expression was elevated in high-grade compared to low-grade carcinoma samples (34.7% vs. 23.4%, respectively) (Figure 1a,b). The immunohistochemical staining of surgically resected specimens from 47 bladder cancer patients showed that positive heparanase expression was observed predominantly in cases exhibiting intravesical relapse ($p < 0.05$) (Figure 1c).

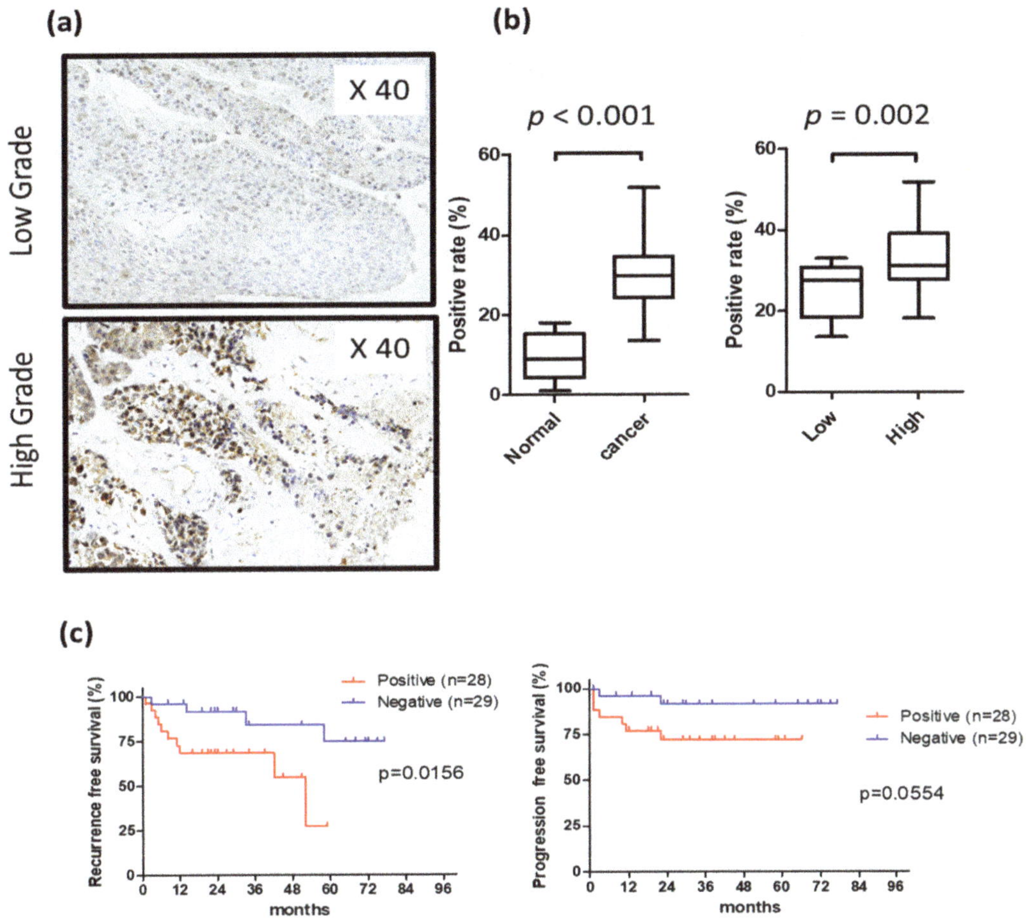

Figure 1. Immunohistological examination of expression of heparanase in bladder tissue; (**a**) positive ratio in low grade bladder cancer and high grade bladder cancer; (**b**) heparanase expression rate; (**c**) Kaplan–Meier curve of intravesical recurrence and invasion.

2.2. Knockdown of Heparanase-Induced Apoptosis in Urothelial Carcinoma Cells

Heparanase expression was studied in the human urothelial cancer cell lines MGH-U3 and T24 and found to increase compared to the normal urothelial cell line (UROtsa). The expression levels of heparanase were similar in MGH-U3 and T24 (Supplementary Figure S1). We first examined the suppression of heparanase protein expression and mRNA expression by knockdown with Si RNA (Supplementary Figure S2). MGH-U3 showed a significant decrease in cell activity due to heparanase knockdown compared to T24. There is a difference that MGH-U3 cells are suppressed by about 15% and T24 cells are suppressed by about 25% by knockdown by Si RNA. Inhibiting the expression of heparanase by siRNA suppressed the proliferative activity of cancer cells strongly, and cytotoxicity was observed (Figure 2a). In the MGH-U3 cell line, proliferation activity was suppressed by approximately 80% compared to approximately 40% in T24 cells. In the UROtsa cell line, heparanase knockdown suppressed growth activity by 15%. Further, heparanase knock-down by siRNA induced apoptosis (Figure 2b).

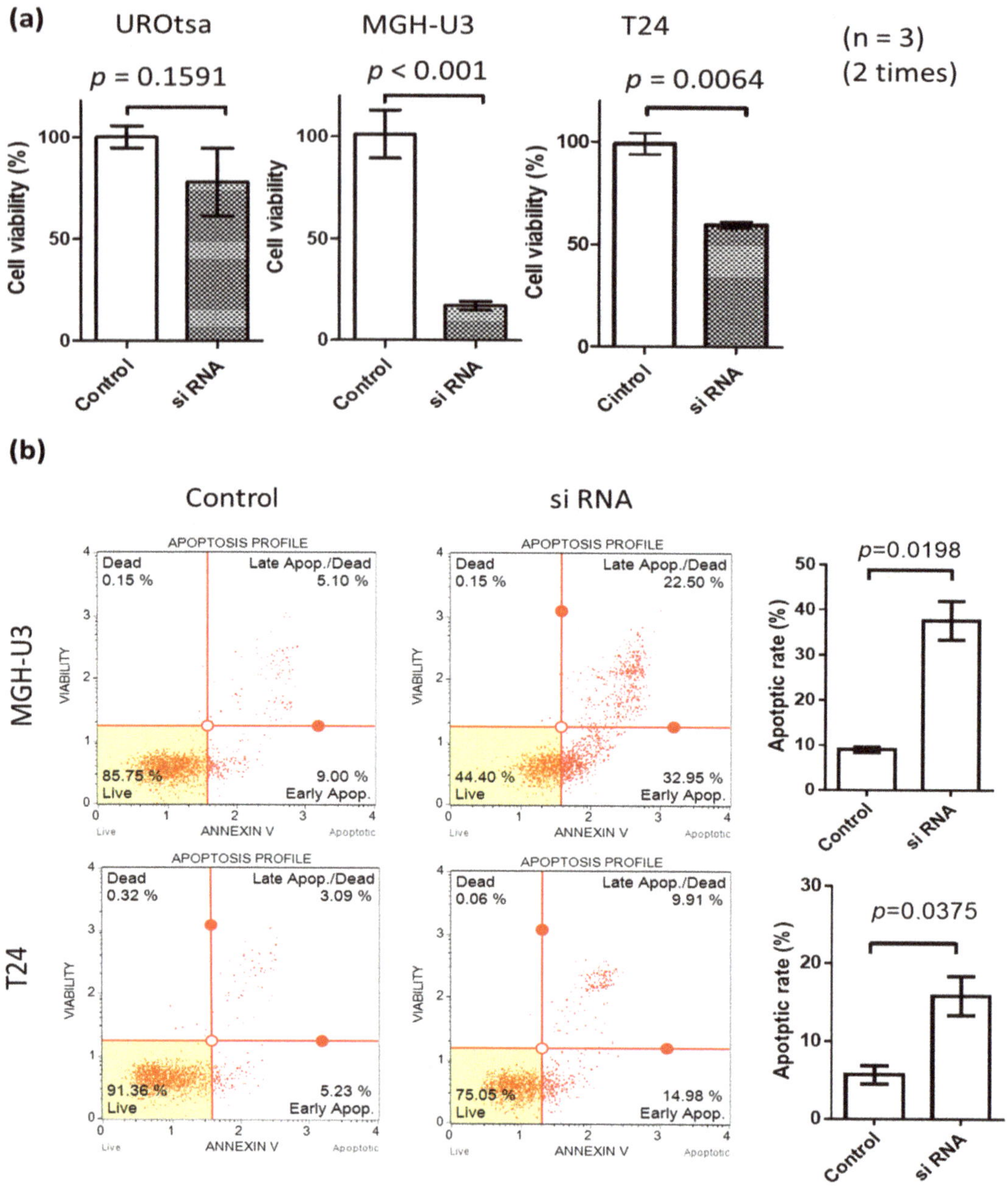

Figure 2. (**a**) Effect of heparanase knockdown on cell survival in urothelial carcinoma cells. Cell viability was assessed by an MTS assay 72 h following transfection; (**b**) 48 h following transfection, cells stained with Annexin V and propidium iodide were analyzed by flow cytometry (upper panels) and the percentages of apoptotic cells (AV[+]/PI[)]) calculated (lower panels). Inset photograph is an immunofluorescence microscopy image showing cells positive for FITC-conjugated Annexin V (AV). Each value is the mean ± standard error. C, control RNA (non-specific siRNA); Si RNA, heparanase siRNA.

2.3. The Multi Enzyme Inhibitor RK-682, Which Is Also a Heparanase Inhibitor, Suppresses Cell Proliferation and Autophagy in Human Urothelial Cancer Cell Lines

RK-682 is an inhibitor of various enzymes including heparanase, phospholipase A_2, HIV-1 protease, some dual-specificity phosphatases (DSP), and a protein tyrosine phosphatase (PTP), CD45. The inhibition of heparanase by RK-682 was examined using MGH-U3 and T24 cell lines. Treatment with RK-682 suppressed heparanase protein expression and mRNA expression in these cells (Supplementary Figure S3). MGH-U3 and T24 cell lines were treated with RK-682 and examined in a cell viability assay to determine cytotoxicity. RK-682-treated MGH-U3 and T24 cells showed a concentration-dependent cytotoxicity (Figure 3a). The half-maximal inhibitory concentration (IC50) of RK-682 was 78.2 nM in

MGH-U3 cells, 43.2 nM in T24 cells, and 145 nM in UROtsa. The cytotoxicity was 2–3 times higher than that of the cancer cell line. UROtsa, which has low expression of heparanae, has an IC50 of RK-682 about 2–3 times higher than that of urothelial carcinoma cell line, MGH-U3 cell line and T24 cell line which has high expression of heparanase. In the heparanse knockdown experiment with Si RNA, the UROtsa cell line showed almost no inhibition of the cell activity, whereas RK-682 inhibited the cell activity of the UROtsa cell line at a high concentration. From this fact, it is considered that RK-682 has an action other than the inhibition of heparanase. The effect of RK-682 treatment was also examined in an invasion migration assay. In MGH-U3 and T24 cell lines, migratory ability decreased by approximately 20% following treatment with RK-682. In RK-682-treated MGH-U3 and T24 cells, invasion ability reduced by 55% and 40%, respectively (Figure 3b). MGH-U3 and T24 cells treated with RK-682 were also tested in an autophagy assay. The expression of autophagy decreased following the treatment with RK-682 (Figure 3c).

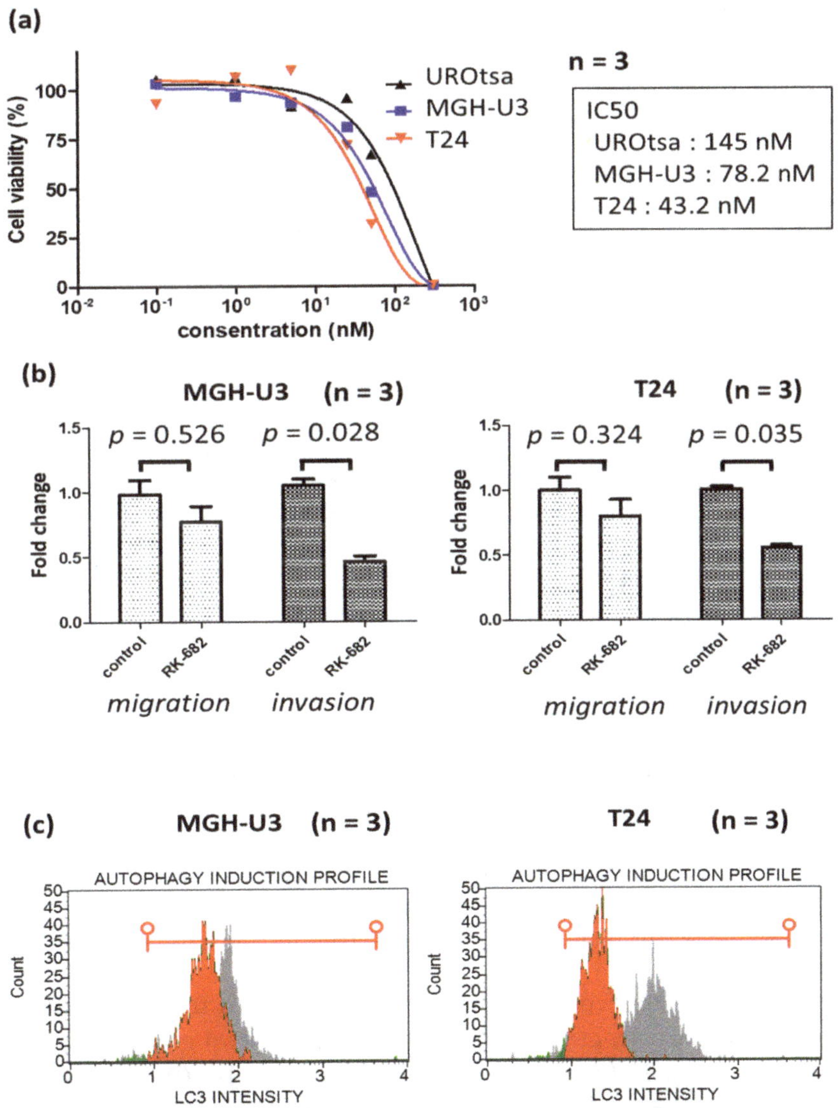

Figure 3. (**a**) Treatment with the multi enzyme inhibitor RK-682 inhibited cell proliferation in MGH-U3, T24 cells and UROtsa. Cells were incubated in serum-free media for 24 h and treated with different concentrations of RK-682 for a further 48 h. The number of viable cells was measured by an MTS assay and expressed as a percentage of viable cells; (**b**) effect of RK-682 on MGH-U3 and T24 cells. RK-682 treatment resulted in a significant inhibition of MGH-U3 and T24 cell invasion ($p < 0.05$); (**c**) 48 h treatment with heparanase inhibitor RK-682 inhibited cell autophagy in MGH-U3 and T24 cells. The red horizontal line shows the range of LC3 intensity after KR-682 treatment.

2.4. In Vivo Growth of Urothelial Carcinoma Is Suppressed by RK-682 in the BBN-Induced Mouse Bladder Cancer Model

The effects of the multi enzyme inhibitor RK-682 were tested using an in vivo model of bladder cancer treated with BBN (Figure 4a). Figure 4a briefly illustrates the experimental protocol for the present study. Six-week-old C57BL/6J mice were orally administered with 0.05% BBN. Bladder cancer-induced mice were prepared in approximately 22 weeks. The animals were divided into two groups, the treatment group ($n = 7$), and the non-treatment group ($n = 5$), totaling $n = 14$ animals. The heparanase inhibitor RK-682 was administered at 2.5 mg/100 μL, into the bladder four times a week through a catheter inserted into the bladder.

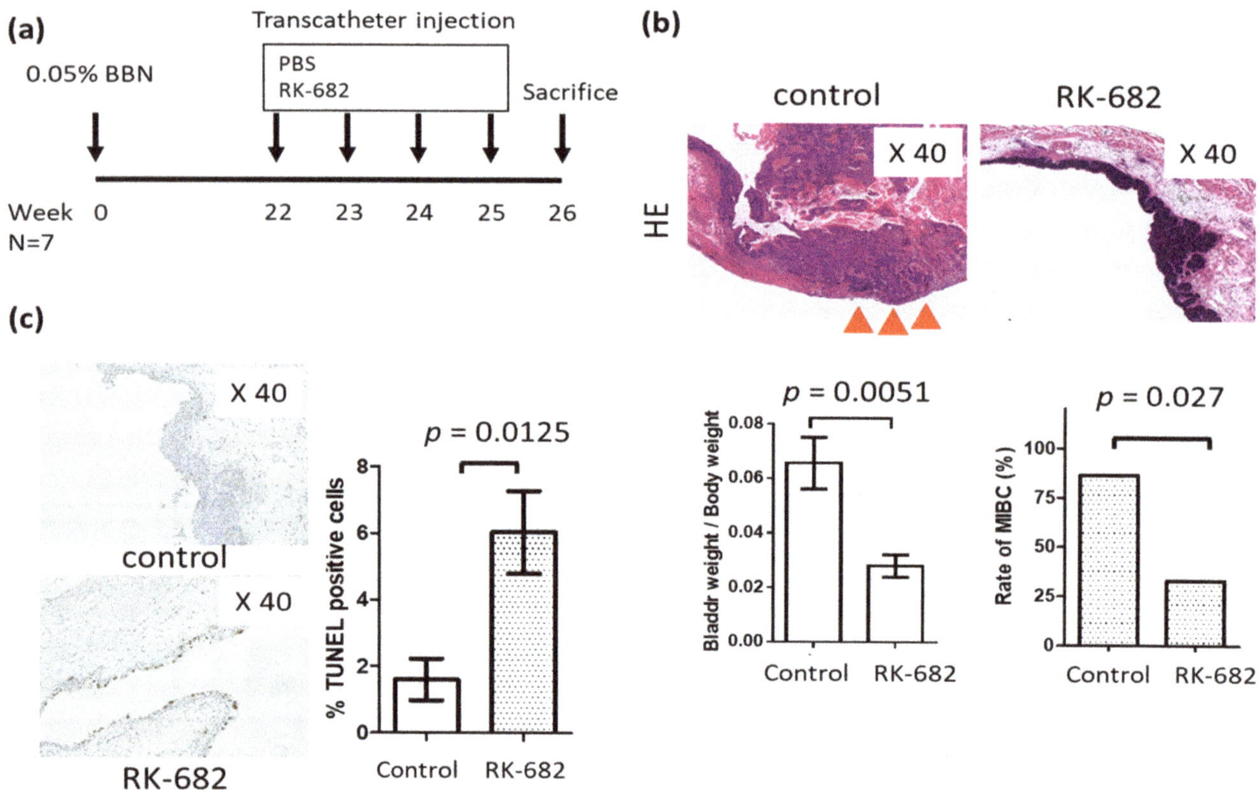

Figure 4. Intravesical injection of RK-682 inhibits in vivo tumor growth in the mouse N-butyl-N-(4-hydroxybutyl) nitrosamine (BBN)-induced bladder cancer implant model. (**a**) Diagrammatic experimental procedure; (**b**) RK-682 or control was transurethrally instilled into the bladder lumen. Bladders were resected post-instillation. Hematoxylin Eosin (HE) staining of bladder, comparison of bladder weight, ratio of muscle layer infiltration. Red triangle indicate images of muscle invasive bladder cancer.; (**c**) the percentage of cells in resected bladder specimens immunoreactive with TUNEL reagent, calculated per 1000 cells/in a high-power field. Each value is the mean ± standard error.

There was no significant difference in body weight between the RK-682-treated group and the control group after the end of treatment. (RK-682 group vs. control group; 24.5 g vs. 25.6 g $p = 0.765$). There was a significant decrease in the bladder weight/body wight, (RK-682 group vs. control group; 0.028 vs. 0.056 $p = 0.0051$) and ratio of infiltrative bladder cancer (RK-682 group vs. control group; 28.6% vs. 85.7% $p = 0.027$) in the RK-682 treatment group compared to the control group (Figure 4b). A TUNEL assay showed that apoptosis was more frequent in the RK-682 treatment group (Figure 4c). IHC studies of the mouse tissue showed decreased expression of Ki67, LC3, and CD31 markers in the specimens from animals treated with RK-682. In contrast, E-cadherin expression level increased after treatment with the inhibitor (Figure 5).

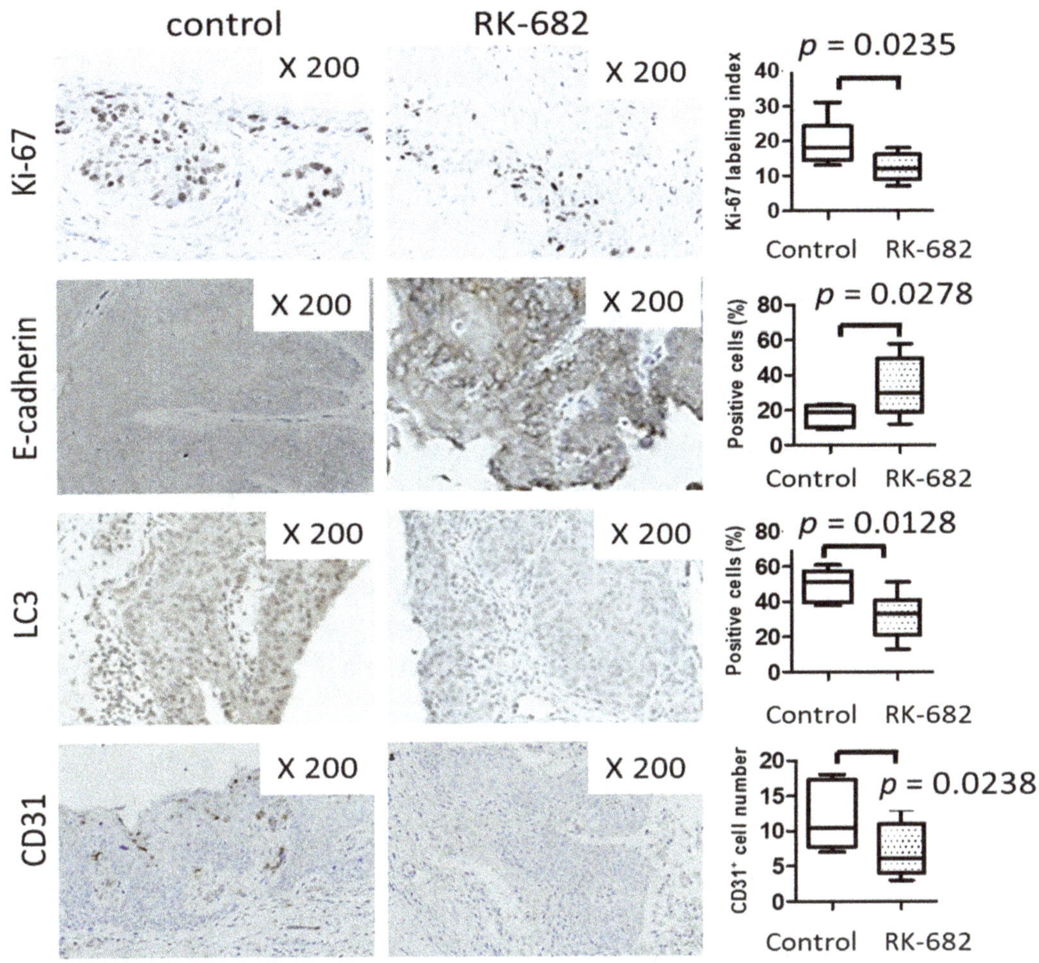

Figure 5. Immunohistochemical analysis of the mouse BBN-induced bladder cancer implant model. Immunohistochemistry for Ki-67, E-cadherin, LC3 and CD31 expression. The percentage of immunopositive cells was determined per 1000 cells in a high-power field.

3. Discussion

Heparanase expression is elevated in many types of tumors and is associated with more aggressive cancer and a poor prognosis [3,13,14,26]. We have previously reported that syndecan-1 is involved in urothelial cancer development through the promotion of angiogenesis [10]. In this study, we investigated heparanase, an activator of syndecan-1, and analyzed its function in urothelial cancer. We have demonstrated that inhibition of heparanase suppresses cell proliferation, epithelial-mesenchymal transition (EMT), autophagy and angiogenesis.

In other cancer types, heparanase activation has been indicated in promoting metastasis and tumor progression. In bladder cancer, Gohji et al. [32] reported that cancer-specific survival rates are significantly lower when heparanase expression is elevated in bladder cancer patients. In our study, increased expression of heparanase in bladder cancer tissue samples correlated with higher recurrence rates within the bladder and progression to muscle-invasive cancer.

Chen et al. [30] suggested an association between heparanase expression and cell adhesion, and metastasis in hepatocellular carcinoma cell lines. Heparanase plays a proadhesive role in cell adhesion and tumor microembolus in hepatocellular carcinoma. In this study, inhibition of heparanase activity significantly reduced the ability of cancer cells to migrate and infiltrate. Furthermore, it was confirmed that the inhibition of autophagy resulted from heparanase inhibition.

Shteingauz et al. [33] reported the regulation of autophagy in normal and malignant cells by heparanse, conferring survival advantages and the development of resistance to chemotherapy. In the spontaneous bladder cancer mouse model, heparanase inhibition significantly suppressed bladder cancer invasion. This study confirmed that the suppression of heparanase induces apoptosis, suppresses cell proliferation and inhibits autophagy.

This report is the first to investigate heparanase inhibition and its effects on the suppression of cancer invasion, autophagy and apoptosis in bladder cancer. Intravesical treatment with a heparanase inhibitor did not result in serious side effects in the in vivo mouse model used here and hence this study was conducted as planned. As a treatment option for bladder cancer, intravesical infusion therapy allows the penetration of a drug directly into cancer cells and has mild side effects. In combination, these observations indicate that heparanase is a potential candidate for targeted therapy in bladder cancer.

This study has limitations. RK-682 is a multi-enzyme inhibitory locus targeting several enzymes including heparanase, protein tyrosine phosphatase (PTP), phospholipase A_2 and other enzymes. The T24 cell line is found to be less sensitive to siRNA inhibition compared with the MGH-U3 cell line, but is more sensitive to RK-682 inhibition. This may explain other effects of RK-682-mediated inhibition observed in this study. In UROtsa cells, the cell activity induced by siRNA was reduced by approximately 20%. However, RK-682 treatment showed cytotoxicity in a dose-dependent manner. The cytotoxicity observed was 2–3 times higher compared to the cancer cell line. Expression analysis shows that RK-682 does have a heparanase inhibitory effect (Supplementary Figure S3). However, heparanase activity alone does explain changes in migration, invasion, and autophagy in bladder cancer cells. Further experiments are required to investigate the molecular function of heparanase.

4. Materials and Methods

4.1. Cell Culture, Plasmids and Chemicals

Human urothelial carcinoma cell lines MGH-U3, T24, and human urothelial cell line (UROtsa) were supplied by American Type Culture Collection (Manassas, VA, USA). MGH-U3 and T24 cells originated from human papillary bladder cancer [34]. T24 cells were cultured in RPMI1640 media supplemented with 10% fetal bovine serum and 50 units/mL penicillin-streptomycin at 37 °C in 5% CO_2.

The antibodies, anti-Ki67, LC3, and CD31, and E-cadherin, were purchased from Abcam (Cambridge, UK). The heparanase inhibitor RK-682 was purchased from Cayman Chemical Company (Ann Arbor, MI, USA). siRNA molecules were purchased from Thermo Fisher Scientific (K.K. Japan).

4.2. siRNA Transfection of Heparanase

For transfection analyses, 10^6 cells from each cell line were seeded into 6-cm dishes. They were transfected with either 100 nM of control RNA (Santa Cruz Biotechnology, Dallas, TX, USA) or with the heparanase siRNA. Transfections were performed with the Lipofectamine system (Invitrogen Japan, Tokyo, Japan) following the manufacturer's protocol.

The primers used were: HPSE sense 5′-AGUACUUGCGGUUACCCUATT-3′; HPSE antisense 5′-UAGGGUAACCGCAAGUACUTG-3′.

Actin sense 5′-CTCTTCCAGCCTTCCTTCCT-3′; Actin antisense 5′-AGCACTGTGTTGGCGTACAG-3′.

Gene expression analysis of cell cycle-related genes was performed by qPCR using the PrimerArray Cell Cycle (Takara, Otsu, Japan).

4.3. Tissue Samples and Immunohistochemistry (IHC)

This study was approved by the Medical Ethics Committee of Nara Medical University. The requirement for informed patient consent was waived due to the retrospective nature of the study (Study ID: NMU 900, July 23, 2013). A total of 57 patients diagnosed with organ-confined urothelial cancer between April 2007 and June 2010 at the Nara Medical University hospital were included in this study. The clinicopathological data and follow-up data were collected via a retrospective chart review. All pathological examinations were performed under the guidance of two pathologists (K.S. and N.K.) according to the 2009 TNM classification system [32]. All patients had bladder cancer and underwent transurethral resection of the bladder tumor (TURBT). IHC staining of 57 TURBT specimens using paraffin-embedded, formalin-fixed tissue blocks was performed as previously described [10,33]. Antibodies against heparinase were used as the primary antibodies at a dilution of 1:500. Staining was scored based on the positive cell ratio using standard light microscopy. Staining outcomes were evaluated by two independent observers (Y.T. and K.S), who were blinded to patient clinicopathological data.

4.4. Cell Proliferation Assay

The CellTiter 96 AQueous One Solution Cell Proliferation Assay (Promega, Madison, WI, USA) was used to measure cell proliferation by MTS assay as previously described [11]. Data were collected from triplicate experiments.

4.5. Apoptosis Detection Assay

Following the transfection with siRNA, cells were stained with propidium iodide (PI) and Fluorescein-5-isothiocyanate (FITC)-conjugated Annexin V (AV) following the manufacturer's protocol (TACS Annexin V-FITC kit; R&D Systems). Apoptotic cells were quantified by calculating the number of cells positive for AV and negative for PI. Experiments were performed a minimum three times of duplicate.

4.6. TdT-Mediated dUTP Nick End Labeling (TUNEL) Assay

Formalin-fixed and paraffin-embedded 5-l-m thick sections of tumor specimens were stained using a TUNEL assay: Tumor TACS in situ apoptosis detection kit (R&D Systems, Minneapolis, MN, USA). The apoptotic index (the number of apoptotic cells per total number of cells) was calculated as per 400 microscopic fields per sample.

4.7. Cell Viability Assay

UROtsa, MGH-U3 and T24 cells were seeded into 96-well plates at 2×10^3 cells/well and incubated overnight. The growth medium was removed, and the cells were washed once with phosphate-buffered saline (PBS). Fresh serum-free medium with or without heparinase inhibitor (RK-682) was applied. Cells were then treated with RK-682 (between 1–1000 nM) for 72 h to evaluate cell viability. The IC50 was determined based on the concentration-effect relationship using PRISM software version 5.00 (GraphPad Software, San Diego, CA, USA). Cell viability was measured using a Cell Counting Kit-8 (Dojindo, Kumamoto, Japan) according to the manufacturer's protocol. Absorbance was measured at 490 nm with a reference at 630 nm using an Infinite 200M PRO microplate autoreader (Tecan, Männedorf, Switzerland).

4.8. Migration Assay

A migration assay was performed using the BD Falcon FluoroBlok Insert System (Becton Dickinson, Franklin Lakes, NJ, USA) according to the manufacturer's instructions. Cells were starved in serum-free media for 24 h, then seeded at a density of 2.5×10^4 cells/well in serum-free media plus RK-682 inhibitor. RPMI1640 media with 10% FBS chemoattractant was contained within the lower wells. The cells were incubated in a humidified environment at 37 °C with 5% CO_2 for 48 h. Cells that were attached to the membrane were stained with the cell viability indicator Calcein AM Fluorescent Dye for 30 min (Promo Kine, Heidelberg, Germany) and quantified with an Infinite 200M PRO microplate spectrophotometer (Tecan, Männedorf, Switzerland) at 495 mm excitation and 515 nm emission. Cells were inspected via fluorescent microscopy.

4.9. Autophagy Assay

Autophagy assays were performed using Muse™ Cell Analyzer from Millipore (Hayward, CA, USA) following the manufacturer's instructions. Following treatment of MGH-U3 and T24 cells with heparinase inhibiter RK-682 (Cayman Chemical Company, Ann Arbor, MI, USA), the treated cells were washed with PBS buffer. The autophagy assays were analyzed using the Muse™ Autophagy LC3-antibody based kit (Millipore) according to the manufacturer's protocol.

4.10. BBN-Induced Mouse Bladder Cancer Model

An in vivo mouse model of bladder cancer was treated with BBN. Fourteen 6-week-old C57BL/6J female mice were obtained from Oriental Bio Service (Kyoto, Japan). All animal studies were approved by Nara Medical University affiliated Frist People's Hospital Committee on Use and Care of Animals and conducted in accordance with local humane animal care standard (Reference Number: 11389). BBN B0938 (Tokyo Chemical Industry, Tokyo, Japan) treated bladder cancer model mice were treated with the heparanase inhibitor RK-682 in the bladder once a week for four weeks by injection. Mice were randomized into a control group (control PBS, $n = 7$) or heparanase inhibitor (RK-682, $n = 7$) treatment group and received a single intravesical treatment instillation that was retained for 1 h with a purse-string suture. Mice were sacrificed (at week 25) after four treatments. Bladders were removed, placed open on filter paper, and fixed in 10% neutral buffered formalin. Bladders were then embedded in paraffin, step-sectioned, and stained with hematoxylin-eosin (H&E) and IHC staining for E-cadherin, Ki67, CD31 and LC3 (Abcam, Tokyo, Japan).

4.11. Statistical Analysis

Differences in cell migration were evaluated with the Student's t-test. The correlation of IHC staining intensity was assessed with the Man–Whitney U test. IBM SPSS Version 21 (SPSS Inc., Chicago, IL, USA) and PRISM software version 5.00 (San Diego, CA, USA) were used for statistical analyses and data plotting, respectively. Statistical significance was set at $p < 0.05$, and all reported p values were two-sided.

5. Conclusions

Heparanase induces invasion and autophagy in urothelial carcinoma. Downregulation of heparanase induces apoptosis. Heparanase may contribute to urothelial carcinoma cell survival and invasion.

Supplementary Materials:
Figure S1: Heparanse protein expression levels and mRNA expression levels in MGH-U3, T24 and U Rotsa cell lines, Figure S2: The suppression of heparanase protein expression and mRNA expression by knockdown with Si RNA MGH-U3, T24 and U Rotsa cell lines, Figure S3: The suppression of heparanase protein expression and mRNA expression by treated with the multi enzyme inhibitor RK-682 in MGH-U3, T24 and U Rotsa cell lines.

Author Contributions: Conceptualization, Y.T. and K.F.; Methodology, Y.T.; Software, Y.T. and T.F.; Validation, Y.T., K.S. and N.K.; Formal analysis, Y.T.; Investigation, Y.T., S.H., Y.M., Y.N., N.K. and K.F.; Resources, Y.T.; Data curation, Y.T., S.H. and Y.M.; Writing—Original draft preparation, Y.T.; Writing—Review and editing, M.M.; Visualization, Y.T.; Supervision, K.S., M.M., S.A., N.T., N.K. and K.F.; Project administration, Y.T., K.S. and M.M.; Funding acquisition, Y.T., N.K. and K.F. All authors have read and agreed to the published version of the manuscript.

Acknowledgments: Editorial support, in the form of medical writing, assembling tables and creating high-resolution images based on authors' detailed directions, collating author comments, copyediting, fact-checking, and referencing, was provided by Editage, Cactus Communications.

Abbreviations

AV	Annexin V
FITC	Fluorescein-5-isothiocyanate
IC50	half-maximal inhibitory concentration
IHC	Immunohistochemistry
PBS	phosphate-buffered saline

PI	propidium iodide
siRNA	Small Interfering Ribonucleic Acid
qPCR	Quantitative Polymerase Chain Reaction
TUNEL	TdT-mediated dUTP nick end labeling
TURBT	Transurethral resection of the bladder tumor

References

1. Sarrazin, S.; Lamanna, W.C.; Esko, J.D. Heparan sulfate proteoglycans. *Cold Spring Harb. Perspect. Biol.* **2011**, *3*, a004952. [CrossRef] [PubMed]
2. Hammond, E.; Khurana, A.; Shridhar, V.; Dredge, K. The Role of heparanase and sulfatases in the modification of heparan sulfate proteoglycans within the tumor microenvironment and opportunities for novel cancer therapeutics. *Front. Oncol.* **2014**, *4*, 195. [CrossRef] [PubMed]
3. Barash, U.; Cohen-Kaplan, V.; Dowek, I.; Sanderson, R.D.; Ilan, N.; Vlodavsky, I. Proteoglycans in health and disease: New concepts for heparanase function in tumor progression and metastasis. *FEBS J.* **2010**, *277*, 3890–3903. [CrossRef]
4. Dhodapkar, M.V.; Abe, E.; Theus, A.; Lacy, M.; Langford, J.K.; Barlogie, B.; Sanderson, R.D. Syndecan-1 is a multifunctional regulator of myeloma pathobiology: Control of tumor cell survival, growth, and bone cell differentiation. *Blood* **1998**, *91*, 2679–2688. [CrossRef]
5. Mahtouk, K.; Cremer, F.W.; Rème, T.; Jourdan, M.; Baudard, M.; Moreaux, J.; Requirand, G.; Fiol, G.; De Vos, J.; Moos, M.; et al. Heparan sulphate proteoglycans are essential for the myeloma cell growth activity of EGF-family ligands in multiple myeloma. *Oncogene* **2006**, *25*, 7180–7191. [CrossRef]
6. Derksen, P.W.; Keehnen, R.M.; Evers, L.M.; Van Oers, M.H.; Spaargaren, M.; Pals, S.T. Cell surface proteoglycan syndecan-1 mediates hepatocyte growth factor binding and promotes Met signaling in multiple myeloma. *Blood* **2002**, *99*, 1405–1410. [CrossRef]
7. Yang, Y.; MacLeod, V.; Dai, Y.; Khotskaya-Sample, Y.; Shriver, Z.; Venkataraman, G.; Sasisekharan, R.; Naggi, A.; Torri, G.; Casu, B.; et al. The syndecan-1 heparan sulfate proteoglycan is a viable target for myeloma therapy. *Blood* **2007**, *110*, 2041–2048. [CrossRef] [PubMed]
8. Nikolova, V.; Koo, C.Y.; Ibrahim, S.A.; Wang, Z.; Spillmann, D.; Dreier, R.; Kelsch, R.; Fischgrabe, J.; Smollich, M.; Rossi, L.H.; et al. Differential roles for membrane-bound and soluble syndecan-1 (CD138) in breast cancer progression. *Carcinogenesis* **2009**, *30*, 397–407. [CrossRef] [PubMed]
9. Shimada, K.; Nakamura, M.; Anai, S.; De Velasco, M.; Tanaka, M.; Tsujikawa, K.; Ouji, Y.; Konishi, N. A novel human AlkB homologue, ALKBH8, contributes to human bladder cancer progression. *Cancer Res.* **2009**, *69*, 3157–3164. [CrossRef]
10. Shimada, K.; Matsuyoshi, S.; Nakamura, M.; Ishida, E.; Konishi, N. Phosphorylation status of Fas-associated death domain-containing protein (FADD) is associated with prostate cancer progression. *J. Pathol.* **2005**, *206*, 423–432. [CrossRef] [PubMed]
11. Shimada, K.; Nakamura, M.; De Velasco, M.A.; Tanaka, M.; Ouji, Y.; Konishi, N. Syndecan-1, a new target molecule involved in progression of androgen-independent prostate cancer. *Cancer Sci.* **2009**, *100*, 1248–1254. [CrossRef] [PubMed]
12. Vlodavsky, I.; Ilan, N.; Naggi, A.; Casu, B. Heparanase: Structure, biological functions, and inhibition by heparin-derived mimetics of heparan sulfate. *Curr. Pharm. Des.* **2007**, *13*, 2057–2073. [CrossRef] [PubMed]
13. Vlodavsky, I.; Elkin, M.; Abboud-Jarrous, G.; Levi-Adam, F.; Fuks, L.; Shafat, I.; Ilan, N. Heparanase: One molecule with multiple functions in cancer progression. *Connect. Tissue Res.* **2008**, *49*, 207–210. [CrossRef]
14. Ilan, N.; Elkin, M.; Vlodavsky, I. Regulation, function and clinical significance of heparanase in cancer metastasis and angiogenesis. *Int. J. Biochem. Cell Biol.* **2006**, *38*, 2018–2039. [CrossRef]
15. Whitelock, J.M.; Iozzo, R.V. Heparan sulfate: A complex polymer charged with biological activity. *Chem. Rev.* **2005**, *105*, 2745–2764. [CrossRef]
16. Maeda, T.; Desouky, J.; Friedl, A. Syndecan-1 expression by stromal fibroblasts promotes breast carcinoma growth in vivo and stimulates tumor angiogenesis. *Oncogene* **2006**, *25*, 1408–1412. [CrossRef]
17. Weissmann, M.; Arvatz, G.; Horowitz, N.; Feld, S.; Naroditsky, I.; Zhang, Y.; Ng, M.; Hammond, E.; Nevo, E.; Vlodavsky, I.; et al. Heparanase-neutralizing antibodies attenuate lymphoma tumor growth and metastasis. *Proc. Natl. Acad. Sci. USA* **2016**, *113*, 704–709. [CrossRef] [PubMed]

18. Zhang, Y.F.; Tang, X.D.; Gao, J.H.; Fang, D.C.; Yang, S.M. Heparanase: A universal immunotherapeutic target in human cancers. *Drug Discov. Today* **2011**, *16*, 412–417. [CrossRef] [PubMed]
19. Chen, T.; Tang, X.D.; Wan, Y.; Chen, L.; Yu, S.T.; Xiong, Z.; Fang, D.C.; Liang, G.P.; Yang, S.M. HLA-A2-restricted cytotoxic T lymphocyte epitopes from human heparanase as novel targets for broad-spectrum tumor immunotherapy. *Neoplasia (N. Y. NY)* **2008**, *10*, 977–986. [CrossRef] [PubMed]
20. Baburajeev, C.P.; Mohan, C.D.; Rangappa, S.; Mason, D.J.; Fuchs, J.E.; Bender, A.; Barash, U.; Vlodavsky, I.; Basappa; Rangappa, K.S. Identification of novel class of triazolo-thiadiazoles as potent inhibitors of human heparanase and their anticancer activity. *BMC Cancer* **2017**, *17*, 235. [CrossRef]
21. Miao, H.Q.; Liu, H.; Navarro, E.; Kussie, P.; Zhu, Z. Development of heparanase inhibitors for anti-cancer therapy. *Curr. Med. Chem.* **2006**, *13*, 2101–2111. [CrossRef] [PubMed]
22. Parish, C.R.; Freeman, C.; Brown, K.J.; Francis, D.J.; Cowden, W.B. Identification of sulfated oligosaccharide-based inhibitors of tumor growth and metastasis using novel in vitro assays for angiogenesis and heparanase activity. *Cancer Res.* **1999**, *59*, 3433–3441. [PubMed]
23. Borsig, L. Antimetastatic activities of modified heparins: Selectin inhibition by heparin attenuates metastasis. *Semin. Thromb. Hemost.* **2007**, *33*, 540–546. [CrossRef] [PubMed]
24. Vlodavsky, I.; Friedmann, Y.; Elkin, M.; Aingorn, H.; Atzmon, R.; Ishai-Michaeli, R.; Bitan, M.; Pappo, O.; Peretz, T.; Michal, I.; et al. Mammalian heparanase: Gene cloning, expression and function in tumor progression and metastasis. *Nat. Med.* **1999**, *5*, 793–802. [CrossRef]
25. Hulett, M.D.; Freeman, C.; Hamdorf, B.J.; Baker, R.T.; Harris, M.J.; Parish, C.R. Cloning of mammalian heparanase, an important enzyme in tumor invasion and metastasis. *Nat. Med.* **1999**, *5*, 803–809. [CrossRef]
26. Parish, C.R.; Freeman, C.; Hulett, M.D. Heparanase: A key enzyme involved in cell invasion. *Biochim. Biophys. Acta* **2001**, *1471*, M99–M108. [CrossRef]
27. Vlodavsky, I.; Friedmann, Y. Molecular properties and involvement of heparanase in cancer metastasis and angiogenesis. *J. Clin. Investig.* **2001**, *108*, 341–347. [CrossRef]
28. Vlodavsky, I.; Beckhove, P.; Lerner, I.; Pisano, C.; Meirovitz, A.; Ilan, N.; Elkin, M. Significance of heparanase in cancer and inflammation. *Cancer Microenviron.* **2012**, *5*, 115–132. [CrossRef]
29. Jung, O.; Trapp-Stamborski, V.; Purushothaman, A.; Jin, H.; Wang, H.; Sanderson, R.D.; Rapraeger, A.C. Heparanase-induced shedding of syndecan-1/CD138 in myeloma and endothelial cells activates VEGFR2 and an invasive phenotype: Prevention by novel synstatins. *Oncogenesis* **2016**, *5*, e202. [CrossRef]
30. Chen, X.-P.; Luo, J.-S.; Tian, Y.; Nie, C.-L.; Cui, W.; Zhang, W.-D. Downregulation of heparanase expression results in suppression of invasion, migration, and adhesion abilities of hepatocellular carcinoma cells. *BioMed Res. Int.* **2015**, *2015*, 241983. [CrossRef]
31. Comperat, E.M.; Burger, M.; Gontero, P.; Mostafid, A.H.; Palou, J.; Roupret, M.; van Rhijn, B.W.G.; Shariat, S.F.; Sylvester, R.J.; Zigeuner, R.; et al. Grading of urothelial carcinoma and the new "world health organisation classification of tumours of the urinary system and male genital organs 2016". *Eur. Urol. Focus* **2019**, *5*, 457–466. [CrossRef] [PubMed]
32. Gohji, K.; Okamoto, M.; Kitazawa, S.; Toyoshima, M.; Dong, J.; Katsuoka, Y.; Nakajima, M. Heparanase protein and gene expression in bladder cancer. *J. Urol.* **2001**, *166*, 1286–1290. [CrossRef]
33. Shteingauz, A.; Boyango, I.; Naroditsky, I.; Hammond, E.; Gruber, M.; Doweck, I.; Ilan, N.; Vlodavsky, I. Heparanase enhances tumor growth and chemoresistance by promoting autophagy. *Cancer Res.* **2015**, *75*, 3946–3957. [CrossRef] [PubMed]
34. Sabichi, A.; Keyhani, A.; Tanaka, N.; Delacerda, J.; Lee, I.L.; Zou, C.; Zhou, J.H.; Benedict, W.F.; Grossman, H.B. Characterization of a panel of cell lines derived from urothelial neoplasms: Genetic alterations, growth in vivo and the relationship of adenoviral mediated gene transfer to coxsackie adenovirus receptor expression. *J. Urol.* **2006**, *175*, 1133–1137. [CrossRef]

Permissions

All chapters in this book were first published by MDPI; hereby published with permission under the Creative Commons Attribution License or equivalent. Every chapter published in this book has been scrutinized by our experts. Their significance has been extensively debated. The topics covered herein carry significant findings which will fuel the growth of the discipline. They may even be implemented as practical applications or may be referred to as a beginning point for another development.

The contributors of this book come from diverse backgrounds, making this book a truly international effort. This book will bring forth new frontiers with its revolutionizing research information and detailed analysis of the nascent developments around the world.

We would like to thank all the contributing authors for lending their expertise to make the book truly unique. They have played a crucial role in the development of this book. Without their invaluable contributions this book wouldn't have been possible. They have made vital efforts to compile up to date information on the varied aspects of this subject to make this book a valuable addition to the collection of many professionals and students.

This book was conceptualized with the vision of imparting up-to-date information and advanced data in this field. To ensure the same, a matchless editorial board was set up. Every individual on the board went through rigorous rounds of assessment to prove their worth. After which they invested a large part of their time researching and compiling the most relevant data for our readers.

The editorial board has been involved in producing this book since its inception. They have spent rigorous hours researching and exploring the diverse topics which have resulted in the successful publishing of this book. They have passed on their knowledge of decades through this book. To expedite this challenging task, the publisher supported the team at every step. A small team of assistant editors was also appointed to further simplify the editing procedure and attain best results for the readers.

Apart from the editorial board, the designing team has also invested a significant amount of their time in understanding the subject and creating the most relevant covers. They scrutinized every image to scout for the most suitable representation of the subject and create an appropriate cover for the book.

The publishing team has been an ardent support to the editorial, designing and production team. Their endless efforts to recruit the best for this project, has resulted in the accomplishment of this book. They are a veteran in the field of academics and their pool of knowledge is as vast as their experience in printing. Their expertise and guidance has proved useful at every step. Their uncompromising quality standards have made this book an exceptional effort. Their encouragement from time to time has been an inspiration for everyone.

The publisher and the editorial board hope that this book will prove to be a valuable piece of knowledge for researchers, students, practitioners and scholars across the globe.

List of Contributors

Sreevidya Santha, Xiang Ling and Jianqun Liao
Department of Pharmacology and Therapeutics, Roswell Park Comprehensive Cancer Center, Elm and Carlton Streets, Buffalo, New York, NY 14263, USA
Canget BioTekpharma, LLC, Buffalo, New York, NY 14203, USA

Ieman A. M. Aljahdali
Department of Pharmacology and Therapeutics, Roswell Park Comprehensive Cancer Center, Elm and Carlton Streets, Buffalo, New York, NY 14263, USA
Department of Cellular & Molecular Biology, Roswell Park Comprehensive Cancer Center, Buffalo, New York, NY 14263, USA

Sailee S. Rasam
Department of Biochemistry, Jacobs School of Medicine, University at Buffalo, State University of New York, Buffalo, New York, NY 14203, USA

Jun Qu
Department of Pharmaceutical Sciences, School of Pharmacy, University at Buffalo, State University of New York, Buffalo, New York, NY 14214, USA

Xue Wang
Department of Pharmaceutical Sciences, School of Pharmacy, University at Buffalo, State University of New York, Buffalo, New York, NY 14214, USA
Department of Cell Stress Biology, Roswell Park Comprehensive Cancer Center, Buffalo, New York, NY 14263, USA

Jue Wang
Department of Interdisciplinary Oncology, University of Arizona Cancer Center, Phoenix Arizona, AZ 85004, USA

Christos Fountzilas
Department of Medicine, Roswell Park Comprehensive Cancer Center, Buffalo, New York, NY 14263, USA

Qingyong Li
College of Pharmaceutical Science, Zhejiang University of Technology, Hangzhou 310014, China

Fengzhi Li
Department of Pharmacology and Therapeutics, Roswell Park Comprehensive Cancer Center, Elm and Carlton Streets, Buffalo, New York, NY 14263, USA
Developmental Therapeutics (DT) Program, Roswell Park Comprehensive Cancer Center, Buffalo, New York, NY 14263, USA

Aikaterini Iliou, Aristeidis Panagiotakis, Dimitra Benaki, Mariangela Kosmopoulou, Evagelos Gikas and Emmanuel Mikros
Section of Pharmaceutical Chemistry, Department of Pharmacy, School of Health Sciences, National and Kapodistrian University of Athens (NKUA), 15701 Athens, Greece

Aikaterini F. Giannopoulou, Athanassios D. Velentzas, Issidora S. Papassideri and Dimitrios J. Stravopodis
Section of Cell Biology and Biophysics, Department of Biology, School of Science, National and Kapodistrian University of Athens (NKUA), 15701 Athens, Greece

Ourania E. Tsitsilonis
Section of Animal and Human Physiology, Department of Biology, School of Science, National and Kapodistrian University of Athens (NKUA), 15701 Athens, Greece

Gerassimos E. Voutsinas
Laboratory of Molecular Carcinogenesis and Rare Disease Genetics, Institute of Biosciences and Applications, National Center for Scientific Research (NCSR) "Demokritos", 15701 Athens, Greece

Eumorphia G. Konstantakou
Harvard Medical School, Massachusetts General Hospital Cancer Center (MGHCC), Charlestown, MA 021004, USA

Juan Carlos Pardo, Andrea Plaja, Olatz Etxaniz and Albert Font
Department of Medical Oncology, Catalan Institute of Oncology, University Hospital Germans Trias i Pujol, Ctra. Can Ruti-Camí de les Escoles s/n, 08916 Badalona, Spain
Catalan Institute of Oncology, Badalona Applied Research Group in Oncology (B·ARGO), Ctra. Can Ruti-Camí de les Escoles s/n, 08916 Badalona, Spain

Vicenç Ruiz de Porras
Catalan Institute of Oncology, Badalona Applied Research Group in Oncology (B•ARGO), Ctra. Can Ruti-Camí de les Escoles s/n, 08916 Badalona, Spain
Germans Trias i Pujol Research Institute (IGTP), Ctra. Can Ruti-Camí de les Escoles s/n, 08916 Badalona, Spain

Cristina Carrato
Pathology Department, Hospital Germans Trias i Pujol, 08916 Badalona, Spain

Oscar Buisan
Urology Department, University Hospital Germans Trias i Pujol, 08916 Badalona, Spain

Sruthi V. Hindupur, Sebastian C. Schmid, Jana Annika Koch, Eva-Maria Baur, Dongbiao Wang, Thomas Horn, Juergen E. Gschwend, Per Sonne Holm and Roman Nawroth
Department of Urology, Klinikum rechts der Isar, Technical University of Munich, 81675 Munich, Germany

Ahmed Youssef
Department of Urology, Klinikum rechts der Isar, Technical University of Munich, 81675 Munich, Germany
Department of Urology, Beni-suef University, Beni Suef 62511, Egypt

Julia Slotta-Huspenina
Department of Pathology, Klinikum rechts der Isar, Technical University of Munich, 81675 Munich, Germany

Toshikazu Tanaka, Daisuke Noro, Kengo Imanishi, Yuta Kojima, Shingo Hatakeyama, Yuki Tobisawa, Kazuyuki Mori, Hayato Yamamoto, Atsushi Imai, Takahiro Yoneyama and Takuya Koie
Department of Urology, Hirosaki University Graduate School of Medicine, Hirosaki 036-8562, Japan

Tohru Yoneyama and Yasuhiro Hashimoto
Department of Advanced Transplant and Regenerative Medicine, Hirosaki University Graduate School of Medicine, Hirosaki 036-8562, Japan

Chikara Ohyama
Department of Urology, Hirosaki University Graduate School of Medicine, Hirosaki 036-8562, Japan
Department of Advanced Transplant and Regenerative Medicine, Hirosaki University Graduate School of Medicine, Hirosaki 036-8562, Japan

Masakazu Tanaka and Shin-Ichiro Nishimura
Graduate School of Life Science, Frontier Research Centre for Advanced Material and Life Science, Hokkaido University, Sapporo 060-0810, Japan

Arnaud Manel
Le Creusot Hospital, 71200 Le Creusot, France

Maria Zvereva
Chair of Chemistry of Natural Compounds, Department of Chemistry, Lomonosov Moscow State University, 119991 Moscow, Russia
International Agency for Research on Cancer (IARC), 69372 Lyon, France

Florence Le Calvez-Kelm
International Agency for Research on Cancer (IARC), 69372 Lyon, France

Eduard Pisarev
Faculty of Bioengineering and Bioinformatics, Lomonosov Moscow State University, 119234 Moscow, Russia

Ismail Hosen
Department of Biochemistry and Molecular Biology, Faculty of Biological Sciences, University of Dhaka, Dhaka 1000, Bangladesh

Olga Kisil
Gause Institute of New Antibiotics, 119021 Moscow, Russia

Simon Matskeplishvili, David Kamalov, Alexander Tivtikyan and Armais Kamalov
Medical Research and Education Center, Lomonosov Moscow State University, 119992 Moscow, Russia

Elena Kubareva
Belozersky Institute of Physico-Chemical Biology, Moscow State University, 119992 Moscow, Russia

Shizuka Kurauchi and Ippei Takahashi
Department of Social Medicine, Hirosaki University Graduate School of Medicine, Hirosaki 036-8562, Japan

Emmanuel Vian
Department of Urology, Protestant Clinic of Lyon, 69300 Lyon, France

Thorsten Ecke
Department of Urology, HELIOS Hospital Bad Saarow, D-15526 Bad Saarow, Germany

Rhiannon V. McNeill, Andrew S. Mason and Jennifer Southgate
Jack Birch Unit for Molecular Carcinogenesis, Department of Biology, York Biomedical Research Institute, University of York, York YO10 5DD, UK

Mark E. Hodson
Department of Environment and Geography, University of York, York YO10 5DD, UK

James W.F. Catto
Academic Urology Unit, University of Sheffield, Sheffield S10 2TN, UK

Karsten Salomo, Ulrike Heberling, Andrea Lohse-Fischer, Romy Fuehrer, Christian Thomas, Michael Froehner, Manfred P. Wirth and Susanne Fuessel
Department of Urology, Technische Universität Dresden, 01307 Dresden, Germany

Kati Erdmann
Department of Urology, Technische Universität Dresden, 01307 Dresden, Germany
National Center for Tumor Diseases (NCT), 01307 Dresden, Germany

Anna Klimova and Ingo Roeder
National Center for Tumor Diseases (NCT), 01307 Dresden, Germany
Institute for Medical Informatics and Biometrics, Technische Universität Dresden, 01307 Dresden, Germany

Hiroshi Fukushima, Kosuke Takemura, Hiroaki Suzuki and Fumitaka Koga
Department of Urology, Tokyo Metropolitan Cancer and Infectious Diseases Center Komagome Hospital, 3-18-22 Honkomagome, Bunkyo-ku, Tokyo 113-8677, Japan

Makito Miyake, Daisuke Gotoh, Sayuri Ohnishi, Takuya Owari, Kota Iida, Kenta Ohnishi, Shunta Hori, Yosuke Morizawa, Yoshitaka Itami, Yasushi Nakai, Takeshi Inoue, Satoshi Anai, Kazumasa Torimoto, Katsuya Aoki, Nobumichi Tanaka and Kiyohide Fujimoto
Department of Urology, Nara Medical University, 840 Shijo-cho, Kashihara-shi, Nara 634-8522, Japan

Yoshihiro Tatsumi
Department of Urology, Nara Medical University, 840 Shijo-cho, Kashihara-shi, Nara 634-8522, Japan
Department of Pathology, Nara Medical University, 840 Shijo-cho, Kashihara-shi, Nara 634-8522, Japan

Keiji Shimada
Department of Pathology, Nara City Hospital, 1501 Higashi kidera-cho, Nara-shi, Nara 630-8305, Japan

Ke-Hung Tsui
Department of Urology, Chang Gung Memorial Hospital-Linkou, Kwei-Shan, Tao-Yuan 33302, Taiwan

Yu-Hsiang Lin and Chen-Pang Hou
Department of Urology, Chang Gung Memorial Hospital-Linkou, Kwei-Shan, Tao-Yuan 33302, Taiwan
Graduate Institute of Clinical Medical Science, College of Medicine, Chang Gung University, Kwei-Shan, Tao-Yuan 33302, Taiwan

Kang-Shuo Chang and Pin-Jung Chen
Department of Anatomy, College of Medicine, Chang Gung University, Kwei-Shan, Tao-Yuan 33302, Taiwan
Graduate Institute of Biomedical Sciences, College of Medicine, Chang Gung University, Kwei-Shan, Tao-Yuan 33302, Taiwan

Horng-Heng Juang
Department of Urology, Chang Gung Memorial Hospital-Linkou, Kwei-Shan, Tao-Yuan 33302, Taiwan
Department of Anatomy, College of Medicine, Chang Gung University, Kwei-Shan, Tao-Yuan 33302, Taiwan
Graduate Institute of Biomedical Sciences, College of Medicine, Chang Gung University, Kwei-Shan, Tao-Yuan 33302, Taiwan

Tsui-Hsia Feng
School of Nursing, College of Medicine, Chang Gung University, Kwei-Shan, Tao-Yuan 33302, Taiwan

Jan Gleichenhagen, Swaantje Casjens, Carmen Meinig, Irina Raiko, Thomas Brüning and Georg Johnen
Institute for Prevention and Occupational Medicine of the German Social Accident Insurance, Institute of the Ruhr-University Bochum (IPA), 44789 Bochum, Germany

Christian Arndt
Department of Urology, Lukaskrankenhaus Neuss, 41464 Neuss, Germany

Holger Gerullis
University Hospital for Urology, Klinikum Oldenburg, 26133 Oldenburg, Germany

Makito Miyake, Shunta Hori, Yosuke Morizawa, Yasushi Nakai, Satoshi Anai, Nobumichi Tanaka and Kiyohide Fujimoto
Department of Urology, Nara Medical University, 840 Shijo-cho, Nara 634-8522, Japan

Keiji Shimada, Tomomi Fujii and Noboru Konishi
Department of Pathology, Nara Medical University, 840 Shijo-cho, Nara 634-8522, Japan

Index

Printed in the USA
CPSIA information can be obtained
at www.ICGtesting.com
LVHW080734221023
761596LV00011B/2122

9 781639 897957